Thyroid Cancer and Other Thyroid Disorders

Editors

KENNETH D. BURMAN
JACQUELINE JONKLAAS

ENDOCRINOLOGY AND METABOLISM CLINICS OF NORTH AMERICA

www.endo.theclinics.com

Consulting Editor
DEREK LeROITH

June 2014 • Volume 43 • Number 2

ELSEVIER

1600 John F. Kennedy Boulevard • Suite 1800 • Philadelphia, Pennsylvania, 19103-2899

http://www.theclinics.com

ENDOCRINOLOGY AND METABOLISM CLINICS OF NORTH AMERICA Volume 43, Number 2
June 2014 ISSN 0889-8529, ISBN-13: 978-0-323-29919-0

Editor: Jessica McCool
Developmental Editor: Susan Showalter

Endocrinology and Metabolism Clinics of North America (ISSN 0889-8529) is published quarterly by Elsevier Inc., 360 Park Avenue South, New York, NY 10010-1710. Months of issue are March, June, September, and December. Periodicals postage paid at New York, NY and additional mailing offices. Subscription prices are USD 330.00 per year for US individuals, USD 581.00 per year for US institutions, USD 165.00 per year for US students and residents, USD 415.00 per year for Canadian individuals, USD 718.00 per year for Canadian institutions, USD 480.00 per year for international individuals, USD 718.00 per year for international institutions, and USD 245.00 per year for international and Canadian and foreign students/residents. To receive student/resident rate, orders must be accompanied by name of affiliated institution, date of term, and the signature of program/residency coordinator on institution letterhead. Orders will be billed at individual rate until proof of status is received. Foreign air speed delivery is included in all *Clinics* subscription prices. All prices are subject to change without notice. **POSTMASTER:** Send address changes to *Endocrinology and Metabolism Clinics of North America*, Elsevier Health Sciences Division, Subscription Customer Service, 3251 Riverport Lane, Maryland Heights, MO 63043. **Customer Service: Telephone: 1-800-654-2452** (U.S. and Canada); **1-314-447-8871** (outside U.S. and Canada). **Fax: 1-314-447-8029. E-mail: journalscustomerservice-usa@elsevier.com** (for print support); **journalsonlinesupport-usa@elsevier.com** (for online support).

Reprints. For copies of 100 or more, of articles in this publication, please contact the Commercial Rights Department, Elsevier Inc., 360 Park Avenue South, New York, NY 10010-1710; phone: +1-212-633-3874; fax: +1-212-633-3820; E-mail: reprints@elsevier.com.

Endocrinology and Metabolism Clinics of North America is covered in *MEDLINE/PubMed (Index Medicus)*, *EMBASE/Excerpta Medica, Current Contents/Clinical Medicine, Current Contents/Life Sciences, Science Citation Index, ISI/BIOMED, BIOSIS*, and *Chemical Abstracts*.

Contributors

CONSULTING EDITOR

DEREK LeROITH, MD, PhD
Director of Research, Division of Endocrinology, Metabolism, and Bone Diseases, Department of Medicine, Mount Sinai School of Medicine, New York, New York

EDITORS

KENNETH D. BURMAN, MD
Chairman, Endocrinology Section, Department of Medicine, Medstar Washington Hospital Center; Professor, Department of Medicine, Georgetown University, Washington, DC

JACQUELINE JONKLAAS, MD, PhD
Associate Professor, Division of Endocrinology, Georgetown University, Washington, DC

AUTHORS

LAURA AGATE, MD
Endocrinology Unit, Department of Clinical and Experimental Medicine, World Health Organization Collaborating Center for the Study and Treatment of Thyroid Diseases and Other Endocrine and Metabolic Disorders, University of Pisa, Pisa, Italy

AGNESE BIAGINI, MD
Endocrinology Unit, Department of Clinical and Experimental Medicine, World Health Organization Collaborating Center for the Study and Treatment of Thyroid Diseases and Other Endocrine and Metabolic Disorders, University of Pisa, Pisa, Italy

HENRY B. BURCH, MD, COL MC U.S. Army
Endocrinology Service, Department of Medicine, Walter Reed National Military Medical Center; Professor of Medicine and Chair, Endocrinology Division, Uniformed Services University of the Health Sciences, Bethesda, Maryland

KENNETH D. BURMAN, MD
Chairman, Endocrinology Section, Department of Medicine, Medstar Washington Hospital Center; Professor, Department of Medicine, Georgetown University, Washington, DC

GLENDA G. CALLENDER, MD
Section of Endocrine Surgery, Department of Surgery, Yale University School of Medicine, New Haven, Connecticut

TOBIAS CARLING, MD, PhD
Section of Endocrine Surgery, Department of Surgery, Yale University School of Medicine, New Haven, Connecticut

EMILY CHRISTISON-LAGAY, MD
Section of Pediatric Surgery, Department of Surgery, Yale University School of Medicine, New Haven, Connecticut

SARA DANZI, PhD
Assistant Professor, Department of Biological Sciences and Geology, Queensborough Community College, Bayside, New York

WILLIAM S. DUKE, MD
Assistant Professor, Department of Otolaryngology; Associate Surgical Director, Georgia Regents University Thyroid Center, Georgia Regents University, Augusta, Georgia

ROSSELLA ELISEI, MD
Endocrinology Unit, Department of Clinical and Experimental Medicine, World Health Organization Collaborating Center for the Study and Treatment of Thyroid Diseases and Other Endocrine and Metabolic Disorders, University of Pisa, Pisa, Italy

GIUSEPPE ESPOSITO, MD
Chief of Nuclear Medicine; Associate Professor, Department of Radiology, Medstar Georgetown University Hospital, Washington, DC

SHEREEN EZZAT, MD, FACP, FRCPC
Endocrine Oncology Site Group, Princess Margaret Hospital, University Health Network, Toronto, Ontario, Canada

JEREMY GILBERT, MD, FRCPC
Division of Endocrinology, Department of Medicine, University of Toronto; Division of Endocrinology, Department of Medicine, Sunnybrook Health Sciences Center, Toronto, Ontario, Canada

JEANNETTE GOGUEN, MD, MEd, FRCPC
Division of Endocrinology, Department of Medicine, University of Toronto; Division of Endocrinology, Department of Medicine, St. Michael's Hospital, Toronto, Ontario, Canada

RACHNA M. GOYAL, MD
Fellow, Division of Endocrinology, Washington Hospital Center; Fellow, Division of Endocrinology, Georgetown University Hospital, Washington, DC

STEVEN P. HODAK, MD
Clinical Associate Professor of Medicine, Division of Endocrinology; Medical Director, Center for Diabetes and Endocrinology, University of Pittsburgh School of Medicine, Pittsburgh, Pennsylvania

MIMI I. HU, MD
Associate Professor, Department of Endocrine Neoplasia and Hormonal Disorders, The University of Texas MD Anderson Cancer Center, Houston, Texas

CAMILO JIMENEZ, MD
Associate Professor, Department of Endocrine Neoplasia and Hormonal Disorders, The University of Texas MD Anderson Cancer Center, Houston, Texas

JENNIFER JONES, PhD
Department of Psychiatry, University of Toronto; Cancer Survivorship Program, Princess Margaret Hospital, University Health Network, Toronto, Ontario, Canada

JACQUELINE JONKLAAS, MD, PhD
Associate Professor, Division of Endocrinology, Georgetown University, Washington, DC

CATHERINE KELLY, MD, FRCPC
Division of Endocrinology, Department of Medicine, University of Toronto; Division of Endocrinology, Department of Medicine, Women's College Hospital, Toronto, Ontario, Canada

IRWIN KLEIN, MD
Professor of Medicine, Department of Medicine and Cell Biology, New York University School of Medicine, New York, New York; Private Office, Great Neck, New York

JULIA LOWE, MBChB, MMedSci
Division of Endocrinology, Department of Medicine, University of Toronto; Division of Endocrinology, Department of Medicine, Sunnybrook Health Sciences Center, Toronto, Ontario, Canada

VINH Q. MAI, DO
Endocrinology Service, Department of Medicine, Walter Reed National Military Medical Center; Assistant Professor, Department of Medicine, Uniformed Services University of the Health Sciences, Bethesda, Maryland

ANTONIO MATRONE, MD
Endocrinology Unit, Department of Clinical and Experimental Medicine, World Health Organization Collaborating Center for the Study and Treatment of Thyroid Diseases and Other Endocrine and Metabolic Disorders, University of Pisa, Pisa, Italy

DONALD S.A. MCLEOD, MBBS, FRACP, MPH
Staff Specialist, Departments of Internal Medicine and Aged Care and Endocrinology, Royal Brisbane & Women's Hospital; PhD Student, Department of Population Health, QIMR Berghofer Medical Research Institute, Herston, Queensland, Australia

ELEONORA MOLINARO, MD
Endocrinology Unit, Department of Clinical and Experimental Medicine, World Health Organization Collaborating Center for the Study and Treatment of Thyroid Diseases and Other Endocrine and Metabolic Disorders, University of Pisa, Pisa, Italy

DENISE P. MOMESSO, MD
Endocrinology Service, Hospital Universitário Clementino Fraga Filho, Universidade Federal do Rio de Janeiro, Rio de Janeiro, Rio de Janeiro, Brazil

SANN YU MON, MD, MPH
Endocrinology Fellow, Division of Endocrinology, University of Pittsburgh School of Medicine, Pittsburgh, Pennsylvania

BECKY T. MULDOON, MD, Endocrinology Service, Department of Medicine, Walter Reed National Military Medical Center; Assistant Professor, Department of Medicine, Uniformed Services University of the Health Sciences, Bethesda, Maryland

ASIMA NAEEM, BSc
Division of Endocrinology, Department of Medicine, University Health Network, Toronto, Ontario, Canada

NISHA NATHAN, MD
Department of Endocrinology, Medstar Georgetown University Hospital and Medstar Washington Hospital Center, Washington, DC

M. SARA ROSENTHAL, PhD
Professor of Bioethics; Director, Program for Bioethics, Departments of Internal Medicine, Pediatrics and Behavioral Science, University of Kentucky, Lexington, Kentucky

MARY H. SAMUELS, MD
Professor of Medicine, Division of Endocrinology, Diabetes, and Clinical Nutrition, Oregon Health & Science University, Portland, Oregon

ANNA M. SAWKA, MD, PhD, FRCPC
Division of Endocrinology, Department of Medicine, University Health Network; Division of Endocrinology, Department of Medicine, University of Toronto, Toronto, Ontario, Canada

PHILIP SEGAL, MD, FRCPC
Division of Endocrinology, Department of Medicine, University Health Network; Division of Endocrinology, Department of Medicine, University of Toronto; Division of Endocrinology, Department of Medicine, Mount Sinai Hospital, Toronto, Ontario, Canada

SHANNON D. SULLIVAN, MD, PhD
Department of Endocrinology, Medstar Georgetown University Hospital and Medstar Washington Hospital Center, Washington, DC

DAVID J. TERRIS, MD, FACS
Porubsky Professor and Chairman, Department of Otolaryngology; Surgical Director, Georgia Regents University Thyroid Center, Georgia Regents University, Augusta, Georgia

R. MICHAEL TUTTLE, MD
Professor of Medicine, Endocrinology, Memorial Sloan Kettering Cancer Center, New York, New York

ROBERT UDELSMAN, MD, MBA
Section of Endocrine Surgery, Department of Surgery; William H. Carmalt Professor of Surgery and Oncology; Surgeon-In-Chief, Yale-New Haven Hospital; Chairman of Surgery, Yale University School of Medicine, New Haven, Connecticut

DAVID VIOLA, MD
Endocrinology Unit, Department of Clinical and Experimental Medicine, World Health Organization Collaborating Center for the Study and Treatment of Thyroid Diseases and Other Endocrine and Metabolic Disorders, University of Pisa, Pisa, Italy

ANITA K. YING, MD
Assistant Professor, Department of Endocrine Neoplasia and Hormonal Disorders, The University of Texas MD Anderson Cancer Center, Houston, Texas

AFSHAN ZAHEDI, MD, FRCPC
Division of Endocrinology, Department of Medicine, University of Toronto; Division of Endocrinology, Department of Medicine, Mount Sinai Hospital; Division of Endocrinology, Department of Medicine, Women's College Hospital, Toronto, Ontario, Canada

Contents

Serum thyroglobulin (sTg) is the marker for monitoring persistence/recurrence of differentiated thyroid cancer, in patients without sTg antibodies. Patients with undetectable basal sTg or peak sTg <2 ng/mL are cured with low risk to recur. Newly detectable level of sTg indicates the recurrence. The significance of increasing sTg in patients treated with emithyroidectomy or total-thyroidectomy but not ablated with radioiodine is undefined. A doubling time <1 year may be a poor prognostic factor, but this is more relevant in cases with high levels of sTg. Because of its sensitivity, neck ultrasound should be performed at any visit, especially when an increased sTg is seen.

Molecular diagnostics offers great promise for the evaluation of cytologically indeterminate thyroid nodules. Numerous molecular genetic and immunohistochemical tests have been developed that may be performed on thyroid specimens obtained during standard fine-needle aspiration, some of which may greatly improve diagnostic yield. A sound understanding of the diagnostic performance of these tests, and how they can enhance clinical practice, is important. This article reviews the diagnostic utility of immunohistochemical and molecular testing for the clinical assessment of thyroid nodules, and makes recommendations about how these tests can be integrated into clinical practice for patients with cytologically indeterminate thyroid nodules.

Thyrotropin (TSH) is the major regulator and growth factor of the thyroid. TSH may be important in the development of human thyroid cancer, with both suggestive animal models and clinical evidence, although definitive proof is still required. Applications for TSH in thyroid cancer management include TSH stimulation of radioiodine uptake, enhancement of biochemical monitoring through thyroglobulin measurement, and long-term suppression of TSH with supraphysiologic levothyroxine. This review synthesizes current knowledge of TSH in both the development and management of differentiated thyroid cancer.

All published guidelines on the use of radioactive iodine for the treatment of well-differentiated thyroid cancer agree that an individualized assessment of the risk of cancer-related mortality and of disease recurrence should direct the decision of whether radioiodine treatment is needed and how much to administer. At the author's institution, they mostly follow the American Thyroid Association's risk stratification system, with the addition of a category of very-low-risk patients that do not receive radioactive iodine.

In this review, we demonstrate how initial estimates of the risk of disease-specific mortality and recurrent/persistent disease should be used to guide initial treatment recommendations and early management decisions and to set appropriate patient expectations with regard to likely outcomes after initial therapy of thyroid cancer. The use of ongoing risk stratification to modify these initial risk estimates is also discussed. Novel response to therapy definitions are proposed that can be used for ongoing risk stratification in thyroid cancer patients treated with lobectomy or total thyroidectomy without radioactive iodine remnant ablation.

Medullary thyroid carcinoma (MTC) is a rare type of thyroid cancer, demonstrating variable behavior from indolent disease to highly aggressive, progressive disease. There are distinguishing phenotypic features of sporadic and hereditary MTC. Activation or overexpression of cell surface receptors and up-regulation of intracellular signaling pathways in hereditary and sporadic MTC are involved in the disease pathogenesis. There has been an exponential rise in clinical trials with investigational agents, leading to approval of 2 medications for progressive, advanced MTC. Developments in understanding the pathogenesis of MTC will hopefully lead to more effective and less toxic treatments of this rare but difficult to treat cancer.

The incidence of thyroid cancer, particularly papillary thyroid cancer, is rising at an epidemic rate. The mainstay of treatment of most patients with thyroid cancer is surgery. Considerable controversy exists about the extent of thyroid surgery and lymph node resection in patients with thyroid cancer. Surgical experience in judgment and technique is required to achieve optimal patient outcomes.

Advances in surgical technology and patient-driven demands have fueled exploration into methods to improve cosmetic outcomes in thyroid surgery. This exploration has produced 2 fundamentally different pathways for reducing the visible thyroidectomy scar. Minimally invasive anterior cervical approaches use small incisions hidden in natural skin creases and reduce the overall extent of dissection required to remove the thyroid. Remote access approaches remove the incision from the anterior neck completely but require more extensive dissection to access the thyroid compartment.

The relevance of persistent posttreatment fatigue (PPF) to thyroid cancer (TC) survivor populations is not known. This article presents a scoping review, which is an overview of published research activity. Uncontrolled data suggest that PPF is one of the most common complaints in TC survivors. Furthermore, statistically significantly worse levels of fatigue were reported in TC survivors, compared with the general population or healthy controls. There was some inconsistency among PPF risk factors. More research is needed on PPF in TC survivors, including long-term prospective cohort studies, research on fatigue severity prevalence, and randomized controlled trials of treatment strategies.

Over the last century, much has been learned about the pathogenesis, manifestations, and management of Graves' disease leading to the establishment of evidence-based clinical practice guidelines. The joint clinical practice guidelines from the American Thyroid Association and the American Association of Clinical Endocrinologists give recommendations on both the diagnosis and treatment of hyperthyroidism. A survey of clinicians performed that same year, however, revealed that current practices diverge from these recently published guidelines in multiple areas. These differences will need to be assessed serially to determine the impact of the guidelines on future clinical practice and perhaps vice versa.

Thyroid hormones, specifically triiodothyronine (T_3), have significant effects on the heart and cardiovascular system. Hypothyroidism, hyperthyroidism, subclinical thyroid disease, and low T_3 syndrome each cause cardiac and cardiovascular abnormalities through both genomic and nongenomic effects on cardiac myocytes and vascular smooth muscle cells. In compromised health, such as occurs in heart disease, alterations in

ENDOCRINOLOGY AND METABOLISM CLINICS OF NORTH AMERICA

FORTHCOMING ISSUES

September 2014
HIV and Endocrine Disorders
Paul Hruz, *Editor*

December 2014
Lipids
Donald A. Smith, *Editor*

March 2015
Pituitary Disorders
Anat Ben-Shlomo and Maria Fleseriu,
Editors

RECENT ISSUES

March 2014
Diabetes Mellitus: Associated Conditions
Leonid Poretsky and Emilia Pauline Liao,
Editors

December 2013
Acute and Chronic Complications of
Diabetes
Leonid Poretsky and Emilia Pauline Liao,
Editors

September 2013
Endocrine and Neuropsychiatric Disorders
Eliza B. Geer, *Editor*

RELATED INTEREST

Emergency Medicine Clinics of North America, Volume 32, Issue 2 (May 2014)
Endocrine and Metabolic Emergencies
George C. Willis and M. Tyson Pillow, *Editors*
Available at: http://www.emed.theclinics.com/

VISIT THE CLINICS ONLINE!
Access your subscription at:
www.theclinics.com

Foreword

Thyroid Cancer and Other Thyroid Disorders

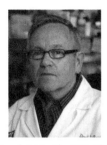

Derek LeRoith, MD, PhD
Consulting Editor

We decided that an update on thyroid disorders would be appropriate since our last thyroid issue a number of years ago. In particular, it is clear that the incidence of thyroid cancer is increasing and there are a number of new modalities to therapy. In addition, there are a number of articles that cover considerations that have not been dealt with previously.

Drs Mon and Hodak discuss the emerging technology of using molecular diagnostic tools in fine-needle aspirations of thyroid nodules. Since up to 40% of the cases remain indeterminate, it is hoped that these molecular tests would result in more definitive results. As they discuss, the specificity and sensitivity are as yet not 100% and therefore not always conclusive.

Dr McLeod discusses how serum thyrotropin (TSH) levels have been associated with thyroid cancer, suggesting a potential causative relationship, although this has never been definitively proven. However, serum TSH levels remain important in the management of thyroid cancer. In particular, in detecting metastatic disease, traditionally thyroid suppression therapy was ceased to induce hypothyroidism and elevate TSH levels prior to isotope studies. Today, with the advent of recombinant TSH availability, it can be administered to elevate circulating levels, without cessation of the thyroid suppression and induction of hypothyroidism.

Thyroid cancer, except in unusual situations, requires thyroid surgery. Drs Callender, Carling, Christison-Lagay, and Udelsman describe in their article that the diagnosis is commonly made on fine-needle aspiration of a nodule greater than 1 cm in diameter. Occasionally, the diagnosis may be made by detecting the BRAF V600E mutation in papillary thyroid cancer or rearranged during transfection (RET) protoncogene mutations in the case of multiple endocrine neoplasia, or familial medullary thyroid carcinoma. Small tumors may suffice with partial thyroidectomy, while those greater than 1 cm require total (or near total) thyroidectomy to reduce recurrence. Central lymph node dissection is critical if lymph nodes are involved or even the absence, if the tumor

Endocrinol Metab Clin N Am 43 (2014) xiii–xvi
http://dx.doi.org/10.1016/j.ecl.2014.03.001
endo.theclinics.com

is large. These and other considerations require a team of thyroid cancer specialists and thus patients should be referred to large academic centers where possible, for the best considerations and care.

Drs Duke and Terris describe alternative approaches to avoiding scarring of the neck following thyroidectomy. Numerous groups have perfected the minimally invasive anterior cervical approach that leaves a limited scar. Recently, the development of remote access approaches has been developed in an attempt to totally avoid the cervical scar. Unfortunately, these approaches from the chest, axilla, breast, and so on, while avoiding the scar, may be extremely problematic given the tissues they traverse and potential harm inflicted, as well as more prolonged postsurgery recovery; perhaps they should be avoided?

Staging of disease in the situation of differentiated thyroid disease has been very useful to decide on appropriate therapy. However, as discussed by Drs Momesso and Tuttle, this staging needs to remain a dynamic process since incomplete responses are common and tumors may change their characteristics. The authors have devised an algorithm based on initial and ongoing outcomes and ranges from those with excellent responses to those with either biochemical or structural incomplete responses. Physicians are encouraged to consider these situations and treat appropriately.

Drs Hu, Ying, and Jimenez describe the underlying oncogenic process in medullary thyroid cancer, an aggressive, often familial and fortunately rare form of thyroid cancer. The RET oncogene is the most common abnormality, due to either germline or somatic mutations that result in an activated RET. Other tyrosine kinase receptors have also been found to be overexpressed but whether they are primary or secondary to RET is unclear. Initial diagnosis is usually made with fine-needle aspiration, but chromogranin A and CEA levels are also useful. At present, there are tyrosine kinase–specific inhibitors that are available for therapeutic use and others in the pipeline. The prognosis in general is still much worse than that of PTC and FTC.

Posttreatment fatigue in survivors of thyroid cancer is apparently a less well-recognized phenomenon. In the article by Sawka and colleagues, a description of the limited published data and their review of the literature are provided. Due to the paucity of data, the authors do not recommend specific interventions, but strongly support the idea of randomized controlled trials, a highly commendable suggestion. One could certainly extrapolate this to other endocrine conditions as well.

Dr Rosenthal discusses, in her article, ethical issues in the management of thyroid diseases. These include informed consent prior to any form of thyroid ablation, whether radioablation or surgery. As she discusses, patients under severe stress or suffering from extremes of the disorders such as hypothyroidism or thyrotoxicosis may not totally comprehend the various therapeutic choices and it behooves the physician to be alert to these possibilities. In addition, there are ethical issues arising from genetic disorders of thyroid disease in terms of confidentiality and testing of family members. Clearly, the use of experimental drugs in clinical trials has its own issues that need addressing. While the article focuses on thyroid disorders, it is clearly important for all medical conditions that we as health care providers are involved in diagnosing and treating.

Since thyroid hormone is critical for normal heart and cardiovascular system physiology, both overt thyroid dysfunction as well as subclinical disease may affect the cardiovascular system. Hyperthyroid-related cardiovascular effects are well known with both classic signs and symptoms, whereas hypothyroidism is associated with more subtle changes; the diagnosis is often established by elevated TSH levels. Of particular concern are the changes in lipid profiles. Drs Danzi and Klein also discuss the precautions needed when starting replacement therapies in the case of hypothyroid-ism, to avoid catastrophes, and further discuss the low T3 syndrome seen in chronic heart disease and amiodarone-induced thyroid dysfunction and how to deal with this problem.

In a similar vein, Dr Samuels discusses the cognitive impairment and other psycho-logical disturbances that are seen in hypothyroidism and thyrotoxic patients. These include anxiety and depression. They may be overt and more severe in classic hypo-thyroid and hyperthyroid patients, whereas they may be more subtle in subclinical forms of these disorders. Nevertheless, the good news is that there is usually signifi-cant improvement when the conditions are treated appropriately.

Pregnancy affects thyroid physiology due to increased thyroid-binding globulin and human chorionic gonadotropin, as well as enhanced iodine metabolism. For these rea-sons, normal reference ranges for thyroid function tests are altered. As Drs Nathan and Sullivan discuss, pregnant women with overt hypothyroidism and those with subclin-ical hypothyroidism but thyroid peroxidase antibody-positive should be treated with levothyroxine to maintain thyroid function in the normal range, specific for each trimester. In regard to treating thyrotoxicosis in pregnancy, thionamides are still the treatment of choice.

Radioisotope use is an important tool in the diagnosis and therapy of well-differen-tiated thyroid cancer and recurrence or distant metastases. Dr Esposito discusses how decisions are made regarding the dosage. In very low-risk patients with confined disease and no lymph node involvement nor distant metastases, a wait and watch approach is justified. In low-risk patients, those under 45 years of age with tumors be-tween 1 and 2 cm, the American Thyroid Association suggests doses of 30 to 100 mCi. For intermediate-risk patients, tumors greater than 2 cm, using up to 100 mCi is sug-gested, whereas for high-risk patients, with residual tumor and lymph node involve-ment or distant metastases, using 150 to 200 mCi is suggested.

While papillary thyroid carcinoma is usually associated with an excellent prognosis, its recurrence often requires additional management. Drs Goyal, Jonklass, and Bur-man discuss how, when cervical lymph nodes are detected after initial surgery as a recurrence, decisions are necessary as whether to use a surgical approach, radioac-tive iodine ablation, percutaneous ethanol injection, or simply observation.

Drs Elisai, Viola, Matorne, Biagini, and Molinaro discuss the value of thyroglobulin (Tg) measurements, particularly in managing and treating recurrences in the case of differentiated thyroid cancer including papillary and follicular subtypes. Since these tu-mors synthesize and secrete Tg, a rising level can be an indication of remnant neck tumor or distant metastases. In follow-up management after surgery, TSH suppres-sion by thyroid hormone often results in undetectable Tg. A rise in Tg suggests recur-rence and requires the search and eradication of the remnant and metastases, usually by careful neck ultrasound and whole radioisotope scans, followed by radioisotope therapy.

Clinical guidelines are developed by appropriate organizations to "guide" physi-cians in the best considered treatment plan for patients with certain disorders. In the case of Graves disease, the American Thyroid Association and the American As-sociation of Clinical Endocrinologists jointly produced these guidelines. However, as detailed by Drs Muldoon, Mai, and Burch, there is a significant discrepancy between the guidelines and actual physician practice. For example, in diagnosing the condition, the guidelines do not recommend routine thyroid scan, uptake, or ultrasound, while between 40% and 50% of physicians still use these tests. Furthermore, thyroid recep-tor antibody, which is not recommended, is used by approximately 60%. In regard to antithyroid drugs, both guidelines suggest and physicians use methylmethimazole preferentially over propylthiouracil, due to potential side effects. Similarly, in regard to thyrotoxicosis and pregnancy, there were discrepancies, while in regard to Graves ophthalmopathy, most physicians followed the guidelines.

I have thoroughly enjoyed reading the articles and hope the readers concur. The articles are written by the experts and cover basic and practical aspects that are important for our daily care of these common disorders. My appreciation to the issue editors, Dr Jonklaas and Burman, and the authors for this excellent compilation.

Derek LeRoith, MD, PhD
Division of Endocrinology, Metabolism, and Bone Diseases
Department of Medicine
Mount Sinai School of Medicine
One Gustave L. Levy Place
Box 1055, Altran 4-36
New York, NY 10029, USA

E-mail address:
derek.leroith@mssm.edu

Preface

Thyroid Cancer and Other Thyroid Disorders

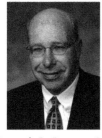 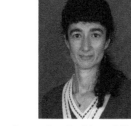

Kenneth D. Burman, MD   Jacqueline Jonklaas, MD, PhD
Editors

The thyroid field has benefited from a wide spectrum of recent advances that have not only allowed us to acquire a better understanding of thyroid diseases but have also permitted refinement of our management strategies. These advances have involved the areas of both benign and malignant thyroid diseases. We are privileged to have a collation of contributions from authors who are well known in their fields, and who have provided us with insightful, stimulating, state-of-the-art analyses of some of the areas affected by these recent advances.

In addition to being clinically relevant, the articles presented are diverse and far-ranging, spanning topics as varied as ethical issues arising during management of thyroid diseases, an update about thyroid cancer staging, a review of the implications of serum TSH concentrations for the diagnosis and management of thyroid cancer, and an examination of fatigue in thyroid cancer survivors. Some of the articles provide much food for thought, as they discuss topics about which the pace of recent advances has been quite rapid and divergent and has thus led to a range of opinions, such as the use of molecular diagnostics for the assessment of indeterminate thyroid nodules, and alternative surgical approaches to the thyroid gland. Some of the material also raises controversial ethical issues that have been subject to debate, and about which differences of opinion persist, such as considering trials of observation in selected patients with thyroid cancer and the topic of universal screening for thyroid disease in pregnancy.

We are especially indebted to the authors who have applied their energy and expertise to their articles and have provided extremely useful clinical and basic science information. We would also like to thank the editorial staff from Elsevier for their proficiency and thoroughness. As guest editors, we have derived significant pleasure and benefit from our interactions with the editors and authors. We have truly learned

Endocrinol Metab Clin N Am 43 (2014) xvii–xviii
http://dx.doi.org/10.1016/j.ecl.2014.03.002
0889-8529/14/$ – see front matter © 2014 Elsevier Inc. All rights reserved.

from reading the contributed articles. We hope that the same will be true for this issue's readership.

Kenneth D. Burman, MD
Endocrinology Section
Department of Medicine
Medstar Washington Hospital Center
110 Irving Street, NW
Washington, DC 20010, USA

Department of Medicine
Georgetown University
4000 Reservoir Road, NW
Washington, DC 20007, USA

Jacqueline Jonklaas, MD, PhD
Division of Endocrinology
Georgetown University
4000 Reservoir Road, NW
Washington, DC 20007, USA

E-mail addresses:
Kenneth.D.Burman@medstar.net (K.D. Burman)
jonklaaj@georgetown.edu (J. Jonklaas)

How to Manage Patients with Differentiated Thyroid Cancer and a Rising Serum Thyroglobulin Level

Rossella Elisei, MD*, Laura Agate, MD, David Viola, MD,
Antonio Matrone, MD, Agnese Biagini, MD,
Eleonora Molinaro, MD

KEYWORDS

- Differentiated thyroid carcinoma • Thyroglobulin • Recombinant human TSH
- Thyroid hormones • 131-iodine

KEY POINTS

- Serum thyroglobulin (Tg) is a very sensitive and specific marker of differentiated thyroid cancer persistence and recurrence; however, before initiating active radiologic surveillance, all possible causes of false-positivity or misinterpretation of the Tg value must be ruled out.
- Once the value is confirmed, a series of imaging procedures should be performed to discover the source of Tg secretion.
- The significance of the trend of an increasing serum Tg level is still unclear.
- Preliminary studies suggest that a Tg doubling time of less than 1 year represents a poor prognostic factor, but this seems to be applicable mainly in advanced cases.
- While awaiting follow-up data, neck ultrasound should be carefully performed any time a suspicious increase of Tg is observed.

INTRODUCTION
Differentiated Thyroid Cancer

Differentiated thyroid cancer (DTC), both papillary (PTC) and follicular (FTC), arise from follicular cells.[1] They are defined well differentiated because they maintain the typical morphologic features and physiologic functions of the normal follicular cells. In

The authors have nothing to disclose.
Endocrinology Unit, Department of Clinical and Experimental Medicine, WHO Collaborating Center for the Study and Treatment of Thyroid Diseases and Other Endocrine and Metabolic Disorders, University of Pisa, Via Paradisa 2, Pisa 56124, Italy
* Corresponding author. Endocrinology Unit, Department of Clinical and Experimental Medicine, University of Pisa, Via Paradisa 2, Pisa 56124, Italy.
E-mail address: rossella.elisei@med.unipi.it

Endocrinol Metab Clin N Am 43 (2014) 331–344
http://dx.doi.org/10.1016/j.ecl.2014.02.002
0889-8529/14/$ – see front matter © 2014 Elsevier Inc. All rights reserved.

endo.theclinics.com

particular, they typically retain (1) sensitivity to thyroid-stimulating hormone (TSH); (2) the ability to trap iodine; and (3) the ability to produce thyroglobulin (Tg). The maintenance of these properties is at least partly responsible for the high survival rate of patients with DTC (ie, 95% for PTC and 80% for FTC after 30–40 years of follow-up).[2] In fact, in many cases, tumor cell growth can be controlled with L-thyroxine (LT4) suppressive therapy, metastatic lesions can be treated successfully with iodine 131 (^{131}I), and recurrences can be discovered through monitoring serum Tg levels.[3] In indirect confirmation of this, evidence shows that 50% of poorly differentiated and anaplastic thyroid cancers, which lose completely or almost completely all of the properties mentioned earlier, are frequently lethal after a mean follow-up time of approximately 5 years and 6 months, respectively.[4,5]

LT4 Therapy in Patients with DTC

LT4 suppressive therapy is an integral part of antineoplastic treatment in patients with both biochemical and metastatic DTC, because it is usually able to reduce the growth of thyroid cancer cells. The optimal dose of LT4 should be able to simultaneously maintain FT4 levels within or near the normal range and TSH at low values (<0.1 μU/mL). Suppressive therapy should be administered until evidence of clinical remission is seen.[6] At this point, to reduce the potential side effects of a chronic LT4 suppressive therapy, the daily dose of LT4 must be reduced to increase the TSH values slightly greater than the lower value of the normal range.[7] During LT4 suppressive therapy, thyroid cell functions are suppressed, such as the ability to take up iodine and secrete Tg.

The Ability to Trap Iodine

Iodine uptake is a very particular function of thyroid cells and is mediated by the membrane sodium-iodine symporter, which is able to actively transfer iodide from the blood pool inside thyroid cells, both benign and malignant.[8] In physiologic states, this function is fundamental for a correct production of mature thyroid hormones, because triiodotironine (T_3) and thyroxine (T_4) require 3 and 4 atoms of iodine, respectively, to be active. A deficiency of iodine leads to decreased production of T_3 and T_4, enlarges the thyroid tissue, and causes the disease known as *goiter*.[9,10] Radioiodine is taken up by thyroid cells through the same mechanism, and more than 50 years ago investigators showed that it can be used not only for the ablation of postsurgical thyroid remnant but also for the treatment of metastatic lesions.[11] To be effective, iodine uptake of both postsurgical remnant thyroid cells and metastatic cells requires TSH stimulation, either endogenous or exogenous.[12]

SERUM TG
Biochemistry and Physiology of Tg

Tg is a big glycoprotein (molecular weight of 660,000) composed of 2 subunits of 330 kDa each. It is almost exclusively produced by thyroid follicular cells (**Fig. 1**), although some evidence suggests that small amounts of Tg can also be produced by the thymus gland.[13,14] Tg protein is not biologically active but is fundamental for the synthesis of T_4 and T_3, which are released after the endocytosis and proteolysis of Tg inside the thyrocytes. The relevance of Tg in producing thyroid hormones is clearly demonstrated by the fact that inborn genetic alterations of Tg DNA are causative of congenital hypothyroidism because the thyroid, although completely developed and well localized in the neck, is unable to produce mature T_3 and T_4 as a consequence of an abnormal or absent Tg.[15,16] Although Tg is secreted and stored in the colloid

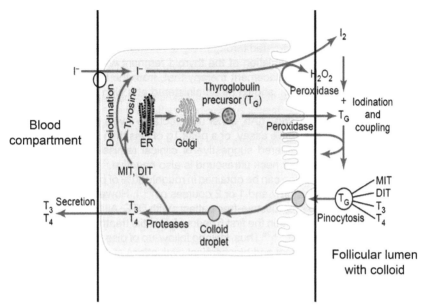

Fig. 1. Schematic representation of thyroid cell showing the process of synthesis of thyroid hormones in which thyroglobulin plays a major role. The relationship is shown between the thyroid cell with the follicular lumen, where the hormones are stored, and the blood compartment, where the hormones are secreted.

of follicular epithelium, thus representing approximately 75% of the total protein contained in thyroid follicles, Tg is also present in the serum of normal individuals and the concentrations are related to thyroid volume and function.[17]

Serum Tg: A Sensitive and Specific DTC Tumor Marker

Serum Tg concentrations are known to be very low or undetectable in athyreotic individuals, and therefore serum Tg is an excellent tumor marker (after total thyroidectomy and remnant ablation) in DTC.[18] Tumoral marker Tg is very sensitive and specific for detecting thyroid cancer recurrence, but 2 limitations must be taken into consideration: (1) the presence of serum Tg antibodies (TgAb) can interfere in the Tg assay by competing with the antibodies used for the measurement,[19,20] and (2) serum Tg secretion is dependent on TSH stimulation also in metastatic cells, and therefore a false-negative value can be obtained if measured when TSH is suppressed by LT4 therapy.[12,21]

The presence of circulating TgAb is an important issue because approximately 25% of patients with DTC usually have TgAbs,[22] and in these cases the sensitivity of Tg measurement is very low or null. Regarding the effect of LT4 suppressive therapy on Tg secretion, currently the possibility of using ultrasensitive Tg assays or the recombinant human TSH (rhTSH) stimulation test allows avoidance of LT4 therapy withdrawal, which was the common practice in the past to have a serum Tg value that was more reflective of the disease status.[23] In this regard, it is important to stress that Tg values measured after endogenous or exogenous TSH stimulation should not be compared with Tg values measured when TSH was normal or low, because TSH stimulation changes the baseline Tg determinations.[21]

follow-up, as shown in 2 different recent series.[34,35] However, assays are well-known to differ in their sensitivity and specificity.[36] Low specificity is the main cause of the large number of patients with low but detectable levels of serum Tg using ultrasensitive assays (ie, >0.1 ng/mL but <1 ng/mL), who currently cannot be defined as disease-free. In these cases, a rhTSH stimulation test can discriminate the real-positive Tg findings (≈25%) from the real-negative findings (≈75%).[20,37] To be useful from a clinical point of view, especially for decision making, ultrasensitive Tg assays require an institutional decisional cutoff likely higher than 0.1 ng/mL.[34,35]

Increasing of Already Detectable Serum Tg: Persistent Disease

The meaning of increasing serum Tg is different from the previously described unexpected evidence of detectable levels of serum Tg in a patient considered disease-free. The presence of detectable levels of serum Tg in the absence of any detectable lesions using common imaging techniques is defined as biochemical disease. Despite industrious attempts to find the source of Tg production, all imaging procedures produce negative results in approximately 10% of patients with detectable levels of either basal or stimulated Tg. Possible ectopic Tg production from residual thymus should be considered in the presence of persistent relatively low detectable levels of serum Tg, especially in young patients.[14] This hypothesis can be supported by a computed tomography (CT) scan of the neck/mediastinum region and the presence of an enlarged thymus. This technique does not prove the thymus is the source of Tg, but raises the suspicion.

In patients with detectable levels of serum Tg, a stable value of serum Tg is considered a favorable finding and indicative of stable disease. The same concept is valid for both patients with biochemical disease and those with an identifiable metastatic disease. Given these comments, no active or aggressive therapies should be prescribed; rather, a "wait and see" strategy should be applied to most of these patients, who must be monitored closely (**Fig. 3**).[6]

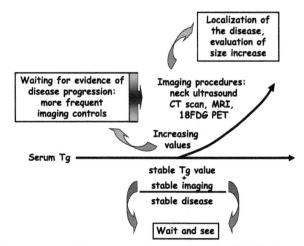

Fig. 3. Serum Tg–based algorithm for following up patients with DTC. When serum Tg is stable in the absence of TgAb, the disease can be considered stable and no active therapies should be initiated, even in the presence of high values of serum Tg. When Tg values begin to increase, a more stringent follow-up protocol should be performed, with imaging procedures every 6 months, and only when authentic disease progression is observed should a new therapeutic strategy be started.

Unfortunately, the quantitative interval Tg increase that should promote further investigation is currently unknown, and only preliminary evidence shows that a serum Tg doubling time less than 1 year, when patients are on LT4 therapy, represents a poor prognostic factor for their cancer-related survival.[38,39] Moreover, the prognostic role of serum Tg doubling time is more relevant for elevated values of serum Tg, especially in advanced cases.

The serum Tg trend analysis is even more important because of the increasing number of low-risk patients with DTC who are not submitted to remnant radioablation and those who are treated with lobectomy alone.[40,41] In these patients, low but detectable levels of serum Tg, especially if monitored with ultrasensitive assays, will be found because of the persistence of residual thyroid tissue, either when it is represented by a small remnant or an entire lobe. Although several studies have been already published on the interpretation of the basal serum Tg values determined with ultrasensitive assays[42,43] no data are currently available for the interpretation of the increasing Tg in patients with DTC treated with a conservative approach. Although these are usually low-risk patients with DTC, they are not free from the risk of recurrence, estimated to be approximately 2% to 3% in this group.[44,45] Because in most cases the tumors recur in the neck area or in the residual lobe, neck ultrasound is significantly helpful in their monitoring.[46,47] Only a long-term follow-up study of these patients could determine the significance and quantitation of the trend of serum Tg increase.

Increasing Serum Tg Levels and Imaging Procedures

The identification of detectable levels of serum Tg after a period of undetectability or the increase of longstanding detectable but stable levels of serum Tg does not provide per se any information on the location of recurring or persistent diseases. Thus, the process of identifying metastases should include further diagnostic procedures to localize the sites of lesions, measure their size, and establish if therapy should be initiated (see **Fig. 3**). Although patients with highly elevated serum Tg levels are expected to have detectable and measurable metastases, those with detectable but low levels of Tg are expected to have negative findings on imaging studies. In the latter case, appropriate imaging techniques should be repeated after any significant increase of serum markers.

Neck Ultrasound

As shown in **Box 2**, both metastatic lymph nodes and local recurrence typically have very peculiar echographic features and can be easily recognized on neck ultrasound.[48] However, when the ultrasound features are doubtful, the malignant nature of the lesions can be confirmed through fine-needle aspiration (FNA), cytology (with or without immunocytochemistry for Tg), and serum Tg measurements in the washout of the needle used for FNA.[49]

Neck ultrasound is one of the most important tools in the management of patients with DTC, because it can reveal unsuspected lymph node metastases and/or local recurrence (**Fig. 4**) even when serum Tg levels are undetectable.[47] For this reason and because of its cost-effectiveness, an annual neck ultrasound control is recommended, even in apparently cured patients with DTC. In particular, neck ultrasound should be immediately performed when an unexpected increase of serum Tg levels is observed and every 6 to 12 months in patients with DTC with persistently elevated serum Tg levels.

In the first few years after surgical treatment, metastases to small lymph nodes in the neck are the most frequent cause of persistent or recurrent disease, especially

Box 2

Echographic features of persistent or recurrent disease in the thyroid bed and of metastatic lateral cervical lymph nodes

A. Suspicious lesions in the thyroid bed (mainly local recurrence)

    1. Ovoid shape in the longitudinal plane but taller than wide in the transverse plane

    2. Hypoechogenicity

    3. Microcalcifications

    4. Irregular borders

    5. Increased vascularization

B. Suspicious lesions in the lateral neck compartment (mainly lymph node metastases)

    1. Round shape

    2. Loss of hilum

    3. Microcalcifications

    4. Hypoechogenicity or cystic features or even hyperechoic tissue looking like thyroid tissue

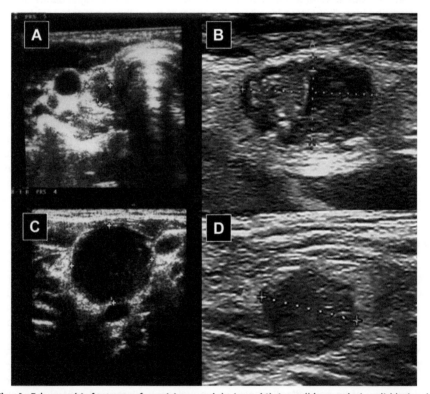

Fig. 4. Echographic features of suspicious neck lesions. (*A*) A small hypoechoic solid lesion is present in the right part of the thyroid bed, likely because of a local recurrence. (*B*) Microcalcifications and irregular borders make this solid lesion highly suspicious for a lymph node metastases. (*C*) This round hypoechoic lesion very close to the carotid and jugular vein is strongly suspicious for lymph node metastases. (*D*) The irregular borders of this solid round lesion are strongly suggestive of malignancy, either local recurrence or lymph node metastases. Cytologic analysis of smears obtained through FNA of these lesions and the Tg measurement in the washout of the needle used for FNA will clarify the nature of these lesions.

in patients affected by PTC, and particularly in children and young adults, even after several local surgical treatments.

CT Scan, MRI, and Bone Scintigraphy

A total body spiral CT scan should be performed when a significant increase of serum Tg is revealed. A spiral chest CT is the most sensitive imaging for lung metastasis, because it can detect lung micronodules as small as 2 mm (**Fig. 5**). The chest CT is usually performed without intravenous radiocontrast if a radioactive iodine scan or treatment is planned in the near future. Magnetic resonance imaging (MRI) is recognized as the most sensitive tool for detecting liver lesions and to distinguish their real nature (ie, angiomas, cysts, metastases, or benign nodules). If the radiologic interpretation of lung or liver lesions is doubtful, the possibility of performing a biopsy should be discussed with the radiologist taking into account the size and the position of the lesions: too small lesions or lesions rather distant form the surface are difficult to be biopsied and theoretically unsuccessful procedures should be avoided. The most traditional but most sensitive imaging technique for identifying bone lesions is bone scintigraphy,[50] which is used during follow-up for patients with PTC and FTC with persistent disease. Whenever possible, a total body MRI of the skeleton can be useful in detecting bone metastatic lesions.[51]

Nuclear Medicine Imaging

Whether an empiric high activity of ^{131}I should be administered solely based on an increase of serum Tg is controversial.[52–55] Diagnostic whole body scan (dWBS) is known to have a low diagnostic sensitivity,[56] whereas a posttherapeutic whole body scan (ptWBS) shows a higher sensitivity[52,53] and can reveal metastatic lesions not detected with dWBS. However, metastatic lesions visible at ptWBS but not at dWBS have been shown to be rarely cured by ^{131}I, thus bringing into questioning the utility of this practice.[57,58]

Administration of an empiric high-activity radioactive iodine dose followed by a ptWBS is also important for planning future therapeutic strategies, because a negative ptWBS, after excluding interfering factors such as iodine contamination, clearly indicates that the tumor has become radiorefractory and other systemic therapies should be considered in the future, such as tyrosine kinase inhibitors, rather than continue

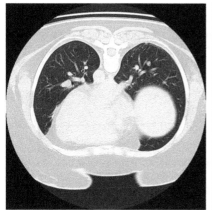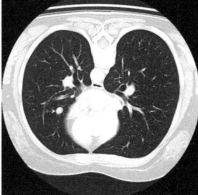

Fig. 5. Chest CT scan of 2 patients with DTC with increasing values of serum Tg; in both cases small multiple lung metastatic lesions are visible.

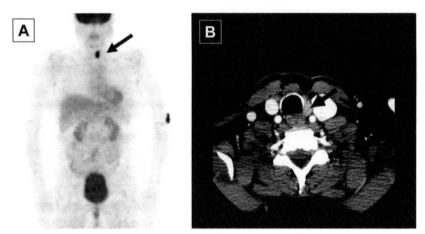

Fig. 6. (*A*) Typical image obtained with FDG-PET/CT in an advanced case of DTC with local recurrence/persistent disease, indicated by the *arrow*. (*B*) The CT scan shows the paratracheal position of the FDG-PET–positive lesion.

with [131]I.[59] Therefore, non–[131]I-based imaging techniques should be used in the follow-up of these patients. However, when the risk of persistent or recurring disease is very high, because of the presence of very high levels of serum Tg while on LT4 therapy, ^{123}I may be used in place of ^{131}I to avoid jeopardizing the efficacy of subsequent ^{131}I therapy. In this case, images are usually acquired 48 hours after intravenous administration of 185 MBq of [123]I[60] and, if positive, the ^{131}I treatment can be performed immediately.

The low biologic aggressiveness of DTC is the major limitation of using 18-fluoro-deoxyglucose positron emission tomography (FDG-PET). Well-differentiated DTC in patients with detectable but low levels of serum Tg is usually not seen on FDG-PET scans, and evidence shows that lesions are rarely detected by FDG-PET in patients with serum Tg levels lower than 10 ng/mL who are on LT4 therapy.[61] FDG-PET combined with a CT scan is of great relevance for better mapping the metastatic lesions (**Fig. 6**).

The prognostic significance of FDG-PET is more relevant because evidence shows that, among patients with metastatic DTC, those with FDG-PET–positive lesions have a worse prognosis than those with FDG-PET–negative lesions.[62] Thus, FDG-PET is particularly indicated in patients with aggressive DTC, especially if they are unable to trap iodine. Although FDG-PET can be performed while a patient is on LT4 treatment, FDG uptake by DTC cells is higher under TSH stimulation that is able to increase the expression of the glucose receptors on cell membranes.[63] Therefore, FDG-PET is recommended after the administration of rhTSH, in accordance with the standard procedure (see **Fig. 2**).

SUMMARY

Serum Tg is a very sensitive and specific marker of DTC persistence and recurrence. However, before initiating active radiologic surveillance, all possible causes of false-positivity or misinterpretation of the Tg value must be ruled out. Once the value is confirmed, a series of imaging procedures should be performed to discover the source of Tg secretion. The success of this search is related to the levels of serum Tg, and results will more likely be positive for higher values of serum Tg.

One issue that remains unclear is the significance of the trend of an increasing serum Tg level. Preliminary studies suggest that a Tg doubling time of less than 1 year represents a poor prognostic factor, but this seems to be applicable mainly in advanced cases. No data are currently available regarding low-risk patients with DTC undergoing conservative treatment and who have low but detectable levels of serum Tg because of the postsurgical unablated remnant or the unresected lobe. While awaiting follow-up data, neck ultrasound should be carefully performed any time a suspicious increase of Tg is observed.

REFERENCES

1. Schlumberger MJ. Papillary and follicular thyroid carcinoma. N Engl J Med 1998;338(5):297–306.
2. Elisei R, Molinaro E, Agate L, et al. Are the clinical and pathological features of differentiated thyroid carcinoma really changed over the last 35 years? Study on 4187 patients from a single Italian institution to answer this question. J Clin Endocrinol Metab 2010;95(4):1516–27.
3. Elisei R, Pinchera A. Advances in the follow-up of differentiated or medullary thyroid cancer. Nat Rev Endocrinol 2012;8(8):466–75.
4. Ibrahimpasic T, Ghossein R, Carlson DL, et al. Poorly differentiated thyroid carcinoma presenting with gross extrathyroidal extension: 1986-2009 Memorial Sloan-Kettering Cancer Center experience. Thyroid 2013;23(8):997–1002.
5. Chiacchio S, Lorenzoni A, Boni G, et al. Anaplastic thyroid cancer: prevalence, diagnosis and treatment. Minerva Endocrinol 2008;33(4):341–57.
6. Cooper DS, Doherty GM, Haugen BR, et al. Revised American Thyroid Association management guidelines for patients with thyroid nodules and differentiated thyroid cancer. Thyroid 2009;19(11):1167–214.
7. Biondi B, Cooper DS. Benefits of thyrotropin suppression versus the risks of adverse effects in differentiated thyroid cancer. Thyroid 2010;20(2):135–46.
8. Levy O, Dai G, Riedel C, et al. Characterization of the thyroid Na+/I- symporter with an anti-COOH terminus antibody. Proc Natl Acad Sci U S A 1997;94(11):5568–73.
9. Zimmermann MB, Andersson M. Assessment of iodine nutrition in populations: past, present, and future. Nutr Rev 2012;70(10):553–70.
10. Aghini Lombardi F, Fiore E, Tonacchera M, et al. The effect of voluntary iodine prophylaxis in a small rural community: the Pescopagano survey 15 years later. J Clin Endocrinol Metab 2013;98(3):1031–9.
11. Frantz VK, Larsen WG, Jaretzki A 3rd. An evaluation of radioactive iodine therapy in metastatic thyroid cancer. J Clin Endocrinol Metab 1950;10(9):1084–91.
12. Sabra MM, Tuttle RM. Recombinant human thyroid-stimulating hormone to stimulate 131-I uptake for remnant ablation and adjuvant therapy. Endocr Pract 2013;19(1):149–56.
13. Spitzweg C, Joba W, Heufelder AE. Expression of thyroid-related genes in human thymus. Thyroid 1999;9(2):133–41.
14. Zanotti-Fregonara P, Keller I, Calzada-Nocaudie M, et al. Increased serum thyroglobulin levels and negative imaging in thyroid cancer patients: are there sources of benign secretion? A speculative short review. Nucl Med Commun 2010;31(12):1054–8.
15. Agretti P, De Marco G, Di Cosmo C, et al. Congenital hypothyroidism caused by a novel homozygous mutation in the thyroglobulin gene. Eur J Pediatr 2013;172(7):959–64.

48. Leboulleux S, Girard E, Rose M, et al. Ultrasound criteria of malignancy for cervical lymph nodes in patients followed up for differentiated thyroid cancer. J Clin Endocrinol Metab 2007;92(9):3590–4.

49. Pacini F, Fugazzola L, Lippi F, et al. Detection of thyroglobulin in fine needle aspirates of nonthyroidal neck masses: a clue to the diagnosis of metastatic differentiated thyroid cancer. J Clin Endocrinol Metab 1992;74(6):1401–4.

50. Giraudet AL, Vanel D, Leboulleux S, et al. Imaging medullary thyroid carcinoma with persistent elevated calcitonin levels. J Clin Endocrinol Metab 2007;92(11): 4185–90.

51. Ribrag V, Vanel D, Leboulleux S, et al. Prospective study of bone marrow infiltration in aggressive lymphoma by three independent methods: whole-body MRI, PET/CT and bone marrow biopsy. Eur J Radiol 2008;66(2):325–31.

52. Pacini F, Lippi F, Formica N, et al. Therapeutic doses of iodine-131 reveal undiagnosed metastases in thyroid cancer patients with detectable serum thyroglobulin levels. J Nucl Med 1987;28(12):1888–91.

53. Pineda JD, Lee T, Ain K, et al. Iodine-131 therapy for thyroid cancer patients with elevated thyroglobulin and negative diagnostic scan. J Clin Endocrinol Metab 1995;80(5):1488–92.

54. Schlumberger M, Arcangioli O, Piekarski JD, et al. Detection and treatment of lung metastases of differentiated thyroid carcinoma in patients with normal chest X-rays. J Nucl Med 1988;29(11):1790–4.

55. Rosario PW, Mourao GF, Santos JB, et al. Is empirical radioiodine therapy still a valid approach in patients with thyroid cancer and elevated thyroglobulin? Thyroid 2014;24:533–6.

56. Pacini F, Capezzone M, Elisei R, et al. Diagnostic 131-iodine whole-body scan may be avoided in thyroid cancer patients who have undetectable stimulated serum Tg levels after initial treatment. J Clin Endocrinol Metab 2002;87(4): 1499–501.

57. Sabra MM, Grewal RK, Tala H, et al. Clinical outcomes following empiric radioiodine therapy in patients with structurally identifiable metastatic follicular cell-derived thyroid carcinoma with negative diagnostic but positive post-therapy 131I whole-body scans. Thyroid 2012;22(9):877–83.

58. Pacini F, Agate L, Elisei R, et al. Outcome of differentiated thyroid cancer with detectable serum Tg and negative diagnostic (131)I whole body scan: comparison of patients treated with high (131)I activities versus untreated patients. J Clin Endocrinol Metab 2001;86(9):4092–7.

59. Schlumberger M, Sherman SI. Approach to the patient with advanced differentiated thyroid cancer. Eur J Endocrinol 2012;166(1):5–11.

60. Urhan M, Dadparvar S, Mavi A, et al. Iodine-123 as a diagnostic imaging agent in differentiated thyroid carcinoma: a comparison with iodine-131 post-treatment scanning and serum thyroglobulin measurement. Eur J Nucl Med Mol Imaging 2007;34(7):1012–7.

61. Lee JW, Lee SM, Lee DH, et al. Clinical utility of 18F-FDG PET/CT concurrent with 131I therapy in intermediate-to-high-risk patients with differentiated thyroid cancer: dual-center experience with 286 patients. J Nucl Med 2013;54(8):1230–6.

62. Robbins RJ, Wan Q, Grewal RK, et al. Real-time prognosis for metastatic thyroid carcinoma based on 2-[18F]fluoro-2-deoxy-D-glucose-positron emission tomography scanning. J Clin Endocrinol Metab 2006;91(2):498–505.

63. Sisson JC, Ackermann RJ, Meyer MA, et al. Uptake of 18-fluoro-2-deoxy-D-glucose by thyroid cancer: implications for diagnosis and therapy. J Clin Endocrinol Metab 1993;77(4):1090–4.

Molecular Diagnostics for Thyroid Nodules

The Current State of Affairs

Sann Yu Mon, MD, MPH[a], Steven P. Hodak, MD[b],*

KEYWORDS

- Molecular diagnosis for thyroid nodules • Immunohistochemical tests
- Genetic mutations in thyroid cancer • Atypia of uncertain significance/
follicular lesion of uncertain significance • Follicular neoplasm/
suspicious for follicular neoplasm • Suspicious for malignant cells

KEY POINTS

- Approximately 10% to 40% of thyroid fine-needle aspirations (FNA) are cytologically indeterminate, and the inability to definitively resolve thyroid nodules as benign or malignant is a substantial clinical problem.
- A growing number of molecular and immunohistochemical tests have been developed, which may be performed on specimens obtained during standard FNA.
- Many molecular markers have been evaluated for their diagnostic performance, but only a few have demonstrated robust and clinically applicable results.
- A better understanding of the diagnostic performance of molecular tests, and how they can enhance clinical management of cytologically indeterminate nodules, is important.

INTRODUCTION

Fine-needle aspiration (FNA) cytology remains the gold standard for the evaluation of thyroid nodules. However, 10% to 40% of thyroid FNAs are cytologically indeterminate.[1] The prevalence of thyroid nodules continues to increase, and in 2012 it is estimated that 450,000 thyroid nodule FNAs were performed in the United States.[2] The prevalence of indeterminate cytology and the inability to definitively resolve thyroid nodules as benign or malignant is therefore a substantial clinical problem. When cytology alone cannot provide a diagnosis, many patients are referred for a diagnostic

The authors have nothing to disclose.
[a] Division of Endocrinology, University of Pittsburgh School of Medicine, 200 Lothrop Street, BST 1140, Pittsburgh, PA 15213, USA; [b] Division of Endocrinology, Center for Diabetes and Endocrinology, University of Pittsburgh School of Medicine, 3601 Fifth Avenue, Suite 587, Pittsburgh, PA 15213, USA
* Corresponding author.
E-mail address: sph12@pitt.edu

Endocrinol Metab Clin N Am 43 (2014) 345–365
http://dx.doi.org/10.1016/j.ecl.2014.02.015
0889-8529/14/$ – see front matter © 2014 Elsevier Inc. All rights reserved.

lobectomy for definitive histologic diagnosis. However, in patients who undergo diagnostic lobectomy, more than 50% have benign histology.[3] In cases where clinically relevant cancers are found at lobectomy, a second definitive procedure (ie, completion thyroidectomy) is usually performed, which conveys additional surgical risks and costs.[4] To address the common problem of indeterminate cytology an increasing number of molecular and immunohistochemical tests have been developed, which may be performed on specimens obtained during standard FNA. Many of these tests improve diagnostic yield and are already being incorporated into standard clinical algorithms as important adjunctive tools for assessing cytologically indeterminate nodules.

Multiple different molecular and immunohistochemical approaches have been developed to improve diagnostic yield in cytologically indeterminate thyroid nodules. Approximately 75% of thyroid cancers harbor at least 1 of a small number of known somatic genetic mutations (ie, not present in germline DNA) that can be used to identify thyroid cancers with high specificity.[5,6] A recently available commercial test (Afirma assay; Veracyte, South San Francisco, CA) takes a unique and alternative approach to analyzing the genetic signature of benign and malignant thyroid nodules to identify lesions with a very low risk of malignancy. MicroRNA (miRNA) profiles allow predictive discrimination between benign and malignant thyroid nodules, and blood testing for mRNA for the thyroid-stimulating hormone receptor (TSHR) has been shown to correlate with malignant thyroid nodules in addition to recurrences in patients treated definitively with thyroidectomy and radioactive iodine. Numerous immunohistochemical tests have also been shown to have variable sensitivity and specificity for thyroid cancer. Although many molecular markers have been evaluated, only a few have demonstrated robust diagnostic performance. This article reviews the diagnostic utility of molecular and immunohistochemical testing for the clinical assessment of thyroid nodules.

IMMUNOHISTOCHEMICAL TESTING FOR THYROID CANCER
Galectin-3

Galectin-3, a galactoside-binding lectin, is involved in the regulation of cell-to-cell and cell-to-matrix interactions, cell growth, neoplastic transformation, and apoptosis.[7] Several studies have suggested that galectin-3 can be used as an immunohistochemical marker to differentiate benign from malignant thyroid nodules[8–10]; however, these studies have reported variable sensitivities and specificities of galectin-3 as a malignant marker in thyroid neoplasms. A meta-analysis of 66 studies published between January 2001 and December 2011 reported that galectin-3 had sensitivity of 82% and specificity of 81% for the diagnosis of malignant thyroid lesions.[11] Despite these findings, the widespread use of galectin-3 alone as a molecular predictor of thyroid cancer has remained limited.

HBME-1

HBME-1 (Hector Battifora mesothelial cell 1) monoclonal antibody is directed against mesothelioma cells. HBME-1 has been shown to be differentially expressed in malignant thyroid cancer in comparison with benign follicular lesions of the thyroid; however, the specificity and the sensitivity of HBME-1 as a diagnostic tumor marker varies from 79% to 87% and 83% to 96%, respectively, in the literature.[11–16] The specificity improves slightly when HBME-1 is used in a panel with other immunohistochemical markers[17]; nevertheless, the utility of HBME-1 as a sole diagnostic marker for thyroid cancer is still limited.

CK-19

CK-19 is a low molecular weight keratin, which is normally expressed in the lining of the gastroenteropancreatic and hepatobiliary tracts where it is responsible for structural integrity of epithelial cells. Although some studies have proposed its usefulness for differentiating malignant from benign thyroid masses, others have shown that CK-19 expression is found in both benign and malignant nodules.[11,12,17–20] A few studies have reported that diffuse expression of CK-19 was associated with papillary thyroid cancer (PTC), whereas focal expression was found in benign nodules.[17,18] Owing to the lack of consistent well-validated data on its sensitivity and specificity, the diagnostic importance of CK-19 staining of FNA cytologic specimens remains controversial.

CXCR-4

CXCR-4 is a G-protein–linked receptor for chemokines that is thought to promote metastasis by acting directly on tumor-cell migration and invasion. Overexpression of CXCR-4 was reported in PTC with a sensitivity of 92% and specificity of 96%.[21] In addition, a correlation between CXCR-4 expression and an increased risk of lymph node metastasis in PTC was also reported.[22] However, these data have not yet been validated by large-scale clinical trials.

Fibronecin-1, CITED-1, CXCL-12

A few small studies have proposed the diagnostic utility of other immunohistochemical tests, such as Fibronection-1, CITED-1, and CXCL-12, in differentiating benign from malignant nodules.[12,18,23,24] However, their use remains limited because of the lack of sufficient research documenting their sensitivity and specificity.

Combined Immunohistochemical Panels

The diagnostic value of combined immunohistochemical panels has been evaluated in several studies. Although different combinations of immunohistochemical markers have been studied, most panels have included Galectin-3, HBME-1, and CK-19. A meta-analysis has demonstrated that a combination of these 3 markers had sensitivity of 85%, specificity of 97%, and a diagnostic odds ratio of 95.1.[11] In a small study of 125 FNA samples of cytologically indeterminate thyroid nodules, the combination of galectin-3 and CK-19 improved both the sensitivity and specificity to 100%.[15] This study suggested that the sequential combination of 2 markers improved the accuracy of the diagnosis of follicular neoplasms, but a combination of 3 or more markers did not further improve diagnostic accuracy. Studies on this topic remain limited in scale, and robust data to support the accuracy and diagnostic performance of such combined panels in screening for thyroid cancer in FNA cytology specimens are still lacking.

GENETIC TESTING FOR THE IDENTIFICATION OF THYROID CANCER
BRAF

The *BRAF* gene, a serine-threonine kinase in the family of *RAF* kinases, is located on chromosome 7, and is mainly involved in transmitting signals from the extracellular space into the nucleus thereby regulating cell proliferation, differentiation, and migration through the mitogen activation protein kinase (MAPK) pathway.[25,26] There are more than 40 mutations in the *BRAF* gene that have been linked to human cancers; however, only a few mutations are found in thyroid cancer. The T1799A point *BRAF* mutation (*BRAF*V600E) is the most common mutation in thyroid cancer,[26] and results from a substitution of glutamic acid for valine at position 600 in the *BRAF* protein,[25] leading to constitutive activation of MAPK and tumorigenesis.[27] It has been reported in approximately 45% of all thyroid cancers, 51% of conventional PTCs, and in 24% of follicular variant PTCs.[26] The *BRAF*V600E mutation is also common in more histologically aggressive cancers, and has been reported in 80% to 83% of tall-cell variant PTC,[28–30] 10% to 15% of poorly differentiated carcinomas, and 20% to 30% of anaplastic carcinomas.[31] *BRAF*V600E has only rarely been reported in follicular thyroid cancers.[26,27,32,33] Numerous studies have identified *BRAF*V600E mutations as an independent risk factor for more advanced disease at presentation, with an increased risk of disease-specific mortality.[34,35] However, other published data call these findings into question.[36] The prognostic value of *BRAF*V600E therefore remains unresolved. A few other *BRAF* mutations, such as the K601E point mutation, small inframe insertions or deletions surrounding codon 600, and the AKAP9/*BRAF* rearrangement are only rarely identified in 1% to 2% of PTCs.[37–41]

Although the prognostic role of *BRAF*V600E mutation in FNA cytology specimens may be unclear, its diagnostic role has been extensively studied, and has repeatedly been shown to improve the accuracy of the cytologic diagnosis of thyroid nodules.[28,42–44] Melck and colleagues[28] summarized the studies evaluating *BRAF* testing of FNA biopsy (FNAB) specimens between 2004 and 2010. The specificity of *BRAF* testing in FNAB specimens for PTC was reported as between 97.3% and 100%, with a positive predictive value (PPV) for PTC between 95.7% and 100%; the negative predictive value (NPV) for PTC was reported to be between 17.9% and 91.8%.[28] A meta-analysis of 18 studies evaluating the diagnostic utility of *BRAF* in a total of 2766 thyroid FNA samples concluded that papillary cancer was confirmed in 580 of 581 *BRAF*-positive cases, providing a PPV of 99.8%.[44]

Although detection of the *BRAF* mutation is highly specific for PTC, it is rarely found in other types of thyroid cancer, especially follicular thyroid cancer.[26,27,32,33] In addition, although *BRAF* mutations can be identified in up to 45% of all thyroid cancers, the prevalence of *BRAF* mutations was only 16% among indeterminate thyroid nodules in the largest study to date.[42] Because up to 55% of all thyroid cancers do not harbor BRAF mutations, its sensitivity is poor and its use as an isolated molecular marker (when negative) has limited value.

RAS

The *RAS* oncogene family consists of 3 genes: *HRAS*, *KRAS*, and *NRAS*. The *RAS* proteins are small guanosine triphosphatase proteins that play an important role in the transduction of mitogenic signals through MAPK, phosphatidylinositol-3-kinase (PI3K)/Akt, and other intracellular signaling pathways responsible for cellular differentiation, proliferation, and survival.[45,46] Point mutations at codons 12, 13, and 61 of the *RAS* genes have been identified in many different types of human cancers. Most human cancers are specific for only 1 of the 3 *RAS* gene mutations, whereas mutations of all 3 *RAS* genes have been reported in thyroid neoplasia.[45] A variable prevalence of *RAS* mutations in thyroid neoplasms has been reported. However, most studies suggest a predominant distribution of 40% to 50% in follicular thyroid cancer,[31,45,47] 10% to 20% in follicular variant PTCs, 35% in poorly differentiated carcinomas, and 55% in anaplastic carcinomas.[31,47] In the largest study reported to date of 68 thyroid FNA aspirates from 66 patients positive for *RAS* mutations, *NRAS* codon 61 mutation was most prevalent and was identified in 72%, whereas *HRAS* codon 61 and *KRAS* codons 12 were identified in 22% and 6% of aspirates, respectively.[48] Recent literature has also described the presence of *RAS* mutations in 68% of *RET*-oncogene–negative sporadic medullary thyroid cancers.[49]

RAS molecular testing in FNA specimens has been shown to have PPV for malignancy ranging from 74% to 88%.[1,6,31,48] In the specific case of cytologically indeterminate thyroid nodules, *RAS* mutations are associated with an 85% to 88% risk of thyroid cancer, depending on Bethesda indeterminate cytology category.[43] Identification of *RAS* mutations are also useful diagnostically because they frequently occur in follicular variant PTC and follicular carcinoma, which are notoriously difficult to diagnose by cytology alone.[31,48] *RAS* mutations are also identified in benign follicular adenomas and hyperplastic nodules, contributing to the approximately 15% false-positive rate.[31,48] However, many investigators propose that *RAS*-positive benign nodules are actually all premalignant clonal adenomas that would eventually transform into *RAS*-positive follicular variant papillary and follicular carcinomas over time.[31,48,50,51]

RET/PTC

The *RET* proto-oncogene codes for a tyrosine kinase receptor protein, which is involved in intracellular signal transduction. Somatic *RET* rearrangements have been identified in thyroid cancer, specifically PTC, and have been thus named *RET/PTC*. These clonal somatic mutations are present only in the thyroid cancer itself and differ from the germline RET-oncogene mutations associated with multiple endocrine neoplasia–2 syndromes. The 2 most common *RET/PTC* rearrangements associated with PTC are *RET/PTC*1 and *RET/PTC*3, both of which have been reported with increased incidence in patients with a history of radiation exposure.[47,52] *RET/PTC* mutations are also prevalent in thyroid cancers that occur in younger patients, and its prevalence is reported in up to 45% of PTCs among the age group of 6 to 21 years.[47,52,53]

RET/PTC rearrangements occur in approximately 10% to 20% of papillary thyroid carcinomas[47,51]; however, their prevalence in sporadic papillary thyroid carcinomas has been reported to range widely from 0% to 61%.[51,52] This variability is thought to arise from inconsistent sensitivities of detection methods in these studies, in addition to evidence suggesting that RET/PTC prevalence may be increased in specific geographic locations such as North America and Australia.[31,54,55] In 2 prospective studies conducted by Nikiforov and colleagues[1] and Cantara and colleagues,[6] all thyroid nodules positive for clonal *RET/PTC* mutations were histologically proved to be papillary carcinomas. However, RET/PTC mutations can be demonstrated in a variety of benign and malignant lesions, usually through the use of ultrasensitive polymerase chain reaction (PCR) techniques.[56] These mutations are nonclonal (ie, they present at low allelic frequency), and are therefore not a marker of a clonally expanded neoplasm derived from a single progenitor cell.[56] Identification of nonclonal *RET/PTC* mutations has no proven diagnostic utility for identifying thyroid cancer.[51] This aspect highlights the importance of using appropriately standardized detection methods to increase the specificity of *RET/PTC* mutations and, in fact, all mutations in detecting thyroid cancer.[31] Although testing for *RET/PTC* is extremely specific for thyroid cancer, the diagnostic utility of this test as an isolated molecular marker is limited because of its low prevalence. In the largest study to date of indeterminate thyroid nodules, prevalence of *RET/PTC* was only 0.83% (1 sample among 121 histologically proven malignant nodules).[43]

PAX8/PPARG

The *PAX8/PPARG* fusion protein is a somatic tumor genetic rearrangement resulting from the chromosomal translocation t(2;3)(q13;p25). This rearrangement leads to a fusion between the *PAX8* gene, which encodes a paired domain transcription factor, and the *PPARG* gene, which encodes the peroxisome proliferator-activated receptor.[57] Although the exact pathogenesis of the *PAX8/PPARG* oncogene in thyroid cancer is still under investigation, it has been shown to occur in about 36% of follicular thyroid cancers, 13% of follicular variant PTCs, and 2% of oncocytic (Hürthle cell) carcinomas and anaplastic thyroid cancers.[58] Although the prevalence of *PAX8/PPARG* has been reported to vary widely from 0% to 55% of follicular adenomas, these studies use different methods for *PAX8/PPARG* detection, which likely accounts for this variability.[58] However, when only nodules with indeterminate cytology are considered, *PAX8/PPARG* has been shown to have a specificity of 100% for thyroid cancer.[1,6,43] Nevertheless, many investigators believe that *PAX8/PPARG*-positive follicular adenomas may also be premalignant lesions that may eventually develop into cancer.[58]

Combined Genetic Analysis

Although many of the individual genetic markers described so far have poor sensitivity (ie, they are frequently absent in cancer), they have high specificity (ie, the presence of a marker is highly correlated with the presence of cancer). Combining multiple markers has been shown to dramatically improve diagnostic yield. The combination of *BRAFV600E*, *NRAS* codon 61, *HRAS* codon 61, *KRAS* codon 12/13 point mutations, and *RET/PTC1*, *RET/PTC3*, and *PAX8/PPARG* rearrangements has been shown to identify up to 70% of all thyroid cancers, and up to 64% of thyroid cancers in cytologically indeterminate nodules, thus improving diagnostic yield in comparison with cytology alone.[1,6,43,59] In the largest report to date, Nikiforov and colleagues[43] evaluated the diagnostic utility of a combined panel of molecular markers including *BRAF*, *RAS*, *RET/PTC*, and *PAX8/PPARG* for analysis of cytologically indeterminate thyroid nodules. If any marker in the panel was positive, the risk of malignancy increased from 14%, 27%, and 54% based on cytology alone to 88%, 87%, and 95% for lesions categorized using the Bethesda System for Reporting Cytopathology as atypia of uncertain significance/follicular lesion of uncertain significance (AUS/FLUS), follicular neoplasm/suspicious for follicular neoplasm (FN/SFN), and suspicious for malignant cells (SMC), respectively.[60] In another large prospective study of 235 cytology samples, Cantara and colleagues[6] studied the combined testing of a panel of molecular tests including *BRAF* point mutations V600E and K601E, *H-K-NRAS* point mutations at codons 12, 13, and 61, *RET/PTC* rearrangements, *TPK*, and *PAX8/PPARG* rearrangements, and showed an improvement in diagnostic accuracy from 83.0% to 93.2% compared with cytology alone. Studies that have incorporated mutations of *BRAF*, *RAS*, *RET/PTC*, and *PAX8/PPARG* in indeterminate nodules have reported specificity between 95% and 100%.[43,61] However, because methodologies varied across these studies, a detailed comparison of the results is challenging. For instance, point mutation analysis was used by Nikiforov and colleagues[43] and Ohori and colleagues,[61] whereas other studies used PCR with direct sequencing methodology.[6,62] Although not all thyroid cancers can be identified by this combined genetic analysis, a positive molecular test result is very helpful, especially in indeterminate cytology results. The 2009 revised American Thyroid Association management guidelines recommend considering the use of molecular markers, such as *BRAF*, *RAS*, *RET/PTC*, *PAX8/PPARG*, and Galectin-3, in cases with indeterminate FNA cytology.[59] This recommendation predates the Veracyte publications.

The cost-effectiveness of the use of the *BRAF*, *RAS*, *RET/PTC*, and *PAX8/PPARG* panel for evaluation of nodules with indeterminate cytology was demonstrated in a recent analysis performed at the authors' institution.[4] This modeling study demonstrated that standard of care for evaluation and treatment of a thyroid nodule costs roughly US$578 per patient, which includes all testing and procedure-related costs. The cost increases by $104 per patient when molecular testing is added. The use of molecular testing resulted in fewer thyroid lobectomies (11.6% in the standard-care group vs 9.7% in the molecular-testing group), allowing a greater number of histologically malignant cases to be managed with upfront total thyroidectomy as the initial surgical procedure. This cost-modeling study demonstrated that although the routine use of molecular testing added a distributed cost of $5031 to the base cost of $11,383 for each total thyroidectomy, the total cost was still lower than the costs associated with the conventional approach of diagnostic lobectomy ($7684) followed by completion thyroidectomy ($11,954). In sensitivity analysis, cost savings were demonstrated if molecular-testing costs were less than $870. This study concluded that molecular testing of cytologically indeterminate FNA can allow cost savings, and improves patient care by providing an indication for optimal initial surgical management with total thyroidectomy when molecular testing is positive. However, the study did not consider additional cost savings that are accrued by deferring surgical management in appropriately selected cytologic AUS/FLUS, a common practice at this center, where the mutation panel has been shown to have an NPV of 94%.[43]

Commercially Available Multigene Mutation Panels from Quest Diagnostics and Asuragen

Quest Diagnostics (Madison, NJ) offers a Thyroid Cancer Mutation Panel, which includes discrete tests for mutations of *BRAF* codons 600 and 601, *PAX8/PPARG*, *RAS* analysis of *HRAS*, *KRAS*, and *NRAS*, and *RET/PTC* rearrangement testing for *RET/PTC1* and *RET/PTC3*. A real-time PCR method is used for all the mutation testing except *RAS*, whereby a pyrosequencing method is used.

The Asuragen (Austin, TX) miRInform thyroid panel is another commercially available panel of molecular markers that can be used in FNA specimens to detect mutations of *BRAF*, *KRAS*, *NRAS*, and *HRAS*, and 3 gene rearrangements: *RET/PTC1*, *RET/PTC3*, and *PAX8/PPARG*. It includes a total of 17 known thyroid cancer mutations and translocations, and uses PCR and real-time PCR combined with bead-binding and fluorescence-based detection using the Luminex system.[63]

Multiple studies have shown that the molecular markers available through Quest Diagnostics and Asuragen have high specificity and PPV for thyroid cancer.[5,6,43,61,62] However, the analytical methods used by Quest Diagnostics and Asuragen and those used in the supporting references are not identical. Therefore, whether and to what degree results obtained by different methods can be directly generalized to the performance of the Quest Diagnostics tests remains unclear. Smith and colleagues[63] verified the diagnostic utility of the Asuragen method for *BRAF* mutation in thyroid nodules. The authors are unaware of any further validation study to date using the specific Asuragen method for any other genes, and are also unaware of any validation study regarding the specific method available from Quest Diagnostics.

Next-Generation Sequencing Expanded Multigene Panel

Recently, Nikiforova and colleagues[64] introduced a custom next-generation sequencing (NGS) panel (ThyroSeq) designed to detect 12 cancer genes with 284 mutational hot spots, allowing simultaneous testing for multiple mutations with high accuracy in both FNA and histologic samples. NGS techniques achieve economies of scale by permitting simultaneous parallel testing of multiple genes in multiple discrete samples. This approach offers advantages over conventional techniques such as Sanger sequencing that require serial direct sequencing of PCR products, each with an associated incremental cost. This technique therefore offers the possibility of a cost-effective method that allows detection of an expanded set of informative point mutations, gene rearrangements, and small insertion/deletion mutations known to occur in thyroid cancer. The mutually exclusive mutations of the MAPK and PI3K pathways (BRAF, RAS, and rearrangements of RET/PTC and PAX8/PPARγ) are present in more than 70% of PTCs and 75% of follicular thyroid carcinomas (FTCs), and can be tested commercially. In addition to these tests, the current version of the ThyroSeq chip also includes mutations of CTNNB1, PIK3CA, PTEN, ACT1, TP53, GNAS, and RET point mutations. These additional DNA mutations increase detection yield of thyroid cancers to 80%, and also allow detection of relatively less prevalent markers of aggressive tumor behavior such as TP53, AKT1, and CTNNB1.[65] Furthermore, 9 of 99 (9%) of the cancers in this study contained more than 1 mutation, including mutations of TP53 and PI3KCA observed to overlap with BRAFV600E, and a tumor with a PI3KCA mutation overlapping with a RAS mutation. Not surprisingly, and as has been previously reported,[65–67] these tumors with overlapping mutations also demonstrated aggressive histologic features.[64] Nikiforov and colleagues also plan to combine this current version of the ThyroSeq chip with a panel of RNA-based tests that will detect multiple gene-fusion mutations that should further increase the diagnostic sensitivity of ThyroSeq (Y.E. Nikiforov, personal communication, 2013).

The combined ability to detect an expanded set of mutations including those associated with histologically aggressive disease, as well as to identify tumors containing multiple and overlapping mutations, suggest that NGS methods such as ThyroSeq will improve not only diagnostic yield but also prognostication for thyroid cancer. Although further studies will be required to validate the diagnostic utility of these NGS multigene panel methods, current data are already encouraging.

The Veracyte Afirma Gene Expression Classifier

The Afirma gene expression classifier (GEC),[68] developed by Veracyte, represents a unique approach to analysis of cytologically indeterminate thyroid nodules. The GEC evaluates expression of 167 genes using mRNA transcripts from FNA specimens, and is designed to identify nodules with benign histology. Many consider the Afirma GEC a "rule-out" test a potentially useful tool in the clinical evaluation of cytologically indeterminate thyroid nodules that are either AUS/FLUS or FN/SFN by Bethesda criteria.[69] The classifier is approved for use only in nodules 1 cm and larger, and Veracyte does not recommend GEC analysis for indeterminate nodules with SMC cytology.

Several primarily industry-sponsored studies initially reported favorable GEC performance for identifying histologically benign thyroid nodules.[70–73] In an industry-sponsored double-blind, prospective, multicenter validation study that included 210 nodules with histologic correlation and cytologically indeterminate aspirates classified as either AUS/FLUS or FN/SFN, the GEC correctly identified 145 of 159 histologically negative nodules as GEC benign and 46 of 51 histologic malignancies as GEC suspicious, yielding 90% sensitivity. The GEC misclassified 5 histologic malignancies as GEC benign, yielding a false-negative rate of 10%; this resulted in negative predictive values (NPVs) of 95% and 94% for nodules classified as AUS/FLUS and FN/SFN, respectively.[70]

Four of the 5 histologic cancers in this group misclassified as GEC benign were attributed to insufficient sampling in post hoc analysis.[70] Most of the missed cancers were conventional and follicular variant PTC. However, this raises a concern. Veracyte currently does not incorporate a method for prospectively detecting and excluding specimens that lack an adequate number of thyroid epithelial cells. Therefore, if an inadequate specimen from a malignant nodule is unknowingly submitted, Veracyte's validation study suggests that a false-negative GEC-benign result will occur for every 4 of 210, or 2%, of cases. The validation study also reported a false-negative GEC-benign result for a 2.9-cm oncocytic (Hürthle cell) carcinoma from an adequately sampled specimen. Regardless of cause, clinicians should be aware that just as with benign cytology, false-negative results do occur, and these can sometimes include histologically aggressive cancers such as oncocytic (Hürthle cell) carcinomas.

An important limitation of the GEC is its poor performance in cytologically suspicious aspirates. Because the NPV was only 85% in SMC nodules, the GEC was not considered to have adequate predictive value for ruling out cancer. Based on this finding, Veracyte no longer recommends GEC analysis for cytologically suspicious aspirates.[74]

In an industry-sponsored study, investigators reported that the finding of a GEC-benign nodule led to a 10-fold reduction in diagnostic surgeries from 76.0% historically to 7.6% on cytologically indeterminate nodules.[72] Because the study could not assess histology among cases that did not go to surgery, whether and to what extent cancers were missed in nodules with GEC-benign results is unknown.

The cost of the GEC test is approximately $3200.[72] However, as many surgeries can be avoided in GEC-benign cases, Markov modeling suggests that substantial cost savings can be accrued by incorporating GEC analysis into the evaluation of FLUS and FL/SFN. By performing this test, unnecessary diagnostic surgeries can be avoided, which would further save costs. The cost of care with current standard-care practices without molecular testing is $12,172 per patient, but with the use of the GEC test this be reduced to $10,719.[2] Avoiding diagnostic surgeries is the major driver of cost savings in this model. However, this comes at the expense of missing histologic cancers that are incorrectly classified as GEC benign. The cost model estimates that 1.4% of malignant nodules are missed with GEC, which is slightly lower than the 2% false-negative rate published by Alexander and colleagues.[70] Moreover, the cost associated with missing nodules such as the 2.9-cm oncocytic carcinoma, which represented 20% of the missed cancers among AUS/FLUS and FN/SFN specimens in the series, is not discussed.[75]

With the exception of several academic institutions that are Veracyte "enabled", the Veracyte pathway requires cytologic evaluation of FNA specimens to be done by its independent industry partner Thyroid Cytopathology Partners (TCP) (Austin, TX). TCP is a high-volume facility, reporting an average monthly case volume of approximately 4000 cases with an approximately 16% rate of cytologically indeterminate cases[76] (S. Thomas Traweek, President, Thyroid Cytopathology Partners, personal communication). However, TCP does not receive histology data that allow calculation of actual cancer prevalence in its cytologically indeterminate cases. This fact has important implications: Bayes' theorem (**Fig. 1**) demonstrates that the NPV of any test depends not only on test sensitivity and specificity but also on disease prevalence in the studied population. Because cancer prevalence in TCP's indeterminate cases is unknown, there is no way to definitely know whether the NPV of a Veracyte

Bayes' Theorem

$$PPV = \frac{(Sensitivity)(Prevalence)}{(Sensitivity)(Prevalence) + (1 - Specificity)(1 - Prevalence)}$$

$$NPV = \frac{(Specificity)(1 - Prevalence)}{(Specificity)(1 - Prevalence) + (1 - Sensitivity)(Prevalence)}$$

Fig. 1. Bayes' theorem. NPV, negative predictive value; PPV, positive predictive value.

GEC-benign result will be similar to the 95% and 94% rates published in the landmark validation trial by Alexander and colleagues[70] for AUS/FLUS and FN/SFN cases, respectively. To correctly understand the true NPV of the Veracyte GEC, users submitting cases to Veracyte would therefore need to know the actual cancer prevalence rate for specimens they submit. It is certainly likely that for users who preferentially select cases with greater clinical risk for GEC evaluation, the population of cancers among cytologically indeterminate cases would be enriched to higher than the 24% and 25% rates published by Alexander and colleagues[70] for AUS and FN cases, respectively, and from which the aforementioned NPVs were calculated. With an increase in disease prevalence, the NPV of the GEC would be lower. Conversely, if disease prevalence was lower than 24% and 25%, the NPV would be better than that suggested by Alexander and colleagues.[70]

Although disease prevalence for cases processed for Veracyte by TCP is unknown, TCP's 16% rate of cytologically indeterminate cases is approximately similar to that of previously published meta-reviews that include a mix of both academic and community-based practices, as well as the Alexander validation study.[70,75,77,78] This result may suggest that the GEC NPV for specimens analyzed through the standard Veracyte pathway is similar to the 95% and 94% rates for AUS/FLUS and FN/SFN specimens. However, only knowledge of true disease prevalence rates would allow such a conclusion to be made with certainty, and the possibility of divergent NPVs, driven by different disease prevalence rates, should be considered by clinicians who use this test.

Alexander and colleagues[79] have also reported a prospective multicenter experience with the Afirma GEC. The 5 included sites were Veracyte-enabled academic centers; that is, cytology evaluation used to trigger the GEC analysis was done locally, and cases were not submitted for cytologic evaluation to TCP. The findings of the study are similar to those of the 2012 New England Journal of Medicine Afirma validation study.[70] The study showed that of 326 evaluated cytologically AUS/FLUS and FN/SFN nodules, 170 (52%) were GEC benign and 139 (43%) were GEC suspicious. Of the GEC-suspicious cases, 23 of 48 operated AUS/SFN (48%) and 24 of 65 operated FN/SFN (37%) were malignant. In this patient cohort from these academic centers the investigators report that the use of the GEC for evaluation of cytologically indeterminate nodules decreased the use of surgical management by 76%. A noteworthy limitation of this study is that the investigators did not know actual cancer prevalence rates in cytologically indeterminate nodules, and instead provided "best estimates" from 5% to 30% for both AUS/FLUS and FN/SFN nodules. Of the 14 of 174 GEC-benign cytologically indeterminate specimens that had surgical correlation, cancer was confirmed in 2 (14%) cases. The number of missed cancers in the remaining 160 GEC-benign cases was not determined. In addition, because the participating academic centers did not use Veracyte's standard pathway that includes having cytology performed by TCP, it is unclear how well these results can be generalized to community-based clinical practice.

Duick and colleagues[72] published a similar study of GEC use in a largely community-based population. Although the study included a minority of patients from Veracyte-enabled sites, most of the study cases did use the standard Veracyte pathway with cytology analysis performed by TCP. Study users of the GEC deferred surgical management nearly 90% of the time when nodules were cytologically indeterminate and GEC benign. However, the study presents no data regarding prevalence of disease in the studied population, surgical outcomes among the relatively few GEC-benign cases taken for surgery, or any way to calculate the NPV of the GEC. Although this study is another interesting attempt to better define the clinical relevance of the Afirma method, these important limitations are noteworthy.

The authors are aware of only a single real-world study describing a community clinical practice's experience using the Afirma GEC that incorporates cytologic evaluation by TCP as part of the standard Veracyte analysis workflow. Harrell and Bimston[80] performed 645 FNAs in 519 patients over 27 months, yielding 58 (9%) cytologically indeterminate cases after cytologic evaluation by TCP. Of these indeterminate cases, 2 had inadequate RNA content for evaluation, 36 (62%) were GEC suspicious, and 20 were GEC benign. Of 30 GEC-suspicious cases referred for surgery, 21 had histologic cancer, including 4 cases of microcarcinoma of dubious clinical significance. Of the 20 GEC-benign cases, 5 were referred to surgery and 2 were confirmed to have histologic cancers. Unique in this group's data is a calculation of the rate of cancer prevalence in their cytologically indeterminate cases, and NPV for the Afirma GEC when applied to their specific patient population. When excluding incidental or clinically irrelevant microcarcinomas, and considering only the 19 clinically relevant cancers (17 from the GEC-suspicious group and 2 [operated] from the GEC-benign group), the investigators calculated a "best-case" cancer prevalence rate of 19 cancers in 58 cases, or 33%. Consistent with Bayes' theorem, the resulting best-case NPV for Afirma performance in this group was 89.6%; that is, a GEC-benign result in this patient population is incorrect in approximately 1 of every 10 cases. This calculation presumes that no further cancers are present in the 15 unoperated GEC-benign and 6 unoperated GEC-suspicious cases. The presence of additional histologic cancers would further increase that population's cancer prevalence rate, and therefore further decrease NPV of the Afirma GEC. It is important to emphasize that these data do not suggest that Afirma worked less well than the Alexander validation study suggested.[70] Rather, these data illustrate the exquisite dependence of predictive value on disease prevalence rates, and why it is imperative that disease prevalence is correctly understood to correctly interpret the significance of a test's NPV and PPV.

Because the diagnostic performance of the GEC in heterogeneous clinical populations is limited, and classifier NPV heavily depends on disease prevalence rates that are often completely unknown or not well characterized among cases submitted for evaluation, clinicians are cautioned to consider how the GEC will perform in their unique patient populations. Despite these limitations, the Afirma GEC remains an intriguing molecular diagnostic tool for evaluation of cytologically indeterminate thyroid nodules. It is hoped that real-world experience with the diagnostic performance of the GEC, which to date remains scant, will continue to be clarified by future studies.

MICROARRAY ANALYSIS
MicroRNA Expression

miRNAs are small, endogenous, noncoding, functional RNAs that regulate gene expression by regulating mRNA translation and degradation.[81] Various miRNAs are reported to be involved in the development of several types of human cancers, and specific miRNAs are associated with distinct histologic subtypes of thyroid cancer.[82] MiRNAs can be detected using several methods, including microassays, bead-based arrays, and quantitative real-time PCR. A study that used the real-time PCR method for the detection of miRNAs in FNA reported that the overexpression of miR-221, miR-222, and miR-181b was associated with PTC.[83] Weber and colleagues[84] used microassay analysis to detect miRNA in a total of 45 primary thyroid samples, which included 23 FTCs, 20 follicular adenomas, and 4 normal (control) thyroid samples. This study suggested that 2 specific miRNAs, miR-197 and miR-346, were significantly overexpressed in FTC.

A recent study analyzing the expression levels of miR-222, miR-328, miR-197, miR-21, miR-181a, and miR-146b in a total of 101 indeterminate FNA samples reported that a panel of 4 miRNAs (miR-222, miR-328, miR-197, and miR-21) had sensitivity of 100%, specificity of 86%, and predictive accuracy of 90% in differentiating malignant from benign nodules.[85] Another recent study, using quantitative PCR in FNA specimens, suggested that a set of 4 miRNAs (miR-146b, miR-221, miR-187, and miR-30d) had a diagnostic accuracy of 85.3% to 93.3%.[86] In addition, the detection of miR-7 in FNA specimens might be useful in differentiating malignant from benign nodules.[87] However, large validation studies are lacking, and an miRNA analysis of FNA specimens is not yet commercially available.

The Cleveland Clinic TSHR mRNA Assay (in Serum)

The TSHR mRNA assay is a quantitative real-time PCR method developed by the Cleveland Clinic to measure thyrotropin receptor mRNA levels from a peripheral blood sample. Its use as a marker for circulating thyroid cancer cells and its clinical utility for differentiating between benign and malignant thyroid nodules have been proposed in a few studies.[88,89] Preoperative TSHR mRNA measurement had sensitivity of 61% and specificity of 83% in differentiating between benign and malignant nodules.[88] In cases with indeterminate FNA, TSHR mRNA correctly diagnosed differentiated thyroid cancers in 16 of 24 (67%) and benign disease in 29 of 39 (74%) cases.[89] The sensitivity improves to 97% with a decline in specificity to 84% when high-quality neck ultrasonography is implemented in addition to TSHR mRNA assay.[88,89] However, because the quality and result of ultrasonography is operator dependent, these findings might not be generalizable in patients when imaging is performed at centers other than the Cleveland Clinic. In addition, these results are single-institution data based only on the experience at the Cleveland Clinic. Widespread validated studies are lacking. This test is commercially available directly through the Cleveland Clinic, and a cost-analysis of the assay has not yet been published.

SUMMARY AND RECOMMENDATIONS

Although FNA remains a valuable approach for evaluating thyroid nodules, indeterminate cytology remains a common clinical problem. Numerous molecular tests that improve diagnostic yield in cytologically indeterminate nodules have been introduced. Many of these tests have been shown to have varying degrees of analytical validation; however, robust clinical validation and sufficient availability are lacking for most of these tests, making them impractical clinical options.

Tests with reasonable availability and validation data include a molecular-panel approach that incorporates the most common mutations in thyroid cancer such as BRAF, RAS, RET/PTC, and PAX8-PPARG, and the GEC approach developed by Veracyte. Performances of these 2 tests for evaluation of cytologically indeterminate nodules are summarized in **Tables 1–3**. Although limitations exist for these methods, both approaches have been shown to offer significant diagnostic improvement over FNA cytology alone if used with appropriate caution. Recommendations for how these 2 tests can be incorporated into a diagnostic approach to nodules with indeterminate cytology are given here.

Nodules with AUS/FLUS Cytology

The authors believe that both the Afirma GEC and the multigene-panel approach (including BRAF, RAS, RET/PTC and PAX8/PPARG) have a robust NPV, and either test can be recommended for evaluation of cytologically AUS/FLUS nodules. As in the case with negative cytology, a small number of cancers will be missed with both approaches. It is therefore reasonable to continue surveillance in AUS/FLUS cases

Table 1 Comparison of test performance for AUS/FLUS nodules							
Test Analysis	Sensitivity (%)	Specificity (%)	NPV (%)	PPV (%)	Histologic Types of Missed Cancers	Intention of the Test	Comments
Afirma GEC[60] N = 129	90	53	95	24	PTC	To avoid unnecessary surgery	10% of histologic cancers will be missed
Mutation panel[39] N = 247	63	99	94	88	PTC	Determines whether diagnostic lobectomy or upfront total thyroidectomy is optimal surgical management	Missed cancers were primarily low-grade PTC without invasion or LN metastasis; watchful waiting rather than diagnostic lobectomy is reasonable in appropriately selected cases

Abbreviations: AUS/FLUS, atypia of uncertain significance/follicular lesion of uncertain significance; GEC, gene expression classifier; LN, lymph node; NPV, negative predictive value; PPV, positive predictive value; PTC, papillary thyroid cancer.

when molecular genetic testing is negative. This monitoring should include annual neck examinations indefinitely and periodic cervical ultrasonography. Recent literature from an academic medical center suggests that surveillance ultrasonography is reasonable 2 to 4 years after a cytologically benign result to identify rare cases of missed cancers attributable to false-negative cytology.[90] Although this recommendation may be reasonable at an academic medical center where the rate of false-negative cytology may be as low as 2%, this rate may reach up to 10% in community practices and 5% to 6% in cytologically AUS/FLUS specimens that are GEC benign and negative on multigene panel.[43,70] The optimum frequency for cervical ultrasonographic surveillance for these lesions is therefore unclear, and must still be based on clinical judgment.

In situations where surgical management is reasonable based on clinical concerns (eg, cases with radiographically worrisome or large thyroid nodules, high-risk patients with a history of ionizing radiation exposure, nodules with clinically significant size increase or associated symptoms), the authors believe that testing with the multigene-panel approach is indicated: the high specificity and very robust PPV of this test provides a compelling indication for initial surgical management with upfront total thyroidectomy (in the case of a positive test result where the likelihood of malignancy is high) rather than a diagnostic lobectomy, which would otherwise be indicated. The need for completion thyroidectomy for cancers found with diagnostic lobectomy can therefore be minimized, as reported by Yip and colleagues.[30]

Nodules with FN/SFN Cytology

Only the Afirma GEC offers a sufficiently robust NPV to recommend its use as a rule-out test for indeterminate nodules in this category. The authors agree that in cases with

Table 2
Comparison of test performance for FN/SFN nodules

Test Analysis	Sensitivity (%)	Specificity (%)	NPV (%)	PPV (%)	Histologic Types of Missed Cancers	Intention of the Test	Comments
Afirma GEC[60] N = 81	90	49	94	37	PTC HCC	To avoid unnecessary surgery	Excellent NPV. However, GEC missed a 2.9-cm adequately sampled oncocytic (Hürthle cell) carcinoma
Mutation panel[39] N = 214	57	97	86	87	PTC HCC	Determines whether diagnostic lobectomy or upfront total thyroidectomy is optimal surgical management	Risk of cancer decreases to 14% in cytologically FN/SFN cases with negative testing, supporting the use of diagnostic lobectomy rather than upfront total thyroidectomy in most cases

Abbreviations: FN/SFN, follicular neoplasm/suspicious for follicular neoplasm; GEC, gene expression classifier; HCC, Hürthle cell carcinoma; NPV, negative predictive value; PPV, positive predictive value; PTC, papillary thyroid cancer.

sufficiently low clinical risk, where evidence to support a decision to defer diagnostic surgery is sought (eg, radiographically low-risk nodules), evaluation with the Afirma GEC is a reasonable option, and a benign GEC result may obviate surgical management. However, the authors remain concerned about the GEC false-negative result from a missed 2.9-cm oncocytic (Hürthle cell) carcinoma in an adequately sampled FN/SFN nodule reported in the Veracyte validation study. Therefore, if the Afirma GEC is used, appropriate clinical judgment should be applied, and the GEC result should not be used as the sole determinant for clinical management. Clinical symptoms and context, nodule size, and radiographic appearance may at times be sufficiently concerning to justify surgical evaluation despite a negative GEC result.

In situations where surgical management is the preferred approach, the robust PPV of the multigene panel informs surgical management, and a positive test result provides a strong indication for upfront total thyroidectomy rather than diagnostic lobectomy as initial surgical management.

Nodules with SMC Cytology

All nodules with SMC cytology should undergo surgical management unless there are compelling clinical concerns that contraindicate surgery. The NPV of the multigene-panel test is insufficient to recommend deferring surgical management. However, the NPV reported by Nikiforov and colleagues[43] makes the likelihood of cancer

Table 3
Comparison of test performance for SMC nodules

Test Analysis	Sensitivity (%)	Specificity (%)	NPV (%)	PPV (%)	Histologic Types of Missed Cancers	Intention of the Test	Comments
Afirma GEC[60] N = 55	94	52	85	76	PTC	To avoid unnecessary surgery	No longer recommended by Veracyte because of poor NPV
Mutation panel[39] N = 52	68	96	72	95	PTC	Determines whether diagnostic lobectomy or upfront total thyroidectomy is optimal surgical management	Risk of cancer decreased to 28% when test was negative with SMC cytology, supporting the use of diagnostic lobectomy rather than upfront total thyroidectomy in most cases

Abbreviations: GEC, gene expression classifier; NPV, negative predictive value; PPV, positive predictive value; PTC, papillary thyroid cancer; SMC, suspicious for malignant cells.

sufficiently low to allow consideration of diagnostic lobectomy rather than upfront total thyroidectomy as initial surgical management in nodules with SMC cytology and a negative multigene-panel test. This approach is used at the authors' center, as the likelihood of cancer in nodules with SMC cytology and a negative multigene test is only 28%.

The NPV of the Afirma GEC, though better than that of the multigene panel, is still too low to recommend deferring surgical management in this cytologic category. Because the GEC is marketed as a test that negates the need for surgery when the result is "benign," Veracyte has elected to defer GEC analysis in nodules with SMC cytology, and this option is therefore unavailable.

Several important caveats should be observed whenever any diagnostic test is used. Clinicians are well advised to consider the important point illustrated by Bayes' theorem (see **Fig. 1**). This formula shows that the NPV and PPV of any diagnostic tests depend not only on test sensitivity and specificity, which are test-specific factors, but also on the prevalence of disease in the tested population. Therefore, actual NPV and PPV may be different if prevalence of disease in a specific population differs from that in published validation trials. Because intraobserver variability in cytologic classification is common and leads to variable disease prevalence, clinicians are cautioned to assess prevalence of disease in their local practice before presuming that test NPV and PPV in their hands will be identical to that found in the literature.[75,91]

Numerous technologies to detect genetic mutations have been developed, such as PCR followed by Sanger sequencing, pyrosequencing, simultaneous amplification and fluorescence detection by using real-time PCR instruments, and, most recently, NGS sequencing.[63,64] Studies evaluating the diagnostic performance of molecular markers continue to emerge, and more recent literature suggests that with the incorporation of

NGS, diagnostic sensitivity of commercially available tests will continue to improve. Nonetheless, clinicians should exercise caution in reviewing and comparing the results in these studies because different methodologies with different test-performance characteristics are frequently used. In some instances, overly sensitive methods have been shown to identify subclonal or nonclonal mutations that have no clinical significance.[56,92] Only the use of well-validated methods that have been shown to have adequate clinical correlation should be used for mutation testing.

Although the number of large multicenter studies examining the clinical utility of molecular testing is increasing, validation data remain limited, and no molecular test has perfect sensitivity and specificity. Nonetheless, clinicians are understandably driven to incorporate molecular tests into their practice algorithms. The authors do not see this as a problem as long as the limitations associated with the numerous tests that are now available, and those that arise in the future, are kept firmly in mind. The authors are optimistic that genetic tests with near-perfect sensitivity and specificity, which will largely obviate cytology and will continue to reduce or entirely eliminate the need for diagnostic surgery, will be available in the near future. Until that time, sound clinical judgment and appropriate critical reasoning must be applied when interpreting results obtained from these exciting but still imperfect tests.

REFERENCES

1. Nikiforov YE, Steward DL, Robinson-Smith TM, et al. Molecular testing for mutations in improving the fine-needle aspiration diagnosis of thyroid nodules. J Clin Endocrinol Metab 2009;94(6):2092–8.
2. Li H, Robinson KA, Anton B, et al. Cost-effectiveness of a novel molecular test for cytologically indeterminate thyroid nodules. J Clin Endocrinol Metab 2011; 96(11):E1719–26.
3. Yassa L, Cibas ES, Benson CB, et al. Long-term assessment of a multidisciplinary approach to thyroid nodule diagnostic evaluation. Cancer 2007;111(6): 508–16.
4. Yip L, Farris C, Kabaker AS, et al. Cost impact of molecular testing for indeterminate thyroid nodule fine-needle aspiration biopsies. J Clin Endocrinol Metab 2012;97(6):1905–12.
5. Moses W, Weng J, Sansano I, et al. Molecular testing for somatic mutations improves the accuracy of thyroid fine-needle aspiration biopsy. World J Surg 2010; 34(11):2589–94.
6. Cantara S, Capezzone M, Marchisotta S, et al. Impact of proto-oncogene mutation detection in cytological specimens from thyroid nodules improves the diagnostic accuracy of cytology. J Clin Endocrinol Metab 2010;95(3):1365–9.
7. Liu FT, Rabinovich GA. Galectins as modulators of tumour progression. Nat Rev Cancer 2005;5(1):29–41.
8. Manivannan P, Siddaraju N, Jatiya L, et al. Role of pro-angiogenic marker galectin-3 in follicular neoplasms of thyroid. Indian J Biochem Biophys 2012; 49(5):392–4.
9. Matesa-Anic D, Moslavac S, Matesa N, et al. Intensity and distribution of immunohistochemical expression of galectin-3 in thyroid neoplasms. Acta Clin Croat 2012;51(2):237–41.
10. Bartolazzi A, Orlandi F, Saggiorato E, et al. Galectin-3-expression analysis in the surgical selection of follicular thyroid nodules with indeterminate fine-needle aspiration cytology: a prospective multicentre study. Lancet Oncol 2008;9(6): 543–9.

11. de Matos LL, Del Giglio AB, Matsubayashi CO, et al. Expression of CK-19, galectin-3 and HBME-1 in the differentiation of thyroid lesions: systematic review and diagnostic meta-analysis. Diagn Pathol 2012;7:97.

12. Scognamiglio T, Hyjek E, Kao J, et al. Diagnostic usefulness of HBME1, galectin-3, CK19, and CITED1 and evaluation of their expression in encapsulated lesions with questionable features of papillary thyroid carcinoma. Am J Clin Pathol 2006; 126(5):700–8.

13. Sack MJ, Astengo-Osuna C, Lin BT, et al. HBME-1 immunostaining in thyroid fine-needle aspirations: a useful marker in the diagnosis of carcinoma. Mod Pathol 1997;10(7):668–74.

14. Cheung CC, Ezzat S, Freeman JL, et al. Immunohistochemical diagnosis of papillary thyroid carcinoma. Mod Pathol 2001;14(4):338–42.

15. Saggiorato E, De Pompa R, Volante M, et al. Characterization of thyroid 'follicular neoplasms' in fine-needle aspiration cytological specimens using a panel of immunohistochemical markers: a proposal for clinical application. Endocr Relat Cancer 2005;12(2):305–17.

16. Fadda G, Rossi ED, Raffaelli M, et al. Follicular thyroid neoplasms can be classified as low- and high-risk according to HBME-1 and Galectin-3 expression on liquid-based fine-needle cytology. Eur J Endocrinol 2011;165(3):447–53.

17. Raphael SJ, McKeown-Eyssen G, Asa SL. High-molecular-weight cytokeratin and cytokeratin-19 in the diagnosis of thyroid tumors. Mod Pathol 1994;7(3): 295–300.

18. Prasad ML, Pellegata NS, Huang Y, et al. Galectin-3, fibronectin-1, CITED-1, HBME1 and cytokeratin-19 immunohistochemistry is useful for the differential diagnosis of thyroid tumors. Mod Pathol 2005;18(1):48–57.

19. Sahoo S, Hoda SA, Rosai J, et al. Cytokeratin 19 immunoreactivity in the diagnosis of papillary thyroid carcinoma: a note of caution. Am J Clin Pathol 2001; 116(5):696–702.

20. Saleh HA, Jin B, Barnwell J, et al. Utility of immunohistochemical markers in differentiating benign from malignant follicular-derived thyroid nodules. Diagn Pathol 2010;5:9.

21. Torregrossa L, Faviana P, Filice ME, et al. CXC chemokine receptor 4 immunodetection in the follicular variant of papillary thyroid carcinoma: comparison to galectin-3 and Hector Battifora mesothelial cell-1. Thyroid 2010;20(5):495–504.

22. Yasuoka H, Kodama R, Hirokawa M, et al. CXCR4 expression in papillary thyroid carcinoma: induction by nitric oxide and correlation with lymph node metastasis. BMC Cancer 2008;8:274.

23. Chung SY, Park ES, Park SY, et al. CXC motif ligand 12 (CXCL12) as a novel diagnostic marker for papillary thyroid carcinoma. Head Neck 2013. [Epub ahead of print].

24. Prasad ML, Pellegata NS, Kloos RT, et al. CITED1 protein expression suggests papillary thyroid carcinoma in high throughput tissue microarray-based study. Thyroid 2004;14(3):169–75.

25. Davies H, Bignell GR, Cox C, et al. Mutations of the BRAF gene in human cancer. Nature 2002;417(6892):949–54.

26. Kebebew E, Weng J, Bauer J, et al. The prevalence and prognostic value of BRAF mutation in thyroid cancer. Ann Surg 2007;246(3):466–70 [discussion: 470–1].

27. Xing M. BRAF mutation in thyroid cancer. Endocr Relat Cancer 2005;12(2): 245–62.

28. Melck AL, Yip L, Carty SE. The utility of BRAF testing in the management of papillary thyroid cancer. Oncologist 2010;15(12):1285–93.

29. Lupi C, Giannini R, Ugolini C, et al. Association of BRAF V600E mutation with poor clinicopathological outcomes in 500 consecutive cases of papillary thyroid carcinoma. J Clin Endocrinol Metab 2007;92(11):4085–90.

30. Yip L, Nikiforova MN, Carty SE, et al. Optimizing surgical treatment of papillary thyroid carcinoma associated with BRAF mutation. Surgery 2009;146(6): 1215–23.

31. Nikiforov YE. Molecular diagnostics of thyroid tumors. Arch Pathol Lab Med 2011;135(5):569–77.

32. Begum S, Rosenbaum E, Henrique R, et al. BRAF mutations in anaplastic thyroid carcinoma: implications for tumor origin, diagnosis and treatment. Mod Pathol 2004;17(11):1359–63.

33. Nikiforova MN, Kimura ET, Gandhi M, et al. BRAF mutations in thyroid tumors are restricted to papillary carcinomas and anaplastic or poorly differentiated carcinomas arising from papillary carcinomas. J Clin Endocrinol Metab 2003;88(11): 5399–404.

34. Xing M. BRAF mutation in papillary thyroid cancer: pathogenic role, molecular bases, and clinical implications. Endocr Rev 2007;28(7):742–62.

35. Kim TH, Park YJ, Lim JA, et al. The association of the BRAF(V600E) mutation with prognostic factors and poor clinical outcome in papillary thyroid cancer: a meta-analysis. Cancer 2012;118(7):1764–73.

36. Li C, Aragon Han P, Lee KC, et al. Does BRAF V600E mutation predict aggressive features in papillary thyroid cancer? Results from four endocrine surgery centers. J Clin Endocrinol Metab 2013;98(9):3702–12.

37. Carta C, Moretti S, Passeri L, et al. Genotyping of an Italian papillary thyroid carcinoma cohort revealed high prevalence of BRAF mutations, absence of RAS mutations and allowed the detection of a new mutation of BRAF oncoprotein (BRAF(V599Ins)). Clin Endocrinol 2006;64(1):105–9.

38. Chiosea S, Nikiforova M, Zuo H, et al. A novel complex BRAF mutation detected in a solid variant of papillary thyroid carcinoma. Endocr Pathol 2009;20(2):122–6.

39. Ciampi R, Knauf JA, Kerler R, et al. Oncogenic AKAP9-BRAF fusion is a novel mechanism of MAPK pathway activation in thyroid cancer. J Clin Invest 2005; 115(1):94–101.

40. Hou P, Liu D, Xing M. Functional characterization of the T1799-1801del and A1799-1816ins BRAF mutations in papillary thyroid cancer. Cell Cycle 2007; 6(3):377–9.

41. Trovisco V, Vieira de Castro I, Soares P, et al. BRAF mutations are associated with some histological types of papillary thyroid carcinoma. J Pathol 2004; 202(2):247–51.

42. Cohen Y, Rosenbaum E, Clark DP, et al. Mutational analysis of BRAF in fine needle aspiration biopsies of the thyroid: a potential application for the preoperative assessment of thyroid nodules. Clin Cancer Res 2004;10(8):2761–5.

43. Nikiforov YE, Ohori NP, Hodak SP, et al. Impact of mutational testing on the diagnosis and management of patients with cytologically indeterminate thyroid nodules: a prospective analysis of 1056 FNA samples. J Clin Endocrinol Metab 2011;96(11):3390–7.

44. Nikiforova MN, Nikiforov YE. Molecular diagnostics and predictors in thyroid cancer. Thyroid 2009;19(12):1351–61.

45. Esapa CT, Johnson SJ, Kendall-Taylor P, et al. Prevalence of Ras mutations in thyroid neoplasia. Clin Endocrinol 1999;50(4):529–35.

46. Fehrenbacher N, Bar-Sagi D, Philips M. Ras/MAPK signaling from endomembranes. Mol Oncol 2009;3(4):297–307.

47. Nikiforov YE. Thyroid carcinoma: molecular pathways and therapeutic targets. Mod Pathol 2008;21(Suppl 2):S37–43.
48. Gupta N, Dasyam AK, Carty SE, et al. RAS mutations in thyroid FNA specimens are highly predictive of predominantly low-risk follicular-pattern cancers. J Clin Endocrinol Metab 2013;98(5):E914–22.
49. Moura MM, Cavaco BM, Pinto AE, et al. High prevalence of RAS mutations in RET-negative sporadic medullary thyroid carcinomas. J Clin Endocrinol Metab 2011;96(5):E863–8.
50. Burns JS, Blaydes JP, Wright PA, et al. Stepwise transformation of primary thyroid epithelial cells by a mutant Ha-ras oncogene: an in vitro model of tumor progression. Mol Carcinog 1992;6(2):129–39.
51. Nikiforov YE, Nikiforova MN. Molecular genetics and diagnosis of thyroid cancer. Nat Rev Endocrinol 2011;7(10):569–80.
52. Tallini G, Asa SL. RET oncogene activation in papillary thyroid carcinoma. Adv Anat Pathol 2001;8(6):345–54.
53. Fenton CL, Lukes Y, Nicholson D, et al. The ret/PTC mutations are common in sporadic papillary thyroid carcinoma of children and young adults. J Clin Endocrinol Metab 2000;85(3):1170–5.
54. Chua EL, Wu WM, Tran KT, et al. Prevalence and distribution of RET/PTC 1, 2, and 3 in papillary thyroid carcinoma in New Caledonia and Australia. J Clin Endocrinol Metab 2000;85(8):2733–9.
55. Nikiforov YE. RET/PTC rearrangement in thyroid tumors. Endocr Pathol 2002; 13(1):3–16.
56. Zhu Z, Ciampi R, Nikiforova MN, et al. Prevalence of RET/PTC rearrangements in thyroid papillary carcinomas: effects of the detection methods and genetic heterogeneity. J Clin Endocrinol Metab 2006;91(9):3603–10.
57. Kroll TG, Sarraf P, Pecciarini L, et al. PAX8-PPARgamma1 fusion oncogene in human thyroid carcinoma [corrected]. Science 2000;289(5483):1357–60.
58. Placzkowski KA, Reddi HV, Grebe SK, et al. The Role of the PAX8/PPARgamma fusion oncogene in thyroid cancer. PPAR Res 2008;2008:672829.
59. Cooper DS, Doherty GM, Haugen BR, et al. Revised American Thyroid Association management guidelines for patients with thyroid nodules and differentiated thyroid cancer. Thyroid 2009;19(11):1167–214.
60. Cibas ES, Ali SZ. The Bethesda System for reporting thyroid cytopathology. Am J Clin Pathol 2009;132(5):658–65.
61. Ohori NP, Nikiforova MN, Schoedel KE, et al. Contribution of molecular testing to thyroid fine-needle aspiration cytology of "follicular lesion of undetermined significance/atypia of undetermined significance". Cancer Cytopathol 2010;118(1): 17–23.
62. Ferraz C, Eszlinger M, Paschke R. Current state and future perspective of molecular diagnosis of fine-needle aspiration biopsy of thyroid nodules. J Clin Endocrinol Metab 2011;96(7):2016–26.
63. Smith DL, Lamy A, Beaudenon-Huibregtse S, et al. A multiplex technology platform for the rapid analysis of clinically actionable genetic alterations and validation for BRAF p.V600E detection in 1549 cytologic and histologic specimens. Arch Pathol Lab Med 2014;138(3):371–8.
64. Nikiforova MN, Wald AI, Roy S, et al. Targeted next-generation sequencing panel (ThyroSeq) for detection of mutations in thyroid cancer. J Clin Endocrinol Metab 2013;98(11):E1852–60.
65. Kondo T, Ezzat S, Asa SL. Pathogenetic mechanisms in thyroid follicular-cell neoplasia. Nat Rev Cancer 2006;6(4):292–306.

66. Garcia-Rostan G, Costa AM, Pereira-Castro I, et al. Mutation of the PIK3CA gene in anaplastic thyroid cancer. Cancer Res 2005;65(22):10199–207.

67. Ricarte-Filho JC, Ryder M, Chitale DA, et al. Mutational profile of advanced primary and metastatic radioactive iodine-refractory thyroid cancers reveals distinct pathogenetic roles for BRAF, PIK3CA, and AKT1. Cancer Res 2009; 69(11):4885–93.

68. Algeciras-Schimnich A, Milosevic D, McIver B, et al. Evaluation of the PAX8/PPARG translocation in follicular thyroid cancer with a 4-color reverse-transcription PCR assay and automated high-resolution fragment analysis. Clin Chem 2010;56(3):391–8.

69. Walsh PS, Wilde JI, Tom EY, et al. Analytical performance verification of a molecular diagnostic for cytology-indeterminate thyroid nodules. J Clin Endocrinol Metab 2012;97(12):E2297–306.

70. Alexander EK, Kennedy GC, Baloch ZW, et al. Preoperative diagnosis of benign thyroid nodules with indeterminate cytology. N Engl J Med 2012;367(8):705–15.

71. Chudova D, Wilde JI, Wang ET, et al. Molecular classification of thyroid nodules using high-dimensionality genomic data. J Clin Endocrinol Metab 2010;95(12): 5296–304.

72. Duick DS, Klopper JP, Diggans JC, et al. The impact of benign gene expression classifier test results on the endocrinologist-patient decision to operate on patients with thyroid nodules with indeterminate fine-needle aspiration cytopathology. Thyroid 2012;22(10):996–1001.

73. Haugen BR, Baloch ZW, Chudova D. Development of a novel molecular classifier to accurately identify benign thyroid nodules in patients with indeterminate FNA cytology. Program of the 14th International Thyroid Congress [Abstract LB-03]. Paris, France, September 15, 2010.

74. Ali SZ, Fish SA, Lanman R, et al. Use of the Afirma(R) gene expression classifier for preoperative identification of benign thyroid nodules with indeterminate fine needle aspiration cytopathology. PLoS Curr 2013;5.

75. Wang CC, Friedman L, Kennedy GC, et al. A large multicenter correlation study of thyroid nodule cytopathology and histopathology. Thyroid 2011;21(3): 243–51.

76. Data on file at Thyroid Cytopathology Partners. 2013. Available at: http://www.thyroidcytopath.com/partner-for-afirma/.

77. Lewis CM, Chang KP, Pitman M, et al. Thyroid fine-needle aspiration biopsy: variability in reporting. Thyroid 2009;19(7):717–23.

78. Cibas ES, Baloch ZW, Fellegara G, et al. A prospective assessment defining the limitations of thyroid nodule pathologic evaluation. Ann Intern Med 2013;159(5): 325–32.

79. Alexander EK, Schorr M, Klopper J, et al. Multicenter clinical experience with the Afirma gene expression classifier. J Clin Endocrinol Metab 2014;99(1):119–25.

80. Harrell RM, Bimston DN. Surgical utility of Afirma: effects of high cancer prevalence and oncocytic cell types in patients with indeterminate thyroid cytology. Endocr Pract 2013;1–16 [Epub ahead of print].

81. Bartels CL, Tsongalis GJ. MicroRNAs: novel biomarkers for human cancer. Clin Chem 2009;55(4):623–31.

82. Nikiforova MN, Tseng GC, Steward D, et al. MicroRNA expression profiling of thyroid tumors: biological significance and diagnostic utility. J Clin Endocrinol Metab 2008;93(5):1600–8.

83. Pallante P, Visone R, Ferracin M, et al. MicroRNA deregulation in human thyroid papillary carcinomas. Endocr Relat Cancer 2006;13(2):497–508.

84. Weber F, Teresi RE, Broelsch CE, et al. A limited set of human MicroRNA is deregulated in follicular thyroid carcinoma. J Clin Endocrinol Metab 2006;91(9):3584–91.
85. Keutgen XM, Filicori F, Crowley MJ, et al. A panel of four miRNAs accurately differentiates malignant from benign indeterminate thyroid lesions on fine needle aspiration. Clin Cancer Res 2012;18(7):2032–8.
86. Shen R, Liyanarachchi S, Li W, et al. MicroRNA signature in thyroid fine needle aspiration cytology applied to "atypia of undetermined significance" cases. Thyroid 2012;22(1):9–16.
87. Kitano M, Rahbari R, Patterson EE, et al. Evaluation of candidate diagnostic microRNAs in thyroid fine-needle aspiration biopsy samples. Thyroid 2012;22(3): 285–91.
88. Milas M, Shin J, Gupta M, et al. Circulating thyrotropin receptor mRNA as a novel marker of thyroid cancer: clinical applications learned from 1758 samples. Ann Surg 2010;252(4):643–51.
89. Chia SY, Milas M, Reddy SK, et al. Thyroid-stimulating hormone receptor messenger ribonucleic acid measurement in blood as a marker for circulating thyroid cancer cells and its role in the preoperative diagnosis of thyroid cancer. J Clin Endocrinol Metab 2007;92(2):468–75.
90. Nou E, Kwong N, Alexander LK, et al. Determination of the optimal time interval for repeat evaluation after a benign thyroid nodule aspiration. J Clin Endocrinol Metab 2014;99(2):510–6.
91. Ohori NP, Schoedel KE. Variability in the atypia of undetermined significance/follicular lesion of undetermined significance diagnosis in the Bethesda System for Reporting Thyroid Cytopathology: sources and recommendations. Acta Cytol 2011;55(6):492–8.
92. Guerra A, Sapio MR, Marotta V, et al. The primary occurrence of BRAF(V600E) is a rare clonal event in papillary thyroid carcinoma. J Clin Endocrinol Metab 2012; 97(2):517–24.

Thyrotropin in the Development and Management of Differentiated Thyroid Cancer

Donald S.A. McLeod, MBBS, FRACP, MPH[a,b,c],*

KEYWORDS

- Thyrotropin • Thyroid cancer • Recombinant human TSH • Thyroid hormone • TSH

KEY POINTS

- Thyrotropin (TSH) is the major growth factor and regulator of the thyroid.
- Further research is required to definitely show that higher serum TSH causes human thyroid cancer, whether prediagnostic serum TSH predicts ultimate prognosis, and how best to use serum TSH in determining which patients with thyroid nodules should undergo biopsy.
- TSH is important in the management of thyroid cancer, with TSH stimulation of thyroid cells (either by thyroid hormone withdrawal or recombinant human [rh]-TSH) facilitating radioiodine uptake and detection of occult persistent thyroid tissue via release of serum thyroglobulin.
- The development of rh-TSH was an important advance in thyroid cancer management, permitting TSH stimulation to occur without hypothyroidism, albeit at greater financial cost.
- Further work is required to prove that rh-TSH is equivalent to thyroid hormone withdrawal in patients with metastatic disease.
- A risk-benefit approach to TSH targets in thyroid cancer management may maximize clinical benefit of this therapy while minimizing complications.

Funding Source: Cancer Council Queensland.
Conflict of Interest: Nil.
[a] Department of Internal Medicine & Aged Care, Royal Brisbane & Women's Hospital, Level 3, Dr James Mayne Building, Herston, Queensland 4029, Australia; [b] Department of Endocrinology, Royal Brisbane & Women's Hospital, Level 1, Dr James Mayne Building, Herston, Queensland 4029, Australia; [c] Department of Population Health, QIMR Berghofer Medical Research Institute, Herston Road, Herston, Queensland 4029, Australia
* Department of Internal Medicine & Aged Care, Level 1, Dr James Mayne Building, Royal Brisbane & Women's Hospital, Herston, Queensland 4029, Australia.
E-mail address: donald.mcleod@qimrberghofer.edu.au

INTRODUCTION

Over the past decade, knowledge of the potential role of TSH in the development of differentiated thyroid cancer has expanded. In addition, the therapeutic role of TSH has continued to evolve. This review synthesizes current knowledge of TSH in both the development and management of differentiated thyroid cancer.

TSH BIOLOGY
History

The crucial role of the anterior pituitary in thyroid growth and function was recognized in the early twentieth century, initially with studies in amphibians,[1–3] followed by demonstration in mammals.[4,5] TSH was identified as a distinct hormone secreted from the anterior pituitary shortly after,[6] although it took until 1971 before its structure was elucidated.[7]

Physiology of TSH

TSH is the major regulator and growth factor of the thyroid. The approximately 28-kDa glycoprotein heterodimer is secreted under negative feedback from thyroid hormone, which occurs at both the levels of the pituitary and the hypothalamus (inhibiting secretion of TSH-releasing hormone, which as the name suggests, prompts release of TSH from the anterior pituitary).[8] TSH controls the processes that lead to increased thyroid hormone production and secretion from follicular thyroid cells. These include increasing the number, size, and secretory activity of thyrocytes; increasing the activity of the sodium-iodide symporter (NIS); increasing the organification of iodide; increasing the cleavage and release of preformed thyroid hormone from thyroglobulin; and increasing thyroid blood flow.[9] TSH does not influence parafollicular C-cells; therefore, it does not affect medullary thyroid cancer cells, and all subsequent discussion of thyroid cancer in this article refers to differentiated thyroid cancer (papillary and follicular thyroid cancer), which develops from thyroid follicular cells.

TSH exerts its effect by binding to the TSH receptor, a G protein–coupled receptor on the thyrocyte surface (**Fig. 1**). Classical TSH actions are mainly mediated through the $G_{\alpha s}$–adenylyl cyclase–protein kinase A–cyclic adenosine monophosphate (cAMP) second messenger system, with some actions through the $G_{\alpha q/11}$-inositol phosphate/diacylglycerol-protein kinase C pathway.[10] It has also been recognized, however, that TSH can cross-talk with many other cell signaling pathways, including those known to be associated with thyroid cancer development, including the mitogen-activated protein (MAP) kinase system[11] and phosphoinositide 3-kinase (PI3-K) system.[11,12]

Other factors may also play a role in regulating thyroid function, at least in experimental models. These include insulin, insulin-like growth factor 1, epidermal growth factor, transforming growth factor β, phorbol esters, fibroblast growth factor, and hepatocyte growth factor.[10]

TSH AND THYROID CANCER DEVELOPMENT

The role of TSH in thyroid biology makes it an appealing candidate as a possible cause of thyroid cancer. Evidence for this has accumulated over the past decade in animal models and human clinical studies.

Animal Model Evidence

Follicular thyroid cancer has been assessed in mice using a knock in mutation to the thyroid hormone receptor-β gene ($TR\beta^{PV}$)[13–16] that causes a dominant negative

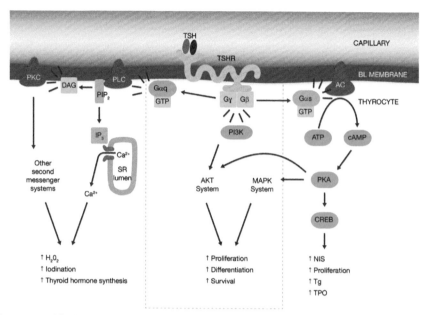

Fig. 1. Simplified model of TSH signaling pathways. TSH binds to its transmembrane receptor, which is coupled to G-protein complexes. Binding of TSH to the receptor leads to transmembrane conformational change, such that GTP binds the G_α, which then dissociates from the complex so it can interact with second messenger targets. The $G_{\alpha s}$–adenylyl cyclase–PKA–cAMP pathway is depicted on the right. Here, the GTP-bound $G_{\alpha s}$ activates the membrane-associated PKA. PKA amplifies the TSH signal by catalyzing the conversion of ATP to cAMP, which in turn activates PKA. Targets of PKA are effectors of many of the classical TSH-dependent actions of thyroid cells. PKA also stimulates with other second messenger systems important in thyroid cancer, including the PI3K/AKT and the MAP kinase systems. The $G_{\alpha q/11}$-IP_3/DAG-PKC pathway is depicted on the left. Here, the $G_{\alpha q}$ activates phospholipase C, which generates 2 second messengers, DAG and IP_3. These in turn activate protein kinase C and release of stored Ca^{2+}, respectively, effecting other TSH-dependent cellular actions. $G_{\beta\gamma}$ also seems to directly stimulate PI3K, hence activating the PI3K/AKT system. AC, adenylyl cyclase; ATP, adenosine triphosphate; BL, basolateral; Ca^{2+}, calcium ions; cAMP, cyclic adenosine monophosphate; CREB, cAMP responsive element binding protein; DAG, diacylglycerol; GTP, guanosine triphosphate; H_2O_2, hydrogen peroxide; IP3, inositol triphosphate; MAPK, mitogen-activated protein kinase; NIS, sodium iodide symporter; P13K, P13 kinase; PIP2, phosphatidylinositol 4,5-biphosphate; PLC, phospholipase C; SR, sarco/endoplasmic reticulum; Tg, thyroglobulin; TPO, thyroid peroxidase; TSH, thyrotropin.

frameshift in TRβ.[17] These mice develop a thyroid hormone resistance syndrome with an elevated non-suppressible TSH, and homozygotes (TRβ$^{PV/PV}$) manifest spontaneous metastatic follicular thyroid cancer.[13] In this model, TSH receptor pathway signaling is necessary for thyroid cancer development, because when TRβ$^{PV/PV}$ mice are crossed with knockout mice for the TSH receptor (TSHR$^{-/-}$), offspring do not develop thyroid cancer.[14] In wild-type mice (ie, no thyroid hormone resistance), however, when TSH is elevated by treatment with propylthiouracil, no metastatic thyroid cancer ensues.[14] Treatment of heterozygous thyroid hormone–resistant mice (TRβ$^{PV/+}$; who do not ordinarily develop cancer) with propylthiouracil generates asymmetric follicular thyroid cancer with frequent metastases.[16] Therefore, TSH is necessary but not sufficient to produce follicular cancer in mice; additional activation of permissive cell signaling pathways is required. In these mice, activating the PI3-K/AKT cascade seems crucial in disease development.[15,18,19]

Animal model evidence also exists for TSH signaling influencing papillary thyroid cancer. Using a mouse model with knock in of BRAF[V600E] (LSL- BRAF[V600E]/TPO-Cre) that produced early and aggressive papillary cancer, Franco and colleagues[20] found that crossing mice with TSHR[−/−] mice led to marked delay in cancer development, with subsequent tumors being indolent. The effect of TSH on cancer development was mediated through the classical $G_{\alpha s}$ pathway, because inhibiting $G_{\alpha s}$ function had similar effects to the TSHR[−/−] experiments. Suppressing TSH with levothyroxine therapy did not revert the BRAF[V600E] phenotype, indicating that TSH signaling was most important in thyroid cancer initiation.

Clinical Evidence

Boelaert and colleagues[21] first reported higher serum TSH concentration predicted human thyroid cancer in 2006 (**Fig. 2**). Since then, many cross-sectional studies have assessed clinical data for an association between serum TSH concentration and thyroid cancer. Most, but not all, studies confirm the association.[22,23] In dose-response meta-analysis, the relationship was present from subnormal levels through the normal range and above.[23] The effect seemed largest at lower TSH levels, with a 3-times greater odds ratio of thyroid cancer between a TSH of 4 mU/L compared with 0 mU/L, although the odds ratio still doubled between 2.2 and 7 mU/L.

Major problems remain, however, with interpreting results of the diagnostic studies: (1) all are cross-sectional and (2) there is often incomplete assessment of potential confounding. Without adequately addressing these issues, it remains unclear whether serum TSH is a cause or simply a predictor of human thyroid cancer. Being a predictor of thyroid cancer diagnosis may have clinical applications (discussed later) but would be

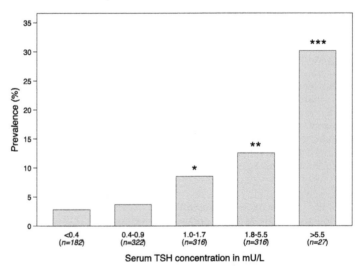

Fig. 2. Prevalence of thyroid cancer from Boelaert and colleagues,[21] according to the serum TSH concentration measured at presentation in 1183 subjects with normal serum free thyroxine concentrations, indicating increased prevalence in those with higher TSH. *, $P = .05$; **, $P = .01$; ***, $P = .001$, compared with TSH <0.4 mU/L. (*From* Boelaert K, Horacek J, Holder RL, et al. Serum thyrotropin concentration as a novel predictor of malignancy in thyroid nodules investigated by fine-needle aspiration. J Clin Endocrinol Metab 2006;91(11):4295–301; with permission.)

less important than proving that increasing serum TSH promotes initiation of human thyroid cancer, like in the animal models. Without confirmation by prospective studies, the relationship seen in the cross-sectional studies may be due to ascertainment bias (ie, higher serum TSH concentration may promote growth of already initiated thyroid cancers so that they are larger and more easily diagnosed). The apparent relationship could also be confounded, for example, by smoking,[24] obesity,[25] or thyroid autoimmunity.[23]

Aside from methodological issues in the literature, there are other gaps and inconsistencies regarding the serum TSH-thyroid cancer hypothesis. Data are rare for patients with thyroid hormone resistance and TSH-secreting pituitary adenomas, although coexisting cancers have been reported.[26,27] Autonomously functioning thyroid nodules are thought uncommonly associated with malignancy,[28] despite the most common cause being activating TSH receptor mutations.[29,30] Thyroid cancer (including aggressive disease), however, can occur in these nodules.[31,32] Thyroid cancer is also highly prevalent in patients with Graves' disease (with its TSH receptor activation),[33] although it is possible that this apparent relationship is due to ascertainment bias.[34] Evidence for increased aggressiveness of thyroid cancer in patients with Graves' disease is mixed, with both suggestive[35–38] and negative[39,40] reports in the literature. Finally, recent genome-wide association studies have reported several single-nucleotide polymorphisms associated with both thyroid cancer and low serum TSH levels (although it does not necessarily follow that patients with the polymorphism who develop thyroid cancer have low serum TSH concentrations themselves; alternatively, it is possible that these genotypes confer increased TSH sensitivity).[41,42]

Serum TSH concentration has also been associated with the aggressiveness of thyroid cancer. Several cross-sectional analyses have documented that increasing serum TSH levels are associated with increasing stage of thyroid cancer.[43–46] This seems to be driven by an increase in extrathyroidal extension and lymph node metastasis with increasing serum TSH, rather than simply tumor size.[46,47] Perhaps it is unsurprising that baseline serum TSH predicts thyroid cancer aggressiveness, because one of the mainstays of long-term thyroid cancer care has been suppression of TSH through supraphysiologic doses of levothyroxine, which has been shown to improve thyroid cancer prognosis, particularly in high-risk patients (discussed later).[48–51]

Future Research Needs and Opportunities

The key task for future research is to perform adequately powered prospective studies assessing the serum TSH-thyroid cancer relationship that adjust for major potential confounders. If a high serum TSH concentration is actually a cause of thyroid cancer, levothyroxine therapy could be indicated as prevention for thyroid cancer in subclinical hypothyroidism and nodular (apparently benign) thyroid disease, or heightened surveillance of patients with previous hypothyroidism could be performed.

For thyroid cancer prediction, serum TSH could potentially form part of nomograms used to determine which patients with thyroid nodules require biopsy. Several equations have been published[21,52] yet have not been externally validated. Whether adding prediagnostic serum TSH concentration to current thyroid cancer staging systems will improve prognostication can only be answered by longitudinal studies, although large patient cohorts and prolonged follow-up will be required.[46]

THYROID CANCER MANAGEMENT
TSH and Radioactive Iodine

Radioactive iodine remains an important element of differentiated thyroid cancer treatment, and to a lesser extent, monitoring of thyroid cancer. Serum TSH enhances radioactive iodine uptake into both benign[53,54] and responsive malignant[55,56] thyroid cells, with the latter observation consistent with the differentiated nature of most thyroid cancers. TSH increases iodine uptake via the NIS, stimulating NIS transcription and translation as well as positioning it on the basolateral thyrocyte membrane.[57] Subsequent organification of the radioiodine (also under TSH control) increases its half-life within the thyroid cells,[58] thereby increasing the effectiveness of the therapy. The traditional TSH concentration for defining adequacy of stimulation was considered 30 mU/L,[59] although more recent evidence suggests that this level of TSH is not necessarily adequate[60] and that maximal saturation of the TSH receptor occurs at TSH concentrations between 51 and 82 mU/L.[61]

The benefits of elevated TSH during radioactive iodine therapy were recognized soon after radioactive iodine had become available in the early 1940s.[62] Bovine TSH injection concomitant with levothyroxine therapy was first reported in 1953,[56] although subsequent use of bovine TSH was beset with problems, including allergic reactions and the development of neutralizing antibodies.[63] The mainstay of TSH stimulation for radioactive iodine therefore became short-term thyroid hormone withdrawal. Thyroid hormone withdrawal may be achieved either through cessation of levothyroxine for 2 to 3 weeks or via substitution of levothyroxine with triiodothyronine for 2 to 4 weeks, followed by 2 weeks off all thyroid hormone treatment.[64]

New gene cloning techniques in the 1980s unlocked the possibility of generating rh-TSH expression in cell lines,[65,66] leading to development of commercially produced rh-TSH (subsequently given the trade name Thyrogen).[67] A phase I/II trial was published in 1994,[68] followed by a phase III study in 1997.[69] The US Food and Drug Administration (FDA) approved rh-TSH for use in diagnostic testing in 1998 and for thyroid remnant ablation therapy in 2007 (2000 and 2005 for European approvals, respectively). Intramuscular rh-TSH (1.1 mg; 0.9 mg/mL rh-TSH reconstituted in 1.2 mL sterile water) is given in 2 injections, 48 hours and 24 hours prior to radioiodine treatment. If rh-TSH is used for diagnostic scanning, this occurs 72 hours after the last rh-TSH dose (48 hours after the radioactive iodine administration).

rh-TSH has comparable effectiveness to thyroid hormone withdrawal for both diagnostic scanning[70,71] and thyroid remnant ablation.[72–74] The 2 most recent multicenter randomized controlled trials also found that in low-risk patients, thyroid remnant ablation success was not compromised by use of rh-TSH, even when using a low administered activity of radioactive iodine (30 mCi; 1.1 GBq).[73,74] Short-term follow-up of observational cohorts[75] and randomized studies[76] have found similar recurrence rates in rh-TSH– and thyroid withdrawal–treated patients undergoing thyroid remnant ablation. Recently, an observational cohort with prolonged follow-up (median 9 years) and a high proportion of intermediate- and high-risk patients confirmed the equivalence of clinical outcomes with either rh-TSH or thyroid hormone preparation for thyroid remnant ablation.[77]

The key advantage of rh-TSH over thyroid hormone withdrawal for TSH stimulation is avoidance of hypothyroidism. Studies have consistently found that rh-TSH prevents degradation in short-term quality of life associated with thyroid hormone withdrawal (**Fig. 3**).[72–74,78–80] Work absenteeism is also reduced by use of rh-TSH.[74,81] Cost is the major disadvantage. In a rigorous cost-utility analysis, the incremental cost utility of rh-TSH was estimated at just over $50,000 per quality-adjusted life-year, although calculations were sensitive to inputs, including patient utility, cost of rh-TSH, days off work, and differences in rates of remnant ablation.[82]

TSH stimulation, regardless of the means used, has some specific risks in thyroid cancer. The most important of these is swelling of metastatic lesions in or near vital organs (eg, brain, spinal cord, and trachea). In circumstances where this is thought

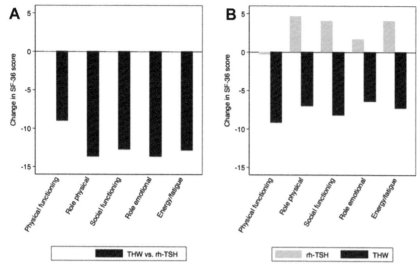

Fig. 3. Quality-of-life impact of rh-TSH versus THW. Results of 2 different studies. (A) Schroeder and colleagues[78] compared health-related quality of life (via SF-36 scale) in 225 patients who underwent both rh-TSH and THW for whole-body scanning and thyroglobulin measurement. The black bars represent the drop in selected SF-36 domains at the time of thyroid hormone withdrawal compared with that during rh-TSH. $P<.0001$ for difference for all. (B) Mallick and colleagues[74] randomized 421 patients to rh-TSH or THW, prior to radioactive iodine thyroid remnant ablation. The bars represent the difference in selected short form (36) health survey scores from time of consent to the day of ablation, with the rh-TSH group represented in gray and THW group in black. $P<.001$ for difference for all except role emotional ($P = .002$). THW, thyroid hormone withdrawal.

possible, external beam radiation and the concomitant use of glucocorticoids is recommended by the American Thyroid Association.[64]

Thus, both TSH withdrawal and rh-TSH are options for preparing patients for radioactive iodine administration, although TSH withdrawal has the attendant complication of hypothyroidism, and rh-TSH is associated with higher cost. Current FDA indications for rh-TSH are listed in **Box 1**. Indications for both techniques largely overlap; however, TSH withdrawal is not successful in secondary hypothyroidism and rh-TSH avoids the risk of frank hypothyroidism when this is medically contraindicated, for example, in patients with unstable cardiac disease or severe psychiatric illness. On the other hand, rh-TSH is not currently approved for use in patients with distant metastatic disease (except for those circumstances where TSH withdrawal can not be

---

Box 1
Current FDA-approved indications for recombinant human TSH use

1. Radioactive iodine remnant ablation

2. Diagnostic whole-body radioiodine scanning assessing for recurrent disease

3. Stimulated thyroglobulin testing assessing for recurrent disease

4. Radioactive iodine for patients with metastatic disease who cannot mount an endogenous TSH response (eg, pituitary disease), or in whom hypothyroidism may be contraindicated (eg, unstable coronary artery disease or psychiatric disease)

used). This reflects the lack of evidence of effectiveness and potential inferiority of rh-TSH in stimulating radioactive iodine uptake within metastases.[83] There is also the possibility of inducing severe hyperthyroidism in the setting of thyroid hormone-producing tumors, although this situation is rare. Other than the lack of symptomatic hypothyroidism, theoretic advantages of rh-TSH include the faster whole-body clearance of radioactive iodine (and thus potential lower toxicity)[84] and shorter period of TSH-induced tumor growth prior to treatment.[85] Although the data are preliminary, evidence is accumulating that rh-TSH can be effective in the setting of metastatic disease as well as being well tolerated.[85–87]

TSH and Monitoring of Thyroid Cancer

Serum TSH concentration is important in interpreting the thyroglobulin level performed in thyroid cancer monitoring. Thyroglobulin is secreted specifically from thyrocytes. Therefore, when all thyroid tissue has been successfully ablated, serum thyroglobulin is absent. If differentiated thyrocytes (either benign or malignant) remain, secretion of thyroglobulin is responsive to serum TSH.[88,89] Suppressed serum TSH concentrations lead to lower or suppressed serum thyroglobulin secretion in residual thyroid tissue, such that serum thyroglobulin may be undetectable in widely available thyroglobulin assays.[64] To overcome this problem, TSH-stimulated thyroglobulin (achieved via thyroid hormone withdrawal or rh-TSH) may be used to detect residual thyroid tissue.

TSH-stimulated thyroglobulin measurement can be performed immediately prior to radioiodine thyroid remnant ablation. The level of thyroglobulin has been shown to predict prognosis, with one study finding a preablative thyroglobulin cutpoint of 27.5 ng/mL the best predictor of both presence of distant metastases and subsequent death.[90] Conceivably, a negative TSH-stimulated thyroglobulin could also be used to identify patients with minimal/absent remnant thyroid tissue who may not receive any additional benefit from remnant ablation. To be practical, however, a rapid turnaround of assay results (or access to multiple courses of rh-TSH) would be required.

In follow-up of patients who have received radioiodine ablation therapy, a detectable stimulated thyroglobulin can either indicate recurrence (either biochemical or structurally identifiable) or persistent thyroid remnants. Haugen and colleagues[70] demonstrated that a stimulated thyroglobulin greater than or equal to 2 ng/mL via either thyroid hormone withdrawal or rh-TSH detected 100% of patients with current metastatic disease. The cutoff of 2 ng/mL has also been shown to predict persistent tumor, whereas in the same study a stimulated thyroglobulin of less than 0.5 ng/mL made recurrence at 3 to 5 years unlikely.[91] More recently, it has been proposed that a stimulated thyroglobulin of less than1 ng/mL, combined with negative neck imaging within the first 2 years after thyroid cancer therapy, can be used to reclassify patients as low risk for future recurrence, even when they were initially at higher risk based on standard clinicopathologic risk markers.[92] In the future, it may not be necessary to measure TSH-stimulated thyroglobulin level as sensitivity of thyroglobulin assays continue to improve.[93]

Knowledge of serum TSH concentration is also crucial when assessing serial serum thyroglobulin levels. Although a rising serum thyroglobulin over time portends worse prognosis,[94] it is important not to overinterpret small rises in serum thyroglobulin from baseline levels in the setting of increased serum TSH (ie, due to poor adherence or changing treatment targets). A detectable serum thyroglobulin clearly indicates residual thyroid tissue and possibly recurrence, yet it does not necessarily mean that the disease itself is progressing if the rising thyroglobulin concentration is due to increased TSH stimulation.

TSH Targets in Long-Term Levothyroxine Treatment

The use of thyroid hormone as a treatment of thyroid cancer was first reported in 1937[95] and was elegantly championed by Crile from the 1950s.[95,96] It was not until the work of Mazzaferri and colleagues[97–99] studying US Air Force recruits, however, that the concept of suppression of TSH with thyroid hormone became widely accepted.

Recent studies have clarified which patients will benefit most from TSH-suppressive therapy with levothyroxine. The National Thyroid Cancer Treatment Cooperative Study (NTCTCS) followed 1548 patients, with inclusion criterion being greater than 50% TSH levels recorded at follow-up.[48] The investigators assigned each patient a TSH score based on mean TSH levels (1 = undetectable, 2 = subnormal, 3 = normal, and 4 = elevated). They found that in patients with high-risk disease (ie, NTCTCS stage III or IV), those with lowest serum TSH levels throughout their follow-up had improved overall and disease-specific survival compared with patients without tight suppression. Although patient numbers were small, those with NTCTCS stage II disease seemed to have higher survival if TSH during follow-up was not high (compared with those with mean TSH score between 3 and 4); there was no evidence that complete suppression of TSH benefited this group. Patients with NTCTCS stage I disease had good prognosis whatever the serum TSH levels were throughout follow-up. These results have been supported in smaller observational studies. In one study of a majority of lower-risk patients, relapse and cause-specific mortality were higher in patients with median TSH concentrations greater than or equal to 2 mU/L compared with less than 2 mU/L,[49] whereas 2 studies of patients with metastatic disease support stringent TSH suppression (ie, <0.1 mU/L).[50,51] One randomized controlled trial has addressed the issue. This Japanese study followed 432 mainly low-risk patients (as defined by the age, metastasis, extension, size [AMES] classification system) for a median of 6.9 years, finding that TSH suppression did not improve disease-free survival.[100] In a subgroup of 50 patients with high-risk disease, no difference was found between TSH suppression and euthyroid patients, although the power to detect any difference in that subgroup was low.

There are potential risks from TSH suppression. Frankly thyrotoxic patients may have impaired quality of life, particularly from adrenergic symptoms.[101] Cardiovascular effects of supraphysiologic thyroid hormone increase with age[102]; the most critical of these is atrial fibrillation.[103] A recent Dutch study has also suggested that stringent TSH suppression is associated with increased mortality, particularly from cardiovascular causes.[104] Although plausible, this study's results require confirmation given previous reassuring studies, which did not suggest altered life expectancy in low-risk patients.[105,106] Finally, bone loss occurs with TSH suppressive treatment, particularly in postmenopausal women.[107]

In deciding which patients should be treated with TSH suppressive therapy, a risk-benefit decision needs to be made. Those at lowest risk of recurrence do not seem to benefit from TSH suppression, at least less than 2 mU/L, so a low-normal serum TSH in these patients is justifiable. Patients with persistent disease or high risk of recurrence have most to gain from TSH suppression, with a target of less than or equal to 0.1 mU/L. The difficult circumstance is a higher-risk patient who is also at risk of (or with current) complications; this is particularly relevant in elderly patients. Here, an individualized decision needs to be made about the specific risks versus benefits and the level of TSH suppression that is most appropriate. A pragmatic solution in these patients could be to have minimal TSH suppression (ie, to a level of 0.1–0.5 m/L). In patients whose disease progresses with less stringent TSH suppression, it is reasonable

Thyroid cancer risk status

		Low	Intermediate/High	Persistent/progressive
Risk of TSH suppression	Low	TSH 0.5-2.0 mU/L	TSH <0.1 mU/L	TSH <0.1 mU/L (if tolerated, proactively managing complications of TSH suppression)
	High	TSH 0.5-2.0 mU/L	TSH 0.1-0.5 mU/L	

Fig. 4. Suggested approach to TSH suppression in differentiated thyroid cancer. Thyroid cancer risk status can be initially assessed through the American Thyroid Association guidelines.[64] Thyroid cancer risk assessment should be a continually dynamic process, with disease-free patients moving to lower risk status if stimulated thyroglobulin testing and neck imaging are negative[92] or after a prolonged disease-free period.[64] Risk of TSH suppression should also be individualized. Treatment risks, in particular atrial fibrillation, increase with age. Patients at high risk of TSH suppression also include those with conditions that may be exacerbated by TSH suppression, such as atrial fibrillation or osteopenia, or current symptomatic intolerance of TSH suppressive therapy.

to reinstitute full TSH suppression with close surveillance and management of thyrotoxic complications. This approach is set out in **Fig. 4**. Although it is likely that in the future all thyroid cancer guidelines will reflect a risk-benefit analysis regarding TSH suppression, only one current guideline specifically advocates taking risks of TSH suppression into account.[108]

SUMMARY

TSH is the major regulator and growth factor of the thyroid. Higher serum TSH is a predictor of differentiated thyroid cancer diagnosis and disease stage. Animal models also suggest TSH plays a role in causing thyroid cancer. Further research is required to definitely show that higher serum TSH causes human thyroid cancer, whether prediagnostic serum TSH predicts ultimate prognosis, and how best to use serum TSH in determining which patients with thyroid nodules should undergo biopsy. TSH is also important in the management of thyroid cancer, with TSH stimulation of thyroid cells (either by thyroid hormone withdrawal or rh-TSH) facilitating radioiodine uptake and detection of occult persistent thyroid tissue via release of serum thyroglobulin. The development of rh-TSH was an important advance in thyroid cancer management, permitting TSH stimulation to occur without hypothyroidism, albeit at greater financial cost. Further work is required to prove that rh-TSH is equivalent to thyroid hormone withdrawal in patients with metastatic disease. Long-term suppression of serum TSH with thyroid hormone improves prognosis in high-risk patients, although there are potential associated harms. A risk-benefit approach to TSH targets in thyroid cancer management may maximize clinical benefit of this therapy while minimizing complications.

REFERENCES

1. Smith PE. Experimental ablation of the hypophysis in the frog embryo. Science 1916;44(1130):280–2.

2. Allen BM. The results of extirpation of the anterior lobe of the hypophysis and of the thyroid of *Rana pipiens* larvae. Science 1916;44(1143):755–8.
3. Smith PE, Smith IP. The repair and activation of the thyroid in the hypophysectomized tadpole by the Parenteral Administration of Fresh Anterior Lobe of the Bovine Hypophysis. J Med Res 1922;43(3):267–284.1.
4. Aron M. Action de la prehypophyse sur le thyroide chez le cobaye. C R Soc Biol (Paris) 1929;102:682–4.
5. Loeb L, Bassett RB. Effect of hormones of anterior pituitary on thyroid gland in the guinea pig. Exp Biol Med 1929;26(9):860–2.
6. Greep RO. Separation of a thyrotropin from the gonadotropic substances of the pituitary. Am J Physiol 1934;110(3):692–9.
7. Liao TH, Pierce JG. The primary structure of bovine thyrotropin. II. The amino acid sequences of the reduced, S-carboxymethyl alpha and beta chains. J Biol Chem 1971;246(4):850–65.
8. Magner JA. Thyroid-stimulating hormone: biosynthesis, cell biology, and bioactivity. Endocr Rev 1990;11(2):354–85.
9. Hall JE. Thyroid metabolic hormones. Guyton and Hall textbook of medical physiology. 12th edition. Philadelphia: Saunders/Elsevier; 2011. p. 907–18.
10. Kimura T, Van Keymeulen A, Golstein J, et al. Regulation of thyroid cell proliferation by TSH and other factors: a critical evaluation of in vitro models. Endocr Rev 2001;22(5):631–56.
11. Stork PJ, Schmitt JM. Crosstalk between cAMP and MAP kinase signaling in the regulation of cell proliferation. Trends Cell Biol 2002;12(6):258–66.
12. Zaballos MA, Garcia B, Santisteban P. Gβγ dimers released in response to thyrotropin activate phosphoinositide 3-kinase and regulate gene expression in thyroid cells. Mol Endocrinol 2008;22(5):1183–99.
13. Suzuki H, Willingham MC, Cheng SY. Mice with a mutation in the thyroid hormone receptor beta gene spontaneously develop thyroid carcinoma: a mouse model of thyroid carcinogenesis. Thyroid 2002;12(11):963–9.
14. Lu C, Zhao L, Ying H, et al. Growth activation alone is not sufficient to cause metastatic thyroid cancer in a mouse model of follicular thyroid carcinoma. Endocrinology 2010;151(4):1929–39.
15. Saji M, Narahara K, McCarty SK, et al. Akt1 deficiency delays tumor progression, vascular invasion, and distant metastasis in a murine model of thyroid cancer. Oncogene 2011;30(42):4307–15.
16. Zhao L, Zhu X, Won Park J, et al. Role of TSH in the spontaneous development of asymmetrical thyroid carcinoma in mice with a targeted mutation in a single allele of the thyroid hormone-beta receptor. Endocrinology 2012;153(10):5090–100.
17. Parrilla R, Mixson AJ, McPherson JA, et al. Characterization of seven novel mutations of the c-erbA beta gene in unrelated kindreds with generalized thyroid hormone resistance. Evidence for two "hot spot" regions of the ligand binding domain. J Clin Invest 1991;88(6):2123–30.
18. Kim CS, Vasko VV, Kato Y, et al. AKT activation promotes metastasis in a mouse model of follicular thyroid carcinoma. Endocrinology 2005;146(10):4456–63.
19. Furuya F, Hanover JA, Cheng SY. Activation of phosphatidylinositol 3-kinase signaling by a mutant thyroid hormone beta receptor. Proc Natl Acad Sci U S A 2006;103(6):1780–5.
20. Franco AT, Malaguarnera R, Refetoff S, et al. Thyrotrophin receptor signaling dependence of Braf-induced thyroid tumor initiation in mice. Proc Natl Acad Sci U S A 2011;108(4):1615–20.

58. Cavalieri RR. Iodine metabolism and thyroid physiology: current concepts. Thyroid 1997;7(2):177–81.
59. Edmonds CJ, Hayes S, Kermode JC, et al. Measurement of serum TSH and thyroid hormones in the management of treatment of thyroid carcinoma with radioiodine. Br J Radiol 1977;50(599):799–807.
60. Valle LA, Gorodeski Baskin RL, Porter K, et al. In thyroidectomized patients with thyroid cancer, a serum thyrotropin of 30 muU/mL after thyroxine withdrawal is not always adequate for detecting an elevated stimulated serum thyroglobulin. Thyroid 2013;23(2):185–93.
61. Torres MS, Ramirez L, Simkin PH, et al. Effect of various doses of recombinant human thyrotropin on the thyroid radioactive iodine uptake and serum levels of thyroid hormones and thyroglobulin in normal subjects. J Clin Endocrinol Metab 2001;86(4):1660–4.
62. Trippel OH, Sheline GE, Moe RH, et al. Clinical applications of radioactive iodine in diseases of the thyroid. Med Clin North Am 1951;35(1):37–50.
63. Hays MT, Solomon DH, Werner SC. The effect of purified bovine thyroid-stimulating hormone in men. II. Loss of effectiveness with prolonged administration. J Clin Endocrinol Metab 1961;21:1475–82.
64. Cooper DS, Doherty GM, Haugen BR, et al. Revised American Thyroid Association management guidelines for patients with thyroid nodules and differentiated thyroid cancer. Thyroid 2009;19(11):1167–214.
65. Watanabe S, Hayashizaki Y, Endo Y, et al. Production of human thyroid-stimulating hormone in Chinese hamster ovary cells. Biochem Biophys Res Commun 1987;149(3):1149–55.
66. Wondisford FE, Usala SJ, DeCherney GS, et al. Cloning of the human thyrotropin beta-subunit gene and transient expression of biologically active human thyrotropin after gene transfection. Mol Endocrinol 1988;2(1):32–9.
67. Cole ES, Lee K, Lauziere K, et al. Recombinant human thyroid stimulating hormone: development of a biotechnology product for detection of metastatic lesions of thyroid carcinoma. Biotechnology (N Y) 1993;11(9):1014–24.
68. Meier CA, Braverman LE, Ebner SA, et al. Diagnostic use of recombinant human thyrotropin in patients with thyroid carcinoma (phase I/II study). J Clin Endocrinol Metab 1994;78(1):188–96.
69. Ladenson PW, Braverman LE, Mazzaferri EL, et al. Comparison of administration of recombinant human thyrotropin with withdrawal of thyroid hormone for radioactive iodine scanning in patients with thyroid carcinoma. N Engl J Med 1997; 337(13):888–96.
70. Haugen BR, Pacini F, Reiners C, et al. A comparison of recombinant human thyrotropin and thyroid hormone withdrawal for the detection of thyroid remnant or cancer. J Clin Endocrinol Metab 1999;84(11):3877–85.
71. Robbins RJ, Tuttle RM, Sharaf RN, et al. Preparation by recombinant human thyrotropin or thyroid hormone withdrawal are comparable for the detection of residual differentiated thyroid carcinoma. J Clin Endocrinol Metab 2001;86(2):619–25.
72. Pacini F, Ladenson PW, Schlumberger M, et al. Radioiodine ablation of thyroid remnants after preparation with recombinant human thyrotropin in differentiated thyroid carcinoma: results of an international, randomized, controlled study. J Clin Endocrinol Metab 2006;91(3):926–32.
73. Schlumberger M, Catargi B, Borget I, et al. Strategies of radioiodine ablation in patients with low-risk thyroid cancer. N Engl J Med 2012;366(18):1663–73.
74. Mallick U, Harmer C, Yap B, et al. Ablation with low-dose radioiodine and thyrotropin alfa in thyroid cancer. N Engl J Med 2012;366(18):1674–85.

75. Tuttle RM, Brokhin M, Omry G, et al. Recombinant human TSH-assisted radioactive iodine remnant ablation achieves short-term clinical recurrence rates similar to those of traditional thyroid hormone withdrawal. J Nucl Med 2008;49(5):764–70.
76. Elisei R, Schlumberger M, Driedger A, et al. Follow-up of low-risk differentiated thyroid cancer patients who underwent radioiodine ablation of postsurgical thyroid remnants after either recombinant human thyrotropin or thyroid hormone withdrawal. J Clin Endocrinol Metab 2009;94(11):4171–9.
77. Hugo J, Robenshtok E, Grewal R, et al. Recombinant human thyroid stimulating hormone-assisted radioactive iodine remnant ablation in thyroid cancer patients at intermediate to high risk of recurrence. Thyroid 2012;22(10):1007–15.
78. Schroeder PR, Haugen BR, Pacini F, et al. A comparison of short-term changes in health-related quality of life in thyroid carcinoma patients undergoing diagnostic evaluation with recombinant human thyrotropin compared with thyroid hormone withdrawal. J Clin Endocrinol Metab 2006;91(3):878–84.
79. Taieb D, Sebag F, Cherenko M, et al. Quality of life changes and clinical outcomes in thyroid cancer patients undergoing radioiodine remnant ablation (RRA) with recombinant human TSH (rhTSH): a randomized controlled study. Clin Endocrinol (Oxf) 2009;71(1):115–23.
80. Lee J, Yun MJ, Nam KH, et al. Quality of life and effectiveness comparisons of thyroxine withdrawal, triiodothyronine withdrawal, and recombinant thyroid-stimulating hormone administration for low-dose radioiodine remnant ablation of differentiated thyroid carcinoma. Thyroid 2010;20(2):173–9.
81. Borget I, Corone C, Nocaudie M, et al. Sick leave for follow-up control in thyroid cancer patients: comparison between stimulation with Thyrogen and thyroid hormone withdrawal. Eur J Endocrinol 2007;156(5):531–8.
82. Wang TS, Cheung K, Mehta P, et al. To stimulate or withdraw? A cost-utility analysis of recombinant human thyrotropin versus thyroxine withdrawal for radioiodine ablation in patients with low-risk differentiated thyroid cancer in the United States. J Clin Endocrinol Metab 2010;95(4):1672–80.
83. Driedger AA, Kotowycz N. Two cases of thyroid carcinoma that were not stimulated by recombinant human thyrotropin. J Clin Endocrinol Metab 2004;89(2):585–90.
84. Hanscheid H, Lassmann M, Luster M, et al. Iodine biokinetics and dosimetry in radioiodine therapy of thyroid cancer: procedures and results of a prospective international controlled study of ablation after rhTSH or hormone withdrawal. J Nucl Med 2006;47(4):648–54.
85. Klubo-Gwiezdzinska J, Burman KD, Van Nostrand D, et al. Radioiodine treatment of metastatic thyroid cancer: relative efficacy and side effect profile of preparation by thyroid hormone withdrawal versus recombinant human thyrotropin. Thyroid 2012;22(3):310–7.
86. Klubo-Gwiezdzinska J, Burman KD, Van Nostrand D, et al. Potential use of recombinant human thyrotropin in the treatment of distant metastases in patients with differentiated thyroid cancer. Endocr Pract 2013;19(1):139–48.
87. Tala H, Robbins R, Fagin JA, et al. Five-year survival is similar in thyroid cancer patients with distant metastases prepared for radioactive iodine therapy with either thyroid hormone withdrawal or recombinant human TSH. J Clin Endocrinol Metab 2011;96(7):2105–11.
88. Uller RP, Van Herle AJ, Chopra IJ. Comparison of alterations in circulating thyroglobulin, triiodothyronine and thyroxine in response to exogenous (bovine) and endogenous (human) thyrotropin. J Clin Endocrinol Metab 1973;37(5):741–5.

89. Schlumberger M, Charbord P, Fragu P, et al. Circulating thyroglobulin and thyroid hormones in patients with metastases of differentiated thyroid carcinoma: relationship to serum thyrotropin levels. J Clin Endocrinol Metab 1980;51(3):513–9.

90. Heemstra KA, Liu YY, Stokkel M, et al. Serum thyroglobulin concentrations predict disease-free remission and death in differentiated thyroid carcinoma. Clin Endocrinol (Oxf) 2007;66(1):58–64.

91. Kloos RT, Mazzaferri EL. A single recombinant human thyrotropin-stimulated serum thyroglobulin measurement predicts differentiated thyroid carcinoma metastases three to five years later. J Clin Endocrinol Metab 2005;90(9):5047–57.

92. Tuttle RM, Tala H, Shah J, et al. Estimating risk of recurrence in differentiated thyroid cancer after total thyroidectomy and radioactive iodine remnant ablation: using response to therapy variables to modify the initial risk estimates predicted by the new American Thyroid Association staging system. Thyroid 2010;20(12):1341–9.

93. Smallridge RC, Meek SE, Morgan MA, et al. Monitoring thyroglobulin in a sensitive immunoassay has comparable sensitivity to recombinant human tsh-stimulated thyroglobulin in follow-up of thyroid cancer patients. J Clin Endocrinol Metab 2007;92(1):82–7.

94. Miyauchi A, Kudo T, Miya A, et al. Prognostic impact of serum thyroglobulin doubling-time under thyrotropin suppression in patients with papillary thyroid carcinoma who underwent total thyroidectomy. Thyroid 2011;21(7):707–16.

95. Hurley JR. Historical note: TSH suppression for thyroid cancer. Thyroid 2011;21(11):1175–6.

96. Crile G Jr. Treatment of cancer of the thyroid with desiccated thyroid. Cleve Clin Q 1955;22(4):161–3.

97. Mazzaferri EL, Young RL, Oertel JE, et al. Papillary thyroid carcinoma: the impact of therapy in 576 patients. Medicine (Baltimore) 1977;56(3):171–96.

98. Mazzaferri EL, Young RL. Papillary thyroid carcinoma: a 10 year follow-up report of the impact of therapy in 576 patients. Am J Med 1981;70(3):511–8.

99. Mazzaferri EL, Jhiang SM. Long-term impact of initial surgical and medical therapy on papillary and follicular thyroid cancer. Am J Med 1994;97(5):418–28.

100. Sugitani I, Fujimoto Y. Does postoperative thyrotropin suppression therapy truly decrease recurrence in papillary thyroid carcinoma? A randomized controlled trial. J Clin Endocrinol Metab 2010;95(10):4576–83.

101. Biondi B, Fazio S, Carella C, et al. Control of adrenergic overactivity by beta-blockade improves the quality of life in patients receiving long term suppressive therapy with levothyroxine. J Clin Endocrinol Metab 1994;78(5):1028–33.

102. Biondi B, Cooper DS. Benefits of thyrotropin suppression versus the risks of adverse effects in differentiated thyroid cancer. Thyroid 2010;20(2):135–46.

103. Sawin CT, Geller A, Wolf PA, et al. Low serum thyrotropin concentrations as a risk factor for atrial fibrillation in older persons. N Engl J Med 1994;331(19):1249–52.

104. Klein Hesselink EN, Klein Hesselink MS, de Bock GH, et al. Long-term cardiovascular mortality in patients with differentiated thyroid carcinoma: an observational study. J Clin Oncol 2013;31(32):4046–53.

105. Links TP, van Tol KM, Jager PL, et al. Life expectancy in differentiated thyroid cancer: a novel approach to survival analysis. Endocr Relat Cancer 2005;12(2):273–80.

106. Eustatia-Rutten CF, Corssmit EP, Biermasz NR, et al. Survival and death causes in differentiated thyroid carcinoma. J Clin Endocrinol Metab 2006;91(1):313–9.

107. Sugitani I, Fujimoto Y. Effect of postoperative thyrotropin suppressive therapy on bone mineral density in patients with papillary thyroid carcinoma: a prospective controlled study. Surgery 2011;150(6):1250–7.
108. Tuttle RM, Ball DW, Byrd D, et al. Thyroid carcinoma v2. 2013; National Comprehensive Cancer Network. Available at: http://www.nccn.org/professionals/physician_gls/pdf/thyroid.pdf. Accessed August 31, 2013.

Initial Radioiodine Administration

When to Use It and How to Select the Dose

Giuseppe Esposito, MD

KEYWORDS

• Radioiodine • Thyroid cancer • Radioactive iodine • Guidelines

KEY POINTS

- All published guidelines on the use of radioactive iodine for the treatment of well-differentiated thyroid cancer agree that an individualized assessment of the risk of cancer-related mortality and of disease recurrence should direct the decision of whether radioiodine treatment is needed and how much to administer.
- With very-low-risk patients, there is no need for radioiodine ablation.
- For low-risk patients, remnant ablation with recombinant human thyroid-stimulating hormone–stimulated diagnostic scan followed by 131-I administration using a fixed empiric activity is recommended.
- For intermediate-risk patients, adjuvant treatment is used with higher activities of 75 to 100 mCi (2.8–3.7 GBq).
- High-risk patients require treatment of residual or metastatic disease; for the treatment of residual or metastatic disease, the author does not exceed 150 mCi (5.5 GBq) unless specifically guided by dosimetry and particularly for elderly patients.

INTRODUCTION AND HISTORICAL FACTS

Radioactive iodine has been used in the management of thyroid cancer since the early 1940s. In 1940, Hamilton and colleagues[1] described the first case of uptake of radioactive iodine by a cancerous thyroid. In 1942, Keston and colleagues[2] described the first cases of uptake by thyroid cancer metastases and noted appreciable accumulation of radioactive iodine in well-differentiated metastatic disease, whereas undifferentiated lesions did not demonstrate significant uptake of radioactivity. These initial observations provided the impetus for the development of treatments that used radioactive iodine, and Seidlin and colleagues[3] performed the first therapeutic administration of 131-I in 1946. Since these initial reports, several other studies have demonstrated that the use of radioactive iodine in thyroid cancer decreases the overall disease-specific mortality as well as the probability of having

Department of Radiology, Medstar Georgetown University Hospital, 3800 Reservoir Road NW, Washington, DC 20007, USA
E-mail address: Exg11@gunet.georgetown.edu

Endocrinol Metab Clin N Am 43 (2014) 385–400
http://dx.doi.org/10.1016/j.ecl.2014.02.003
0889-8529/14/$ – see front matter © 2014 Elsevier Inc. All rights reserved.

disease recurrence.[4,5] Treatment with 131-I radioactive iodine represents today an essential component of individualized, risk-adjusted management of well-differentiated thyroid cancer. A growing body of scientific evidence provides a solid foundation that can be used as a reference by practitioners involved in the management of thyroid cancer. The use of radioactive iodine as one of the available therapies is discussed in the thyroid cancer guidelines developed by the American Thyroid Association (ATA),[6] by the National Comprehensive Cancer Network,[7] and by the European Consensus on Thyroid Cancer.[8] This article provides an overview of the current status of the use of radioactive iodine for the treatment of thyroid cancer after the initial thyroidectomy and reviews the current clinical guidelines, with the intent to provide a reference framework for an individualized use of radioactive iodine in the management of well-differentiated thyroid cancer. Areas of controversy are explored.

Patient follow-up after the initial radioiodine treatment and repeated radioiodine treatments are beyond the scope of this article and are not discussed.

DEFINITION AND OVERVIEW OF RADIOACTIVE IODINE TREATMENT

Radioactive iodine therapy is performed as an adjunct to total thyroidectomy in patients with well-differentiated (papillary and follicular) thyroid cancer. Radioactive iodine in the form of 131-I sodium iodide is administered orally, usually 4 to 6 weeks after total thyroidectomy. The radionuclide 131-I is a β- and γ-emitting radionuclide with a physical half-life 8.1 days. The principal γ-ray of 364 keV is used for imaging. The principal β-particle emission has therapeutic effect with a maximum energy of 0.61 MeV, an average energy of 0.192 MeV, and a mean range in tissue of 0.4 mm.[9] Treatment with radioactive iodine requires a well-coordinated multidisciplinary effort that involves surgeons, pathologists, endocrinologists, radiologists, nuclear medicine physicians, and physicists (**Fig. 1**). The initial disease staging is performed at the time of total thyroidectomy. Subsequent patient management and completion of staging requires the collaborative efforts of endocrinologists and nuclear medicine physicians so that residual thyroid tissue and/or disease is adequately stimulated via thyroid hormone withdrawal or the administration of recombinant thyroid-stimulating hormone (rTSH) for imaging and, when indicated, treatment with radioiodine. These initial steps in the management of thyroid cancer provide an estimate of the individual patient risk for cancer-related mortality and for disease recurrence that will guide the choice of the amount of 131-I to administer to each patient. Several systems have been developed to stratify patients prognostically, according to the estimated risk of disease recurrence and disease-specific mortality; these are discussed later. Risk estimation allows a targeted, individualized selection of the amount of radioactive iodine to administer to each patient so that the most appropriate radiation dose is delivered to the target tissue while minimizing the dose to normal radiosensitive tissues and, therefore, the possibility of side effects. When indicated, the intent of radioactive iodine treatment can

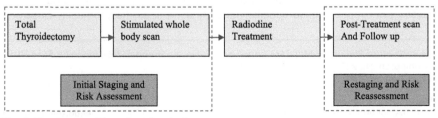

Fig. 1. Treatment with radioactive iodine.

be classified in 3 main categories depending on the patients' estimated risk: (1) remnant ablation, (2) adjuvant therapy, (3) therapy for known persistent disease (**Box 1**, **Table 1**, ATA's guidelines).

Remnant Ablation

Remnant ablation refers to the elimination of residual macroscopic normal thyroid tissue. Thus, this procedure would typically be performed in low-risk patients who have no evidence of local or distant metastases, no aggressive histologies, no locoregional invasion of surrounding tissues, and no vascular invasion. Destruction of normal tissue facilitates the detection of recurrent disease during follow-up by increasing specificity and sensitivity for measurements of the tumor marker thyroglobulin, by improving the sensitivity of follow-up scans to detect residual metastatic disease, and by improving the initial staging of disease because the whole-body scan that is performed after the administration of 131-I for remnant ablation has better sensitivity for detecting disease compared with the lower activity administered for the pretreatment whole-body scan. In addition, ablation of residual thyroid tissue minimizes the risk of developing new cancers in those patients with risk factors or with macroscopic multifocal disease that may harbor additional sites of cancer in the residual thyroid tissue.

Adjuvant Therapy

Adjuvant therapy has the objective of destroying possible but unproven residual or metastatic disease with the ultimate goal of decreasing the risk of disease recurrence. These patients have at least an intermediate risk for disease recurrence (microscopic

---

Box 1
ATA's risk stratification for disease recurrence

Low Risk

  All of the following

    No local or distant metastases

    All microscopic tumor resected

    No invasion of locoregional tissue or structures

    No aggressive histology (eg, insular, columnar, tall cell variants) or vascular invasion

    No uptake outside the thyroid bed on the posttreatment scan if 131-I treatment is given

Intermediate Risk

  Any of the following

    Microscopic invasion of the perithyroidal tissues

    Cervical lymph node metastases or 131-I uptake outside the thyroid bed on the posttreatment scan

    Aggressive histology or vascular invasion

High Risk

  Any of the following

    Macroscopic tumor invasion

    Incomplete tumor resection

    Distant metastases

    Thyroglobulin levels out of proportion to what is seen on the posttreatment scan

Table 1
ATA's guidelines for the treatment of patients with thyroid cancer

Type of 131-I Treatment	Purpose	Effect	Typical Dose		Postoperative Scan	Empiric vs Dosimetry
Ablation	Destroy normal tissue	Better Tg accuracy to detect recurrent disease	30–50 mCi	(1.11–1.85 GBq)	No	E
		Better scan accuracy to detect recurrent disease				
		Minimize risk of new cancers in at-risk patients				
Adjuvant	Destroy possible residual/metastatic disease	Decrease risk of recurrence	50–100 mCi (1.85–3.7 GBq)		Yes	E
Known disease	Treat residual/metastatic disease	Decrease risk of recurrence	150 mCi (5.55 GBq) and greater		Yes	E if 150–200 mCi (5.55–7.4 GBq) D if ≥200 mCi (>7.4 GBq)

Abbreviations: D, dosimetry; E, empiric; Tg, thyroglobulin.

invasion of perithyroidal tissues, cervical lymph node metastases N1, vascular invasion, or tumors with aggressive histologies).

Therapy for Known Residual or Metastatic Disease

Therapy for known residual or metastatic disease has the objective of decreasing the
risk of disease recurrence and of disease-specific mortality. This therapy would be
used in patients with known macroscopic tumor invasion, incomplete tumor resection,
thyroid metastases, and thyroglobulin levels out of proportion to what is seen on postoperative pretreatment imaging.[10]

Although the lower levels of 131-I activity needed to achieve remnant ablation are
associated with only a small probability of experiencing side effects, the larger
amounts of 131-I needed for adjuvant therapy or to treat known residual disease
have a greater probability of developing side effects. For every patient being considered for radioactive iodine treatment, and particularly when using larger amount of
131-I, it is very important to conduct a careful assessment of the (1) individual
cancer-related risk, (2) factors that may affect the delivery of the intended dose,
and (3) probability of delivering excess radiation to normal tissues with resulting
side effects. Radioactive iodine should only be used for those patients that are
more likely to benefit from treatment, and the administered activity should be tailored
according to the individual cancer-related risk while minimizing side effects. Particularly when higher 131-I activities are being contemplated, a more complex approach
to calculate the radiation dose delivered to the more radiosensitive normal tissues
should be considered so that the therapeutic yield is maximized while side effects
are minimized. Please see the later discussion on empiric versus dosimetric approach
to the radioactive iodine treatment of thyroid cancer. The next section presents an
overview of the current classifications and implications for 131-I treatment of well-
differentiated thyroid cancer.

RISK ASSESSMENT OF WELL-DIFFERENTIATED THYROID CANCER: INITIAL STAGING AND IMPLICATIONS FOR RADIOIODINE TREATMENT

Clinical and pathologic disease staging together with other factors, such as most
importantly age at diagnosis, are at the basis of the initial prognostic stratification of patients with well-differentiated thyroid cancer and of an individualized, risk adapted use
of radioactive iodine as an adjunct to surgery for the management of the disease.
Several retrospective studies have suggested that treatment with radioactive iodine
decreases the 10-year risk of tumor recurrence and mortality,[4,11] and this has been
confirmed by a meta-analysis of several retrospective studies.[12–14] Further analyses
suggest, however, that the benefit in mortality is seen only for patients with larger tumor
(at least 1.0–1.5 cm in size), for cases with cervical lymph node metastases, or with perithyroidal tissue invasion.[4] Several systematic reviews have also pointed out that low-
risk patients as defined by the ATA may not benefit in terms of disease recurrence
and disease-specific mortality from radioiodine treatment.[15,16] More robust data
from the prospective collection of patient data under the National Thyroid Cancer Treatment Cooperative Study Group (NTCTCSG[17]) showed a mortality benefit from the use
of radioactive iodine treatment in the higher-risk patients (stage III and IV according to
the group criteria) but not for patients at low risk. Patients with stage II cancer treated
with radioactive iodine had a better overall survival, although no difference in disease-
specific survival or disease-free survival. No benefits from radioactive iodine were
observed for patients with stage I cancer. More recently, the results of a retrospective
analysis from the Memorial Sloan-Kettering Cancer Center have showed that low-risk

patients according to the ATA's classification had low rates of recurrence and high rates of survival when managed without radioactive iodine treatment.[18] Several staging systems are in use for thyroid cancer. The TNM is the most commonly used system,[19] and the American Joint Commission on Cancer (AJCC) has adopted the TNM system together with age for the initial staging of thyroid cancer. Higher disease stage and increasing age are associated with worse disease-specific mortality. Other staging systems include the MACIS system (metastasis, age, completeness of resection, invasion, size) developed for papillary[20] and follicular cancers[21] and the NTCTCSG system.[22] Several other variables affect the probability of patients having recurrence of thyroid cancer. More aggressive histologic subtypes (eg, tall cell, insular, columnar cell carcinoma), the presence of vascular invasion, tumor multifocality, as well as the initial TNM stage and the outcome of initial surgery (incomplete tumor resection) all play a role in the probability of developing tumor recurrence and/or of dying of thyroid cancer. As a whole, up to 30% of the patients with well-differentiated thyroid cancer may develop recurrence over several decades from diagnosis according Mazzaferri and Jhiang,[4] who found that more than 66% of the recurrences occur within the first decade from diagnosis and more frequently in cervical lymph nodes (74%), in thyroid remnants (20%), and in distant metastases (21% of the recurrences, mostly in the lungs). Neck recurrence is usually not fatal for thyroid cancer but, nevertheless, must be considered as a sign of a potentially fatal outcome.[23,24] In the aforementioned study by Mazzaferri and Jhiang,[4] 50% of the patients with distant metastases died of thyroid cancer. Systems that combine the estimation of risk for disease-specific mortality with that for disease recurrence are, therefore, preferred. The ATA's guidelines[6] have divided patients into low-, intermediate-, and high-risk categories for risk of disease recurrence and cancer-related mortality based on a system that combines the AJCC-approved TNM staging with other factors, such as documented surgical resection of all macroscopic tumor, aggressive histologic variants (eg, insular, columnar cell, tall cell, Hurtle cell, follicular carcinomas), vascular invasion, and 131-I uptake outside the thyroid bed on the posttreatment scan.

The Use of Radioiodine Scans for Initial Staging

Whole-body planar or tomographic (single-photon emission computed tomography [SPECT]) postoperative studies can be performed before treatment with radioactive iodine to verify the presence of uptake in the thyroid bed and to quantify the amount of uptake as a measure of the amount of postoperative residual functioning thyroid tissue. In addition, radioiodine scans are used to look for the presence of local cervical lymph node or distant functioning metastases. Diagnostic scans are typically performed using low doses of either 131-I or 123-I (typically between 2 and 5 mCi [0.074 and 0.185 GBq]). The use of higher activities can increase scan sensitivities but could induce stunning of the functioning thyroid tissue, which is then less able to accumulate the treatment dose. The presence of stunning is, however, controversial in the literature, is probably negligible when the low diagnostic doses of radioiodine mentioned earlier are used, and is probably less frequent with the use of 123-I.[25,26] Scanning with 123-I is probably superior to 131-I for diagnostic purposes.[27] At the author's institution, they use 2 mCi (0.074 GBq) of 123-I for the initial diagnostic scan performed before ablation. As the cost of 123-I has decreased significantly in the last few years, the author's institution now prefers to use 123-I also for the follow-up scans because this provides better image quality and less radiation exposure with no need to follow radiation safety guidelines.

There are discordant opinions in the literature as to whether a diagnostic scan is needed before radioiodine treatment. Some omit the pretreatment diagnostic scan and administer empiric therapeutic doses of 131-I followed by a posttreatment scan.[28] Although no approach has been demonstrated to be superior, omitting the pretreatment diagnostic scan may potentially have the disadvantage of undertreating patients with metastases recognizable only with the diagnostic scan. In addition, sometimes surgeons are able to remove all thyroid tissue with no residual uptake identified on the diagnostic scan; these patients can be safely spared a 131-I treatment dose. Van Nostrand and colleagues[29] found that 53% of 355 patients had findings on the pretreatment scan that might have altered management. In patients with very low risk for metastatic disease whereby remnant ablation is the goal of 131-I treatment, it might be reasonable to omit the pretreatment scan. The ATA's guidelines recommend diagnostic scanning if the results of the scan would change the decision to treat with radioiodine or the administered activity. More recently, several studies have found that the adoption of new SPECT/CT technology has advantages over planar wholebody scans.[30] Avram and colleagues[31] found that diagnostic SPECT/CT scans performed in 320 patients detected regional metastases in 35% of patients and distant metastases in 8% of patients. Information acquired with the SPECT/CT scans changed staging in 4% of younger and 25% of older patients. The researchers concluded that preablation scans with SPECT/CT contribute to staging of thyroid cancer. Identification of regional and distant metastases before radioiodine therapy has significant potential to alter patient management.

FACTORS AFFECTING DELIVERY OF RADIOACTIVE IODINE
Patient Preparation

Adequate stimulation of the uptake of radioiodine by thyroid tissue and welldifferentiated thyroid cancer cells can be achieved by one of 2 methods for increasing TSH levels: thyroid hormone withdrawal or administration of recombinant human TSH (rhTSH).

Thyroid hormone withdrawal remains the standard approach for patients with known local residual tumor or metastatic disease. After thyroidectomy, withdrawal from thyroid hormones increases the production of TSH, which stimulates functioning thyroid tissue and well-differentiated cancer cells. An adequate stimulation is thought to occur when the serum TSH levels reach a minimum of 25 to 30 mU/L.[32]

rTSH-rhTSH

This approach is typically used for remnant ablation and follow-up imaging. In the absence of long-term data on disease recurrence and disease-specific survival from randomized trials, many centers consider rhTSH ablation for low-risk patients only, whereas hormone withdrawal is used for patients at higher risk of recurrence or death from disease (adjuvant treatment and treatment of known residual disease). Many institutions, however, also offer the rhTSH approach for intermediate-risk patients (adjuvant treatment). A randomized prospective study found that there was no difference in the ablation effectiveness between the rhTSH approach and hormone withdrawal[33] at an ablation dose of 100 mCi (3.7 GBq), and a more recent study found similar results for 50-mCi (1.85 GBq) ablation doses.[34] Another prospective study found that there was no difference in successful ablation between the 2 approaches, but rhTSH stimulation showed a favorable 33% lower whole-body radiation dose.[35] A meta-analysis of these studies confirmed the equivalence of the 2 approaches for low ablation doses.[36] For those patients that have contraindications to induced hypothyroidism (eg, the elderly, depression, congestive heart failure), rTSH may be administered. The ATA's guidelines recommend remnant ablation with the doses of 30 to 100 mCi

(1.11 to 3.7 GBq) with hormone withdrawal or rhTSH. Of note, another multicenter trial including 438 patients with low-risk differentiated thyroid cancer (TNM stage T1 to T3) but also with possible lymph node involvement (N0, NX, N1) but no distant metastases (M0) and no microscopic residual disease showed similar successful ablation rates whether patients were assigned to low- or high-dose radioiodine (30 vs 100 mCi [1.1 vs 3.7 GBq]), each combined with rhTSH or thyroid hormone withdrawal. Successful ablation was obtained in 87.2% and 86.8% for those who received rhTSH versus thyroid hormone withdrawal.[37] A similar study in a larger cohort of 684 patients also found that there was no difference in successful ablation rates between thyroid tissue stimulation with rhTSH versus hormone withdrawal or between doses of 1.1 GBq versus 3.7 GBq of 131-I.[38]

Long-term outcome data obtained in 2 studies, one including low-risk patients followed for 10 years[39] and the second[40] also including intermediate- and high-risk patients, showed similar effectiveness of withdrawal and rhTSH methods. The rhTSH approach has also been successful in patients with microscopic cervical lymph node or pulmonary metastases,[13,14] and one study also including macroscopic lung metastases[41] suggests that the rhTSH approach is also affective for metastatic disease.

Low-Iodine Diet

Most centers agree that patients should follow a low-iodine diet for 1 to 2 weeks before and for at least 1 day after 131-I is administered, as also recommended by the ATA's guidelines.

MINIMIZATION OF SIDE EFFECTS

The use of radioactive iodine for treatment purposes has been associated with several short-term and long-term side effects that are related to radiation-induced damage of the structures that normally accumulate or excrete 131-I.[42] The most common short-term side effects are typically caused by radiation-induced sialoadenitis, thyroiditis of the residual tissue, and nausea caused by inflammation of the gastric mucosa. Several measures can reduce the likelihood of developing side effects. Hydration with large volumes of fluids facilitates the rapid renal excretion of the radioactive iodine; antiemetics are recommended before treatment administration. Several patients experience sialoadenitis, xerostomia related to decreased production of saliva, and transient change in taste. The use of sialagogues, such as lemon juice or lemon candies, is controversial because some studies have found it to be beneficial, other studies have found it to be useful only with specific timing of administration,[43–46] whereas others have found it to be harmful[45] for the salivary glands during administration of radioactive iodine. The radioprotectant amifostine administered before 131-I administration seems to decrease symptoms and can be useful particularly for repeated treatments.[47] Temporary oligospermia has been found after the administration of higher activities of 131-I but there is no evidence of effects on fertility or on offspring.[48] A minority of women treated with radioactive iodine experience brief amenorrhea with no long-term effects, however, on fertility or on outcomes of pregnancy.[49,50] Hydration with large amount of fluids and frequent voiding of the bladder is helpful to minimize radiation dose to the gonads.

Several studies have reported an excess risk of secondary malignancies in patients treated with radioactive iodine. A large epidemiologic study conducted in the United States by the National Cancer Institute[51] reported an excess of 6.39 cases every 10,000 person-years in the absolute risk for secondary malignancies among more than 30,000 patients treated with radioactive iodine and followed for up to 30 years. A second large epidemiologic study conducted in Europe[52] found a greater relative risk for developing secondary malignancies of the soft tissues, bones, female genital organs, leukemia, and central nervous system among 6840 patients treated for thyroid cancer with a mean cumulative administered activity of 162 mCi (6 GBq). A meta-analysis of these 2 large studies confirmed a 1.19 excess risk of secondary malignancies in patients treated with radioactive iodine.[53] In the subset of the patients of the National Cancer Institute's study with low-risk disease, the excess risk for secondary malignancies was lower than for the entire group (4.6 cases per 10,000 person-years) but still significant. Although statistically significant in these epidemiologic studies, it must be pointed out that the increase in risk for secondary malignancies remains relatively small. Those clinicians involved in the therapeutic administration of radioactive iodine need to be conscious that there is a dose-related incidence of side effects; therefore, for each individual patient, a careful assessment of the benefits versus risks of radioactive iodine treatment must be conducted. This point is particularly important for low-risk patients and when considering repeated treatments in patients with residual or recurrent disease. Measures that promote rapid washout of radioactive iodine from the normal tissues help minimize exposure to radiation and side effects, but even more important is a careful analysis of the patients' cancer-specific risk and of other biologic factors to select the lowest possible dose that achieves the desired therapeutic effect while minimizing short- and long-term side effects. The ATA's 6 guidelines recommend that "the minimum activity necessary to achieve successful remnant ablation should be chosen, particularly for low risk patients." However, the ATA's 6 guidelines also recommend that "if residual microscopic disease is suspected or documented or if there is a more aggressive tumor histology, then higher activities may be given," as is usually the case for patients with intermediate or high risk.

USE OF EMPIRIC OR DOSIMETRIC METHODS

Selection of the appropriate amount of radioactive iodine usually follows one of 2 methods: empiric or dosimetric. The empiric approach is probably the most used method[54–56] and uses a fixed dosage of radioiodine that is modified according to several factors and most importantly disease stage and intent of treatment, remnant ablation versus treatment of suspected or proven residual disease. Other factors that may affect the administered activity are the amount of residual thyroid tissue, the number of cervical lymph nodes involved, the number and location of distant metastases, and the type and extent of lung involvement when present. The empiric method has several advantages: (1) simple, easier, and less expensive process for the health care provider and for the patients (2) extensive scientific evidence from prior studies with fairly established frequency and severity of complications. Because the amount of 131-I is essentially fixed within a specific disease stage, some think that the pretreatment scans are unnecessary, although this remains controversial (see the ATA's and the European guidelines).[57–59] The major limitations of the empiric approach is that it does not estimate the amount of the radiation dose delivered to the normal tissues and to the cancer and it does not assess whether the given dose maximizes the therapeutic yield while remaining less than the tolerable radiation dose to critical organs, such as the lungs or bone marrow. The whole-body dosimetry was initially described by Benua and colleagues[60] and focuses on the maximum tolerable 131-I activity that can be administered without exceeding the maximum tolerable radiation dose to the bone marrow or lungs. The dosimetric approach typically uses more than one whole-body radioiodine scan to study the individual patient kinetics of radioiodine and to calculate the maximum radioiodine activity, also known as maximum tolerable activity (MTA), that can be administered without exceeding a toxic dose to the lungs and bone marrow, the maximum tolerable dose (MTD). The MTD is typically 200 rad (cGy) to the blood, which is used as a surrogate for the bone marrow dose. By maximizing the amount of 131-I that can be administered, the dosimetric approach should minimize the need for repeated treatments. A potential advantage of the dosimetric approach is that when a given empiric dose is not effective and more doses are needed, the fractionation of doses over time may not be as effective as a single dosimetrically determined radioiodine administration. Lesional dosimetry[61,62] determines the amount of radioiodine needed to deliver a sufficient radiation dose to destroy a metastatic lesion. The advantages of dosimetry are (1) the possibility of improving outcomes by selecting and administering higher radioiodine dosages with a greater chance of having a tumoricidal effect and (2) potentially administering lower and safer radioiodine dosages that will still have a tumoricidal effect while minimizing adverse effects. It is important to note that with whole-body dosimetry it is possible to identify up to 20% of patients in which an empiric fixed dosage may exceed the MTA.[63,64] The disadvantages of the dosimetric approach include higher cost and greater patient inconvenience during the lengthier dosimetry procedures. In addition, methodological and technical limitations still create uncertainties in the possibility of performing accurate lesional dosimetry for locoregional and distant metastases. It must be pointed out that there is no consistent evidence in the literature to demonstrate better outcomes with the use of dosimetrically determined dosages of radioiodine relative to empiric dosages. One recent study by Klubo-Gwiezdzinska and colleagues[65] showed that dosimetric therapy in high-risk patients provides much improved outcomes for those with locoregional spread of disease with a similar safety profile to that seen with empiric dosage. The researchers suggested that dosimetric dosages should be used. There are, however, no definitive studies evaluating outcomes of empiric versus dosimetric dosages for the treatment of distant metastases.

SUMMARY AND SELECTION OF 131-I ACTIVITY

All published guidelines on the use of radioactive iodine for the treatment of well-differentiated thyroid cancer agree that an individualized assessment of the risk of cancer-related mortality and of disease recurrence should direct the decision of whether radioiodine treatment is needed and how much to administer. At the authors' institution, they mostly follow the ATA's risk stratification system (see **Box 1**), with the addition of a category of very-low-risk patients that do not receive radioactive iodine. The author's algorithm is explained later and is illustrated in **Fig. 2**.

Very-Low-Risk Patients

There is no need for radioiodine ablation. These patients have cancer that is less than 1 cm with no capsular or vascular invasion, no aggressive histology, and no lymph node or distant metastases. The ATA's and the European guidelines agree that this group does not need radioactive iodine treatment.

Low-Risk Patients

Remnant ablation. rhTSH-stimulated diagnostic scan is typically used, followed by administration of 131-I treatment using a fixed empiric activity, typically between 30 and 50 mCi (1.1 and 1.8 GBq). The ATA's updated guidelines recommend using

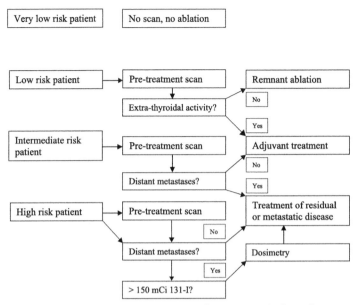

Fig. 2. The author's algorithm for the treatment of patients with thyroid cancer.

the minimal activity (30–100 mCi [1.1–3.7 GBq]) necessary to achieve successful abla-tion. After 2 recent prospective studies have demonstrated the equivalence in suc-cessfully ablating thyroid tissue of 30 and 100 mCi doses (1.1 and 3.7 GBq, respectively),[37,38] at the author's institution they have decided to use 30 to 50 mCi (1.1–1.8 GBq) of 131-I for lower-risk patients (patients younger than 45 years with tu-mors between 1 and 2 cm confined to the thyroid gland).

Intermediate-Risk Patients: Adjuvant Treatment

The author uses higher activities of 75 to 100 mCi (2.8–3.7 GBq) 131-I for patients at an intermediate risk (microscopic capsular invasion, aggressive histology, T >2 cm with no capsular invasion). Dosimetry studies are typically not needed for these low-risk patients for whom doses that are most likely well less than the expected maximal toler-able dose are administered.

High-Risk Patients: Treatment of Residual or Metastatic Disease

Patients at higher risk for local disease recurrence or death that have macroscopic re-sidual disease or distant metastases typically receive doses between 150 and 200 mCi (5.6–7.4 GBq). These patients will receive a pretreatment scan, typically with rhTSH or hormone withdrawal. For those patients with scan evidence of residual postoperative disease in the thyroid bed or in cervical lymph nodes, the author treats with approxi-mately 150 mCi 131-I (5.550 GBq), usually as a result of an empiric approach. Patients that demonstrate a large amount of lymph node disease should be referred back to the surgeon for possible completion of neck dissection. Radioiodine treatment would then follow 6 to 8 weeks after surgery. These patients typically do not need dosimetry because activities of approximately 150 mCi (5.5 GBq) rarely exceed the maximum tolerable dose to the bone marrow of 200 rad. For patients with pulmonary metastases and/or skeletal metastases the administration of activities of 200 mCi (7.4 GBq) using the empiric approach may exceed the maximum tolerable doses as predicted by dosimetry especially in the elderly.[63,64] Therefore, for the treatment of residual or metastatic disease, the author does not exceed 150 mCi (5.5 GBq) unless specifically guided by dosimetry and particularly for elderly patients. A special case is illustrated by patients with diffuse lung metastases whereby pulmonary fibrosis could complicate treatment with radioactive iodine. In these patients also, activities less than 200 mCi (7.4 GBq) could exceed the maximum tolerable lung activity of 80 mCi (2.96 GBq) at 48 hours. A dosimetry-directed activity that does not exceed this threshold greatly minimizes pulmonary injury as demonstrated by Benua and colleagues[60] in their early work.

REFERENCES

1. Hamilton JG, Soley M, Eichorn K. Deposition of radioactive iodine in human thyroid tissue. Los Angeles (CA): Univ Calif Publ Pharmacol; 1940. p. 339–68.
2. Keston AS, Ball RP, Frantz VK. Storage of radioactive iodine in a metastasis from thyroid carcinoma. Science 1942;95(2466):362–3.
3. Seidlin SM, Marinelli LD, Oshry E. Radioactive iodine therapy; effect on functioning metastases of adenocarcinoma of the thyroid. J Am Med Assoc 1946; 132:838–47.
4. Mazzaferri EL, Jhiang SM. Long-term impact of initial surgical and medical therapy on papillary and follicular thyroid cancer. Am J Med 1994;97:418–28.
5. Samaan NA, Schultz PN, Hickey RC, et al. The results of various modalities of treatment of well differentiated thyroid carcinomas: a retrospective review of 1599 patients. J Clin Endocrinol Metab 1992;75:714–20.
6. American Thyroid Association (ATA) Guidelines Taskforce on Thyroid Nodules and Differentiated Thyroid Cancer, Cooper DS, Doherty GM, et al. Revised American Thyroid Association management guidelines for patients with thyroid nodules and differentiated thyroid cancer. Thyroid 2009;19:1167–214.
7. Thyroid carcinoma. National Comprehensive Cancer Center Network (NCCN) clinical practice guidelines in oncology. 2013.
8. Pacini F, Schlumberger M, Dralle H, et al, European Thyroid Cancer Taskforce. European consensus for the management of patients with differentiated thyroid carcinoma of the follicular epithelium. Eur J Endocrinol 2006;154:787–803.
9. Eckerman K, Endo A. MIRD: radionuclide data and decay schemes. Reston (VA): Society of Nuclear Medicine; 2008.
10. Kim TY, Kim WB, Kim ES, et al. Serum thyroglobulin levels at the time of 131I remnant ablation just after thyroidectomy are useful for early prediction of clinical recurrence in low-risk patients with differentiated thyroid carcinoma. J Clin Endocrinol Metab 2005;90:1440–5.
11. DeGroot LJ, Kaplan EL, McCormick M, et al. Natural history, treatment, and course of papillary thyroid carcinoma. J Clin Endocrinol Metab 1990;71:414–24.
12. Sawka AM, Thephamongkhol K, Brouwers M, et al. Clinical review 170: a systematic review and metaanalysis of the effectiveness of radioactive iodine remnant ablation for well-differentiated thyroid cancer. J Clin Endocrinol Metab 2004;89:3668–76.
13. Tuttle RM, Lopez N, Leboeuf R, et al. Radioactive iodine administered for thyroid remnant ablation following recombinant human thyroid stimulating hormone preparation also has an important adjuvant therapy function. Thyroid 2010;20: 257–63.
14. Tuttle RM, Tala H, Shah J, et al. Estimating risk of recurrence in differentiated thyroid cancer after total thyroidectomy and radioactive iodine remnant

ablation: using response to therapy variables to modify the initial risk estimates predicted by the new American Thyroid Association staging system. Thyroid 2010;20:1341–9.

15. Sacks W, Fung CH, Chang JT, et al. The effectiveness of radioactive iodine for treatment of low-risk thyroid cancer: a systematic analysis of the peer-reviewed literature from 1966 to April 2008. Thyroid 2010;20:1235–45.

16. Sawka AM, Brierley JD, Tsang RW, et al. An updated systematic review and commentary examining the effectiveness of radioactive iodine remnant ablation in well-differentiated thyroid cancer. Endocrinol Metab Clin North Am 2008;37: 457–80, x.

17. Jonklaas J, Sarlis NJ, Litofsky D, et al. Outcomes of patients with differentiated thyroid carcinoma following initial therapy. Thyroid 2006;16:1229–42.

18. Vaisman F, Shaha A, Fish S, et al. Initial therapy with either thyroid lobectomy or total thyroidectomy without radioactive iodine remnant ablation is associated with very low rates of structural disease recurrence in properly selected patients with differentiated thyroid cancer. Clin Endocrinol (Oxf) 2011;75(1):112–9.

19. Edge SB, Byrd DR, Compton CC, et al. AJCC cancer staging manual. 7th edition. New York: Springer; 2010.

20. Hay ID, Bergstralh EJ, Goellner JR, et al. Predicting outcome in papillary thyroid carcinoma: development of a reliable prognostic scoring system in a cohort of 1779 patients surgically treated at one institution during 1940 through 1989. Surgery 1993;114:1050–7 [discussion: 1057–8].

21. D'Avanzo A, Ituarte P, Treseler P, et al. Prognostic scoring systems in patients with follicular thyroid cancer: a comparison of different staging systems in predicting the patient outcome. Thyroid 2004;14:453–8.

22. Sherman SI, Brierley JD, Sperling M, et al. Prospective multicenter study of thyroiscarcinoma treatment: initial analysis of staging and outcome. National Thyroid Cancer Treatment Cooperative Study Registry Group. Cancer 1998;83:1012–21.

23. Newman KD, Black T, Heller G, et al. Differentiated thyroid cancer: determinants of disease progression in patients <21 years of age at diagnosis: a report from the Surgical Discipline Committee of the Children's Cancer Group. Ann Surg 1998;227:533–41.

24. Robie DK, Dinauer CW, Tuttle RM, et al. The impact of initial surgical management on outcome in young patients with differentiated thyroid cancer. J Pediatr Surg 1998;33:1134–8 [discussion: 1139–40].

25. Hilditch TE, Dempsey MF, Bolster AA, et al. Self-stunning in thyroid ablation: evidence from comparative studies of diagnostic 131I and 123I. Eur J Nucl Med Mol Imaging 2002;29:783–8.

26. Silberstein EB. Comparison of outcomes after (123)I versus (131)I pre-ablation imaging before radioiodine ablation in differentiated thyroid carcinoma. J Nucl Med 2007;48:1043–6.

27. Mandel SJ, Shankar LK, Benard F, et al. Superiority of iodine-123 compared with iodine-131 scanning for thyroid remnants in patients with differentiated thyroid cancer. Clin Nucl Med 2001;26:6–9.

28. Salvatori M, Perotti G, Rufini V, et al. Are there disadvantages in administering 131I ablation therapy in patients with differentiated thyroid carcinoma without a preablative diagnostic 131I whole-body scan? Clin Endocrinol (Oxf) 2004; 61:704–10.

29. Van Nostrand D, Aiken M, Atkins F, et al. The utility of radioiodine scans prior to iodine 131 ablation in patients with well-differentiated thyroid cancer. Thyroid 2009;19:849–55.

30. Chen L, Luo Q, Shen Y, et al. Incremental value of 131I SPECT/CT in the management of patients with differentiated thyroid carcinoma. J Nucl Med 2008;49: 1952–7.

31. Avram AM, Fig LM, Frey KA, et al. Preablation 131-I scans with SPECT/CT in postoperative thyroid cancer patients: what is the impact on staging? J Clin Endocrinol Metab 2013;98:1163–71.

32. Edmonds CJ, Hayes S, Kermode JC, et al. Measurement of serum TSH and thyroid hormones in the management of treatment of thyroid carcinoma with radioiodine. Br J Radiol 1977;50:799–807.

33. Pacini F, Ladenson PW, Schlumberger M, et al. Radioiodine ablation of thyroid remnants after preparation with recombinant human thyrotropin in differentiated thyroid carcinoma: results of an international, randomized, controlled study. J Clin Endocrinol Metab 2006;91:926–32.

34. Chianelli M, Todino V, Graziano FM, et al. Low-activity (2.0 GBq; 54 mCi) radioiodine post-surgical remnant ablation in thyroid cancer: comparison between hormone withdrawal and use of rhTSH in low-risk patients. Eur J Endocrinol 2009;160:431–6.

35. Pilli T, Brianzoni E, Capoccetti F, et al. A comparison of 1850 (50 mCi) and 3700 MBq (100 mCi) 131-iodine administered doses for recombinant thyrotropin-stimulated postoperative thyroid remnant ablation in differentiated thyroid cancer. J Clin Endocrinol Metab 2007;92:3542–6.

36. Ma C, Xie J, Liu W, et al. Recombinant human thyrotropin (rhTSH) aided radioiodine treatment for residual or metastatic differentiated thyroid cancer. Cochrane Database Syst Rev 2010;(11):CD008302.

37. Mallick U, Harmer C, Yap B, et al. Ablation with low-dose radioiodine and thyrotropin alfa in thyroid cancer. N Engl J Med 2012;366:1674–85.

38. Schlumberger M, Catargi B, Borget I, et al, Tumeurs de la Thyroïde Refractaires Network for the Essai Stimulation Ablation Equivalence Trial. Strategies of radioiodine ablation in patients with low-risk thyroid cancer. N Engl J Med 2012;366: 1663–73.

39. Molinaro E, Giani C, Agate L, et al. Patients with differentiated thyroid cancer who underwent radioiodine thyroid remnant ablation with low-activity ^{131}I after either recombinant human TSH or thyroid hormone therapy withdrawal showed the same outcome after a 10-year follow-up. J Clin Endocrinol Metab 2013;98: 2693–700.

40. Hugo J, Robenshtok E, Grewal R, et al. Recombinant human thyroid stimulating hormone-assisted radioactive iodine remnant ablation in thyroid cancer patients at intermediate to high risk of recurrence. Thyroid 2012;22:1007–15.

41. Tala H, Robbins R, Fagin JA, et al. Five-year survival is similar in thyroid cancer patients with distant metastases prepared for radioactive iodine therapy with either thyroid hormone withdrawal or recombinant human TSH. J Clin Endocrinol Metab 2011;96:2105–11.

42. Van Nostrand D, Freitas J. Side effects of 131-I ablation and treatment of well differentiated thyroid carcinoma, in: Thyroid cancer: a comprehensive guide to clinical management. Totowa (NJ): Humana Press Inc; 2006.

43. Kulkarni K, Van Nostrand D, Atkins F, et al. Does lemon juice increase radioiodine reaccumulation within the parotid glands more than if lemon juice is not administered? Nucl Med Commun 2014;35(2):210–6.

44. Malpani BL, Samuel AM, Ray S. Quantification of salivary gland function in thyroid cancer patients treated with radioiodine. Int J Radiat Oncol Biol Phys 1996; 35:535–40.

45. Nakada K, Ishibashi T, Takei T, et al. Does lemon candy decrease salivary gland damage after radioiodine therapy for thyroid cancer? J Nucl Med 2005;46: 261–6.
46. Van Nostrand D, Bandaru V, Chennupati S, et al. Radiopharmacokinetics of radioiodine in the parotid glands after the administration of lemon juice. Thyroid 2010;20:1113–9.
47. Mendoza A, Shaffer B, Karakla D, et al. Quality of life with well-differentiated thyroid cancer: treatment toxicities and their reduction. Thyroid 2004;14: 133–40.
48. Rosário PWS, Barroso AL, Rezende LL, et al. Testicular function after radioiodine therapy in patients with thyroid cancer. Thyroid 2006;16:667–70.
49. Bal C, Kumar A, Tripathi M, et al. High-dose radioiodine treatment for differentiated thyroid carcinoma is not associated with change in female fertility or any genetic risk to the offspring. Int J Radiat Oncol Biol Phys 2005;63: 449–55.
50. Sawka AM, Lakra DC, Lea J, et al. A systematic review examining the effects of therapeutic radioactive iodine on ovarian function and future pregnancy in female thyroid cancer survivors. Clin Endocrinol (Oxf) 2008;69: 479–90.
51. Brown AP, Chen J, Hitchcock YJ, et al. The risk of second primary malignancies up to three decades after the treatment of differentiated thyroid cancer. J Clin Endocrinol Metab 2008;93:504–15.
52. Rubino C, de Vathaire F, Dottorini ME, et al. Second primary malignancies in thyroid cancer patients. Br J Cancer 2003;89:1638–44.
53. Sawka AM, Thabane L, Parlea L, et al. Second primary malignancy risk after radioactive iodine treatment for thyroid cancer: a systematic review and meta-analysis. Thyroid 2009;19:451–7.
54. Brown AP, Greening WP, McCready VR, et al. Radioiodine treatment of metastatic thyroid carcinoma: the Royal Marsden Hospital experience. Br J Radiol 1984; 57:323–7.
55. Menzel C, Grünwald F, Schomburg A, et al. "High-dose" radioiodine therapy in advanced differentiated thyroid carcinoma. J Nucl Med 1996;37: 1496–503.
56. Schlumberger M, Challeton C, De Vathaire F, et al. Radioactive iodine treatment and external radiotherapy for lung and bone metastases from thyroid carcinoma. J Nucl Med 1996;37:598–605.
57. Chen MK, Yasrebi M, Samii J, et al. The utility of I-123 pretherapy scan in I-131 radioiodine therapy for thyroid cancer. Thyroid 2012;22:304–9.
58. Schlumberger MJ, Pacini F. The low utility of pretherapy scans in thyroid cancer patients. Thyroid 2009;19:815–6.
59. Van Nostrand D, Atkins F, Moreau S, et al. Utility of the radioiodine whole-body retention at 48 hours for modifying empiric activity of 131-iodine for the treatment of metastatic well-differentiated thyroid carcinoma. Thyroid 2009;19:1093–8.
60. Benua RS, Cicale NR, Sonenberg M, et al. The relation of radioiodine dosimetry to results and complications in the treatment of metastatic thyroid cancer. Am J Roentgenol Radium Ther Nucl Med 1962;87:171–82.
61. Maxon HR, Thomas SR, Hertzberg VS, et al. Relation between effective radiation dose and outcome of radioiodine therapy for thyroid cancer. N Engl J Med 1983; 309:937–41.
62. Thomas SR, Maxon HR, Kereiakes JG. In vivo quantitation of lesion radioactivity using external counting methods. Med Phys 1976;03:253–5.

63. Kulkarni K, Van Nostrand D, Atkins F, et al. The relative frequency in which empiric dosages of radioiodine would potentially overtreat or undertreat patients who have metastatic well-differentiated thyroid cancer. Thyroid 2006;16: 1019–23.
64. Tuttle RM, Leboeuf R, Robbins RJ, et al. Empiric radioactive iodine dosing regimens frequently exceed maximum tolerated activity levels in elderly patients with thyroid cancer. J Nucl Med 2006;47:1587–91.
65. Klubo-Gwiezdzinska J, Van Nostrand D, Atkins F, et al. Efficacy of dosimetric versus empiric prescribed activity of 131I for therapy of differentiated thyroid cancer. J Clin Endocrinol Metab 2011;96:3217–25.

Update on Differentiated Thyroid Cancer Staging

Denise P. Momesso, MD[a], R. Michael Tuttle, MD[b],*

KEYWORDS

- Risk stratification • Differentiated thyroid cancer • Response to therapy

KEY POINTS

- An initial assessment of the risk of disease-specific mortality and the risk of persistent/recurrent disease is required to guide initial treatment and early follow-up and to set appropriate patient expectations with regard to likely outcomes after initial therapy.
- Although the American Joint Committee on Cancer/Union for International Cancer Control and MACIS (Metastases, Age, Completeness of Resection, Invasion, Size) staging systems provide valuable information regarding disease-specific survival, they do not adequately predict the risk of recurrent/persistent disease for individual patients; therefore, additional staging systems specifically developed to predict the risk of recurrent/persistent disease should be used to augment the information provided by staging systems designed to predict the risk of dying from thyroid cancer.
- Because all initial staging systems provide only a static initial risk assessment, ongoing management requires that these initial risk estimates continually be modified based on the biological behavior of the disease and the subsequent response to therapy.
- Although the dynamic risk assessment approach was originally proposed and validated in patients treated with total thyroidectomy and radioactive iodine (RAI) remnant ablation, by simply modifying the specific definitions of the response to therapy outcomes (excellent, indeterminate, and biochemically incomplete and structurally incomplete responses), we show how this same ongoing risk stratification approach can be applied to patients who have thyroid cancer treated with lobectomy or total thyroidectomy without RAI ablation.

INTRODUCTION

The last decade has seen a renewed interested in a risk-adapted approach to the management of differentiated thyroid cancer (DTC), in which specific treatment and follow-up recommendations are tailored to individualized estimates of risk.[1–4] This customized management ensures that intensive treatment and follow-up studies are

Disclosures: The authors have no relevant conflicts of interests to disclose.
[a] Endocrinology Service, Hospital Universitário Clementino Fraga Filho, Universidade Federal do Rio de Janeiro, Rua Eduardo Guinle, 20/904 Rio de Janeiro, RJ 22260-090, Brazil; [b] Endocrinology, Memorial Sloan Kettering Cancer Center, Zuckerman Building, Room 590, 1275 York Avenue, New York, NY 10065, USA
* Corresponding author.
E-mail address: tuttlem@mskcc.org

Endocrinol Metab Clin N Am 43 (2014) 401–421
http://dx.doi.org/10.1016/j.ecl.2014.02.010
0889-8529/14/$ – see front matter © 2014 Elsevier Inc. All rights reserved.

recommended for high-risk patients, who are most likely to benefit from an aggressive management approach, whereas low-risk patients are managed with a more conservative approach, designed to identify clinically important persistent/recurrent disease and to avoid exposure to the potential complications and side effects of excessive surgery, radioactive iodine (RAI) ablation, and subclinical hyperthyroidism. Therefore, the keystone for optimal management of DTC is accurate, real-time risk stratification.

From a practical clinical management standpoint, an initial assessment of the risk of dying from thyroid cancer and the risk of having persistent/recurrent disease is required to guide initial treatment, early follow-up and to set appropriate patient expectations with regard to likely outcomes after initial therapy.[1–4] Recent studies have emphasized the need for dynamic risk stratification during follow-up, in which the various clinical important risk estimates are modified over time as additional data are obtained during follow-up.[5–9] These modified risk estimates reflect both the underlying biology of the disease and the response to initial (and subsequent) treatments and provide real-time risk estimates during follow-up, which may differ substantially from the initial risk estimates based only on clinicopathologic features available at the time of diagnosis and initial therapy.

In this review, the critical clinicopathologic risk factors commonly used in our modern staging systems are reevaluated and we then demonstrate how they are used to predict the risk of disease-specific mortality and recurrence is discussed. The concept and practical implementation of dynamic risk assessment are reviewed to explain our approach to long-term management. In previous work, this response to therapy evaluation system has been applied exclusively to patients who had total thyroidectomy and RAI ablation. In this review, this concept is expanded to include patients who did not require RAI ablation and those who were treated with less than total thyroidectomy.

Initial Risk Stratification

Initial risk stratification requires a detailed histologic description of the primary tumor and metastatic foci removed at the time of initial surgery and also a thorough understanding of other important preoperative and intraoperative findings (**Table 1**).[10,11] These findings include preoperative evidence of gross extrathyroidal extension (hoarseness/stridor, fixation to surrounding structures), extensive locoregional metastases (clinical N1 disease), and distant metastases (symptomatic or incidentally found on preoperative imaging). Just as critical are the intraoperative findings of gross extrathyroidal extension (defined by involvement of the surrounding subcutaneous soft tissues, larynx, trachea, esophagus, or recurrent laryngeal nerve) and completeness of surgical resection, which can be major risk factors and are often not readily apparent in the written pathology report.[12–18]

Therefore, accurate initial risk stratification not only requires excellent, detailed histopathology reports but also relies on effective communication of critical findings among all members of the disease management team.[10]

Initial Estimates of Disease-Specific Mortality

A wide variety of staging systems have been used to predict the risk of death from DTC.[19–30] These staging systems take into account a relatively small set of clinicopathologic factors available at the time of initial therapy (**Table 2**). Nearly all of the staging systems use age at diagnosis, tumor size, the presence/absence of gross extrathyroidal extension and distant metastases as the primary variables. The extent of lymph node metastases is included in some of these systems and seems to convey an increased risk of mortality only in the setting of clinically significant metastatic lymphadenopathy (clinical N1 disease) in older patients.[16]

Table 1		
Major factors in initial risk stratification		
Preoperative	Physical examination	Clinical N1 disease
		Hoarseness/stridor
		Fixation to surrounding structures
	Historical features	Unexplained bone pain
		Suspicion of distant metastases
	Imaging findings	Ultrasonography
		Computed tomography
		Magnetic resonance imaging
		[^{18}F]Fluorodeoxyglucose positron emission tomography
Intraoperative	Clinical findings	Extent of thyroid surgery
		Description of gross extrathyroidal extension
		Completeness of resection
		Extent of lymph node dissection
		Resection of major structures
		Surgical complications
Postoperative	Histology/molecular	Pathology report
	Clinical findings	Molecular profile
		Serum thyroglobulin
		Serum antithyroglobulin antibodies
		Serum TSH
		Postoperative ultrasonography

Adapted from Carty SE, Doherty GM, Inabnet WB, et al, for the Surgical Affairs Committee of the American Thyroid Association. American Thyroid Association Statement on the essential elements of interdisciplinary communication of perioperative information for patients undergoing thyroid cancer surgery. Thyroid 2012;4:395–9; with permission.

Although no staging system has been shown to be clearly superior to the others, the most commonly used are the American Joint Committee on Cancer (AJCC)/Union for International Cancer Control (UICC) TNM and the MACIS (Metastases, Age, Completeness of Resection, Invasion, Size) systems. These systems consistently provide the highest proportion of variance explained (PVE, a statistical measure of how well a staging system can predict the outcome of interest[31]) when applied to many patients in different series (**Fig. 1**).[30,32–39]

However, the inability of the current staging systems to account for no more than 30% of the observed variance in disease-specific mortality means that these initial risk stratification systems suboptimally classify individual patients over time with regard to their individual risk of dying from thyroid cancer.

Furthermore, none of the commonly used initial staging systems incorporates specific genetic abnormalities. Identification of the BRAF V600E mutation in DTC is significantly associated with tumor aggressiveness and with increased cancer-related recurrence and mortality.[40–42] In clinical practice, it often seems that the BRAF tumors that are the most aggressive and the most likely to cause disease-specific mortality usually have other clinical features (gross extrathyroidal extension, high-grade tumor histology, extensive lymph node metastases) that already classify them as high-risk tumors. Therefore, additional studies are needed to determine when the presence of the BRAF mutation (or other specific mutational profiles), independent of other high-risk clinical features, should be used to classify a patient as having a high risk of disease-specific mortality.

The AJCC/UICC[19] staging system is recommended for all patients with DTC by the published guidelines of the American Thyroid Association (ATA), the Latin American

Table 2
Staging systems for DTC and their different clinicopathologic variables

	TNM AJCC	MACIS	AGES	AMES	EORTC	MSKCC	UAB/MDACC	Clinical Class	Munster	NTCTCS	OSU	Noguchi
Age	X	X	X	X	X	X	X			X		X
Sex					X	X						X
Tumor size	X	X	X	X	X	X	X		X	X	X	X
Tumor grade			X									
Histologic subtype						X				X		
Lymph node metastases	X				X	X		X		X	X	X
Distant metastases	X	X		X	X	X	X	X	X	X	X	
Complete tumor resection		X										
Extrathyroid extension	X	X	X	X	X	X	X	X	X		X	
Multifocality						X				X		

Abbreviations: AGES, age, grade, extent, size; AMES, age, metastases, extrathyroid extension, size; EORTC, European Organization for Research and Treatment of Cancer; MSKCC, Memorial Sloan Kettering Cancer Center; NTCTCS, National Thyroid Cancer Treatment Cooperative Study; OSU, Ohio State University;[29] Noguchi; TNM AJCC, Tumor–Node–Metastasis Staging System/American Joint Committee on Cancer; UAB/MDACC, University of Alabama at Birmingham/MD Anderson Cancer Center, Clinical Class University of Chicago, Munster University.
Data from Refs.[19–30]

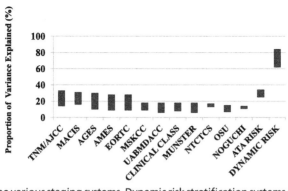

Fig. 1. PVE by the various staging systems. Dynamic risk stratification systems provide a higher PVE than any of the initial, static staging systems. AGES, age, grade, extent, size; AMES, age, metastases, extrathyroid extension, size; ATA, American Thyroid Association; EORTC, European Organization for Research and Treatment of Cancer; MSKCC, Memorial Sloan Kettering Cancer Center; NTCTCS, National Thyroid Cancer Treatment Cooperative Study; OSU, Ohio State University,[29] Noguchi; TNM AJCC, Tumor–Node–Metastasis Staging System/American Joint Committee on Cancer; UABMDACC, University of Alabama at Birmingham/MD Anderson Cancer Center, Clinical Class University of Chicago, Munster University. (*Data from* Refs.[5,9,32–35])

Thyroid Society (LATS), and the European Thyroid Association (ETA), based on its usefulness in predicting disease mortality and its requirement for cancer registries.[43–45]

Initial Staging System Used to Predict Risk of Persistent/Recurrent Disease

Although the AJCC/UICC staging system provides a useful stratification with regard to disease-specific mortality, the risk of having persistent/recurrent disease does not correlate with AJCC stage, as shown in **Fig. 2**.[5]

To better predict the risk of recurrence, the ATA, ETA, and LATS guidelines developed additional staging systems designed to predict the risk of persistent/recurrent disease.[43–45] The proposed risk of recurrence stratification systems from the ATA,

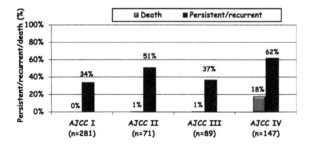

Fig. 2. Initial risk estimates of persistent/recurrent disease and disease-specific mortality within the 4 stages of the TNM/AJCC system. Although the TNM/AJCC system can reliably risk stratify with respect to disease-specific mortality, the risk of recurrent/persistent disease does not significantly differ across the various stages. (*From* Tuttle RM, Tala H, Shah J, et al. Estimating risk of recurrence in differentiated thyroid cancer after total thyroidectomy and radioactive iodine remnant ablation: using response to therapy variables to modify the initial risk estimates predicted by the new American Thyroid Association Staging System. Thyroid 2010;20:1341–9; with permission.)

ETA, and LATS all rely on a common set of clinicopathologic features.[43–45] Nevertheless, there are some differences in the specific definitions of the risk categories between the systems (**Table 3**). In each of the systems, recurrent disease is defined as identification of new biochemical (increased serum thyroglobulin [Tg]) or structural disease after having achieved a disease-free status (no evidence of disease [NED]).[5] Biochemical or structural disease identified in patients who were never rendered disease free is classified as persistent disease.[5–7]

Multiple studies (**Table 4**) have validated the ATA risk of recurrence stratification system in cohorts of patients treated with total thyroidectomy with or without RAI ablation.[5–9,46–48] In addition to predicting the likelihood of having persistent/recurrent disease, the ATA risk stratification system also predicts the likelihood of achieving clinical remission (NED) (see **Table 4**). However, the ATA risk stratification system showed a PVE of only 25% to 34%,[5,9] once again indicating suboptimal long-term risk stratification for individual patients with regard to predicting risk of recurrent/persistent disease.

Table 3
Comparison of risk of recurrent/persistent disease staging systems

Risk	ATA	ETA	LATS
Very low	—	All of the following: Unifocal <1 cm N0M0, no ETE	All of the following: Unifocal <1 cm N0M0, no ETE
Low	All of the following: Any size, intrathyroidal N0M0 All macroscopic tumor resected No ETE No aggressive histology No vascular invasion No ^{131}I uptake outside thyroid bed on the posttreatment scan, if performed	All of the following: Unifocal/multifocal 1–4 cm, intrathyroidal N0M0 No ETE No aggressive histology No vascular invasion No ^{131}I uptake outside thyroid bed on the posttreatment scan, if performed	All of the following: 1–4 cm intrathyroidal N0M0
Intermediate	Any of the following: N1 Minor ETE Tumor with aggressive histology Vascular invasion ^{131}I uptake outside thyroid bed on the posttreatment scan, if performed	—	—
High	Any of the following: Incomplete tumor resection Macroscopic ETE Distant metastases Inappropriate postoperative Tg	Any of the following: N1 >4 cm Macroscopic ETE Distant metastases	Any of the following: N1 >4 cm (>45 y) Macroscopic ETE (>45 y) Residual disease Distant metastases Aggressive histology

Aggressive histology: tall cell, insular, columnar cell carcinoma, Hurthle cell carcinoma, follicular thyroid cancer.
Abbreviation: ETE, extrathyroidal extension.

Table 4					
ATA initial risk stratification systems and clinical outcomes					
ATA Risk	Initial Treatment	Study	NED (%)	Persistent/ Recurrent[a] (%)	Dead (%)
Low	TT and RAI	Tuttle et al,[5] 2010	86	14	0
		Castagna et al,[9] 2011	91	9	0
		Vaisman et al,[6] 2012	88	12	0
		Pitoia et al,[8] 2013	78	22	0
	TT or TL No RAI	Vaisman et al,[46] 2011	99	1	0
		Schvartz et al,[47] 2012	99	1	0
		Durante et al,[48] 2012	99	1	0
Intermediate	TT and RAI	Tuttle et al,[5] 2010	57	43	0
		Vaisman et al,[6] 2012	63	36	1
		Pitoia et al,[8] 2013	52	48	0
	TT or TL No RAI	Vaisman et al,[46] 2011	92	8	0
High	TT and RAI	Tuttle et al,[5] 2010	14	68	18
		Vaisman et al,[6] 2012	16	68	16
		Pitoia et al,[8] 2013	31	69	0[b]

Abbreviations: RAI, RAI remnant ablation; TL, thyroid lobectomy; TT, total thyroidectomy.
 [a] Recurrent/persistent disease: clinical status other than NED.
 [b] The lack of deaths in this study is probably related to small number of very high-risk patients in this cohort and a median follow-up of only 4 years.

The risk of persistent and recurrent disease in patients defined as low risk by the ETA system was 6.1% and 2.5%, respectively; whereas in patients with high risk it was 32.8% and 2.8%, respectively.[9] Using the LATS staging risk system, the risk of biochemical and structural persistent disease in very low risk was 9% and 0%, respectively; in low risk, it was 7% and 7%, respectively; and in high risk, 7% and 23%, respectively.[8]

The ATA, ETA, and LATS staging systems all provide valuable risk stratification information that can be used to provide initial estimates of the risk of recurrent/persistent disease and the likelihood of rendering the patient NED with initial therapy. When used in conjunction with the AJCC/TNM or MACIS systems, accurate initial risk estimates of recurrence and disease-specific mortality enable the clinician to better tailor initial therapy and follow-up recommendations to the expected outcomes in individual patients. However, the ability of these various staging systems to account for less than 30% of the observed variance indicates that additional information is required during follow-up to further modify these initial risk estimates for individual patients.

RESTRATIFICATION OVER TIME: RESPONSE TO THERAPY ASSESSMENT
Response to Therapy Definitions

Initial staging systems are static predictions of risk based on clinicopathologic features available at the time of initial evaluation and therefore cannot adequately account for the subsequent biological behavior of the disease or the individual response to therapy. Accurate ongoing risk estimation requires a system that allows clinicians to modify these initial risk estimates as new data are accumulated during follow-up. For example, an ATA intermediate-risk patient would have an initial risk of recurrent/persistent disease estimate of 40% to 50% (see Table 4). However, if during follow-up, that same ATA intermediate-risk patient shows a normal postoperative neck ultrasonography

(US) result and thyroid-stimulating hormone (TSH) stimulated Tg less than 1 ng/mL, the subsequent risk of recurrence decreases to 1% to 4%.[5–9] Conversely, an ATA low-risk patient who shows an increasing serum Tg level over time or has metastatic disease identified during follow-up would no longer be considered to be a low-risk patient.

To distinguish ongoing (dynamic) risk stratification from the initial risk estimates (low, intermediate, high risk), we developed a novel nomenclature to describe the clinical status of the patient during follow-up in terms of the individual response to therapy[5,7]:

- Excellent response: no clinical, biochemical, or structural evidence of disease
- Biochemical incomplete response: abnormally increased serum Tg or increasing anti-Tg antibody (TgAb) levels in the absence of localizable disease
- Structural incomplete response: persistent or newly identified locoregional or distant metastases with or without abnormal Tg or TgAb
- Indeterminate response: nonspecific biochemical or structural findings, which cannot be confidently classified as either benign or malignant; this response includes patients without localizable disease who have low-level detectable serum Tg values after total thyroidectomy and RAI remnant ablation (nonstimulated Tg of 0.2–1.0 ng/mL or TSH stimulated Tg of 1–10 ng/mL) and patients with stable or declining TgAb levels (see later discussion and **Table 5**)

To classify a patient as having either (1) biochemical incomplete response to therapy, or (2) indeterminate response to therapy, it is important to ensure that risk-appropriate cross-sectional or functional imaging has been completed. For example, ATA low-risk/intermediate-risk patients who have papillary thyroid cancer with nonstimulated serum Tg values less than 5 ng/mL that are stable or declining over time require only cross-sectional imaging of the neck (neck US ± neck computed tomography (CT)/magnetic resonance imaging [MRI]), because non-RAI avid distant metastases are unlikely to be found in this setting. However, after total thyroidectomy and RAI ablation, ATA low-risk/intermediate-risk patients with nonstimulated serum Tg levels greater than or equal to 5 ng/mL (or increasing Tg values over time) require additional cross-sectional imaging to rule out distant metastases (primarily pulmonary metastases). Because the magnitude of increased serum Tg levels generally correlates with the site of distant metastases in both papillary and follicular thyroid cancers, additional cross-sectional and functional imaging tests are needed to rule out distant metastases in patients with very highly increased Tg values.[49] Because of the increased risk of distant metastases and the relatively poor production of serum Tg that can be seen in ATA high-risk patients, extensive imaging, which usually includes CT or MRI of the brain, neck, chest, abdomen, and pelvis (preferably with fluorodeoxyglucose positron emission tomography imaging) and RAI diagnostic studies are needed to rule out structural disease before classifying them as having either a biochemical incomplete or indeterminate response to therapy.

The response to therapy assessment restaging systems have been validated in patients submitted to total thyroidectomy and RAI by several studies, with a PVE range of 62% to 84%, higher than the PVE observed when the ATA risk staging system is used alone.[5–9] Because response to therapy assessments provide a more accurate, dynamic, real-time individualized risk estimate, they can be used to guide critical management issues that arise during follow-up, including the optimal degree of TSH suppression and appropriate frequency and types of surveillance assessments.[1–4]

As originally conceived and validated,[5–7] these response to therapy definitions described the best response to total thyroidectomy and RAI ablation during the first 2 years of follow-up. However, it is apparent that these response to therapy categories can be used to describe the clinical status of a patient at any point during follow-up

Table 5 Response to therapy definitions based on initial therapy			
	Initial Therapy		
	Total Thyroidectomy and RAI Ablation	**Total Thyroidectomy Without RAI Ablation**	**Lobectomy**
Excellent response	Nonstimulated Tg level <0.2 ng/mL[a] or Stimulated Tg level <1 ng/mL[a] and Undetectable TgAb and Negative imaging	Nonstimulated Tg level <0.2 ng/mL[a] or Stimulated Tg level <2 ng/mL[a] and Undetectable TgAb and Negative imaging	Stable, nonstimulated Tg level <30 ng/mL[a] and Undetectable TgAb and Negative imaging
Biochemical incomplete response	Nonstimulated Tg level >1 ng/mL[a] or Stimulated Tg level >10 ng/mL[a] or Increasing TgAb levels and Negative imaging	Nonstimulated Tg level >5 ng/mL[a] or Stimulated Tg level >10 ng/mL[a] or Increasing Tg values over time with similar TSH levels or Increasing TgAb levels and Negative imaging	Nonstimulated Tg level >30 ng/mL[a] or Increasing Tg level values over time with similar TSH levels or Increasing TgAb levels and Negative imaging
Structural incomplete response	Structural or functional evidence of disease regardless of Tg or TgAb	Structural or functional evidence of disease regardless of Tg or TgAb	Structural or functional evidence of disease regardless of Tg or TgAb
Indeterminate response	Nonspecific findings on imaging studies or Faint uptake in thyroid bed on RAI scanning or Nonstimulated Tg level 0.2–1 ng/mL[a] or Stimulated Tg level 1–10 ng/mL[a] or TgAb levels stable or declining in the absence of structural or functional disease	Nonspecific findings on imaging studies or Faint uptake in thyroid bed on RAI scanning or Nonstimulated Tg level 0.2–5 ng/mL[a] or Stimulated Tg level 2–10 ng/mL[a] or TgAb levels stable or declining in the absence of structural or functional disease	Nonspecific findings on imaging studies or TgAb levels stable or declining in the absence of structural or functional disease

[a] In the absence of interfering anti-TgAb.

and also in patients treated with lobectomy or total thyroidectomy without RAI ablation. As described later, the specific definitions of the response-to-therapy categories need to be slightly modified based on the extent of initial surgery and whether or not RAI ablation was used, but the basic concepts remain valid and useful. For example, serum Tg values used to differentiate excellent response from biochemical incomplete response and indeterminate response differ based on the extent of initial surgery and the use of RAI ablation, but once appropriately defined, an excellent response still conveys a low risk of recurrence without regard to the extent of initial therapy. (See **Table 5** for specific definitions of response to therapy variables based on the extent of initial therapy.)

USING THE RESPONSE-TO-THERAPY RECLASSIFICATION SYSTEM TO PREDICT SUBSEQUENT OUTCOMES AND GUIDE LONG-TERM FOLLOW-UP AFTER TOTAL THYROIDECTOMY AND RAI ABLATION
Excellent Response to Therapy

Patients with an excellent response to therapy have no clinical, biochemical, or structural evidence of disease on risk-appropriate follow-up studies. After total thyroidectomy and RAI remnant ablation, an excellent response was originally defined as a stimulated Tg level less than 1 ng/mL, in the absence of TgAb or structural evidence of disease, and was associated with a risk of recurrence over 5 to 10 years from 1% to 4% in several studies.[5–7,9,50–66] Similar very low recurrence rates were also reported when excellent response to therapy was defined using either a TSH stimulated Tg before RAI ablation or highly sensitive Tg assays without TSH stimulation at various time points after initial therapy.[52,56,57,67,68]

ATA low-risk and intermediate-risk patients who are subsequently classified as having an excellent response to therapy can be reclassified as having a very low risk of recurrence and even lower risk of disease-specific mortality. Based on these revised risk estimates, we decrease the intensity of TSH suppression (new goal approximately 1 mIU/L) and decrease the frequency of follow-up visits (every 12–18 months) and follow-up neck US (every 3–5 years or less). In our practice, these patients are transferred into the thyroid cancer survivorship clinic and transferred back to follow-up with their local endocrinologists. We are more cautious with the few ATA high-risk patients who achieve an excellent response, because the risk of recurrence in this cohort is slightly higher, at 5% to 15%.[9] In these patients, we often continue mild TSH suppression (0.1–0.4 mIU/L) and continue with appropriate cross-sectional imaging for at least 3 to 5 years after they achieve an excellent response.

Biochemical Incomplete Response to Therapy

After total thyroidectomy and RAI ablation, we previously defined biochemical incomplete response as a nonstimulated Tg level greater than 1 ng/mL or TSH stimulated Tg levels greater than 10 ng/mL or increasing TgAb levels in association with negative cross-sectional and functional imaging.[5–7] This finding is observed in 11% to 19% of ATA low-risk, 21% to 22% of ATA intermediate-risk, and 16% to 18% of ATA high-risk patients.[5–7]

Despite the biochemical evidence of persistent disease, the clinical outcomes are very good. Over 5 to 10 years of follow-up, previous studies reported no deaths, only 8% to 17% of structural identifiable disease progression, 19% to 27% persistent stable biochemical evidence of disease, and 56% to 68% became NED.[5–7] Of these patients, 34% evolved to NED without any additional treatment.[7] Further evidence corroborates that serum Tg values can gradually decline over time without any additional therapy, in the absence of structural identifiable disease.[7,55,65,69–74] On the contrary, a progressive increase in Tg values is observed in a small percentage of patients. In these cases, clinically significant increase in nonstimulated Tg (Tg doubling time <1 year) may identify patients at increased risk of developing structural locoregional or distant metastases.[75,76]

A biochemical incomplete response to therapy does not necessarily mean that the patient has persistent thyroid cancer. In some cases, an incomplete thyroidectomy results in persistent measureable low-level Tg values arising from normal thyrocytes. So, this term is used simply to signify the presence of serum Tg in the absence of identifiable structural disease and may or may not indicate the presence of persistent disease.

In our practice, a biochemical incomplete response to therapy manifest by stable or declining serum Tg levels leads to ongoing observation with mild TSH suppression (0.1–0.4 mIU/L) with appropriate cross-sectional or function imaging based on the magnitude of the Tg level and, more importantly, the doubling time of the Tg determined over time.[68] We seldom recommend empirical therapy in patients with biochemical incomplete response (either surgery or RAI therapy), because the outcomes in this cohort are excellent and Tg levels so often decline over time without any additional therapy.

Structural Incomplete Response to Therapy

Structural incomplete response to therapy is defined by evidence of locoregional or distant metastases regardless of the corresponding Tg or TgAb levels.[5–7] It includes both patients with biopsy proven disease and patients in whom structural or functional disease is identified that is highly likely to be metastatic disease based on the clinical scenario and radiologic context.

A locoregional structural incomplete response is associated with 11% disease-specific mortality whereas distant metastases are associated with 57% mortality.[6,7] Even with additional therapy, most patients who show an initial structural incomplete response to therapy have persistent biochemical or structural evidence of disease.[5–7] In patients with locoregional disease, remission rates of 29% to 51% after surgical intervention have been described.[77–79] Therefore, because most additional treatments are not curative, it is critical that the risks of interventions be appropriately balanced with potential benefits.

The management of patients with a structural incomplete response to therapy must be individualized based on the specific features of the case. In most cases, we continue TSH suppression (approximately 0.1 mIU/L), unless there are specific contraindications. Patients with rapidly progressive structural disease are candidates for appropriate additional therapies (such as RAI therapy, surgical resection, external beam irradiation, systemic therapy). Patients with small volume, persistent cervical lymph node metastases can be considered for observation, because appropriately selected patients usually have relatively stable disease for years.[80,81] Additional RAI can be considered if the structural disease is RAI avid but is seldom helpful if the diagnostic scan fails to show RAI avid disease.[11] Ideally, these complex patients are managed by a multidisciplinary team, which can appropriately weigh the risk and benefits of potential therapies and guide care.

Indeterminate Response to Therapy

In clinical practice, we not infrequently encounter patients with biochemical, structural, or functional findings that cannot be confidently classified as either benign or malignant.[5–7,80] To accommodate these patients, we defined an indeterminate response to therapy category in patients submitted to total thyroidectomy and RAI, which includes:

- Nonspecific findings on imaging studies including
  - Subcentimeter avascular thyroid bed nodules
  - Atypical cervical lymph nodes likely to be reactive

- ○ Faint uptake in the thyroid bed on RAI imaging
- ○ Nonspecific pulmonary nodules
- Nonstimulated Tg levels that are detectable but less than 1 ng/mL in the absence of structural disease
- Stimulated Tg levels that are detectable but less than 10 ng/mL in the absence of structural disease
- TgAb that are stable or declining in the absence of structural disease

An indeterminate response to therapy is observed in 12% to 29% of ATA low-risk patients, 8% to 23% of ATA intermediate-risk patients, and 0% to 4% of ATA high-risk patients.[5–7] The clinical outcomes in these patients are intermediate between patients with excellent response and those with incomplete response to therapy. Most remain free of disease over time, but up to 20% of them are reclassified as having either biochemical or structural incomplete response, as additional data is obtained over the years.[5–7]

Therefore, patients with an indeterminate response are followed with yearly follow-up visits with serum Tg and TgAb measurements, maintaining a TSH level in the range of 0.5 to 1.0 mIU/L. Cross-sectional imaging of indeterminate radiologic findings is performed at 1-year to 2-year intervals, depending on the specific findings and likelihood that these areas represent persistent disease. Once we are confident that the nonspecific findings do not represent persistent disease, they are reclassified as excellent response and followed appropriately. Conversely, if it becomes clear that the indeterminate findings represent persistent disease, they are reclassified as having either biochemical or structural incomplete response and evaluated appropriately.

MODIFICATION OF THE RESPONSE-TO-THERAPY RECLASSIFICATION SYSTEM DEFINITIONS FOR USE IN PATIENTS WHO DID NOT RECEIVE RAI ABLATION

Although the dynamic risk stratification system was proposed and validated on cohorts of patients who had received total thyroidectomy and RAI ablation, it is also important to be able to perform ongoing risk stratification in patients treated with either thyroid lobectomy or total thyroidectomy without RAI ablation. Although the nomenclature remains the same (excellent, biochemical incomplete, structural incomplete, or indeterminate), application to patients who did not receive RAI ablation requires slight modifications of the definitions to account for the differences in Tg values that should be considered excellent or biochemical incomplete during follow-up.

Total Thyroidectomy Without RAI Ablation

Total thyroidectomy (without RAI ablation) achieves stimulated Tg value less than 1 ng/mL in more than 50% of patients (**Table 6**). Furthermore, nonstimulated Tg values are less than 0.2 ng/mL in 50% of patients and less than 1 ng/mL in more than 90% of patients.[48,53,63,66,68,82–90] Obviously, the postoperative serum Tg value achieved with surgery alone is a reflection of both persistent thyroid cancer and residual normal thyroid tissue remaining. Nonetheless, an appropriate total thyroidectomy achieves very low suppressed and stimulated Tg values in most patients.

The predictive value of the postoperative Tg level is influenced by a variety of factors, including the amount of residual thyroid cancer or normal thyroid tissue, the TSH level, the functional sensitivity of the assay, the individual risk of having RAI avid locoregional metastasis, and the time elapsed since total thyroidectomy.[91] The half-life of serum Tg disappearance is usually 1 to 2 days (ranges from 1–6 days),[92,93] and the postoperative Tg should reach its nadir by 3 to 4 weeks postoperatively in

Table 6
Prevalence of postoperative Tg values in different series

Reference		Risk Stratification[a]	Prevalence (%)
Stimulated postoperative Tg value (ng/mL)			
<1.0	Pelttari et al,[53] 2010	Finland N = 468	Low risk	47
	Rosario et al,[82] 2005	Brazil N = 212	Low risk	50
	Rosario et al,[83] 2011	Brazil N = 237	Low risk	56
	Vaisman et al,[84] 2010	Canada N = 104	Low risk	56.7
	Durante et al,[48] 2012	Italy N = 290	Low risk	60
	Schlumberger et al,[85] 2012	France N = 729	Low risk	95
	Nascimento et al,[66] 2011	France N = 242	Low intermediate risk	24
<1.5	Phan et al,[86] 2008	Netherlands N = 94	Low risk 32% High risk 68%	27
<2.0	Mallick et al,[87] 2012	UK N = 438	Low intermediate risk	25.3
	Kim et al,[88] 2005	Korea N = 268	Low risk	47
	Piccardo et al,[63] 2013	Italy N = 243	High risk	33
<10.0	Webb et al,[68] 2012	Meta-analysis 15 studies, N ~ 4000	Variable	70
Nonstimulated postoperative Tg value (ng/mL)			
<0.1	Nascimento et al,[89] 2013	France N = 86	Low risk	62
<0.2	Giovanella et al,[90] 2008	Italy N = 126	Low intermediate risk 95%	50
<1.0	Nascimento et al,[89] 2013	France N = 86	Low risk	91
<2.0	Nascimento et al,[89] 2013	France N = 86	Low risk	96

[a] Risk stratification as described by the individual authors, which may not correspond to ATA risk classification definitions.

nearly all patients. Thus, the appropriate time for Tg measurement should be after 4 to 6 weeks after thyroidectomy.

Furthermore, multiple studies have reported a close relationship between the postoperative TSH stimulated Tg level (before ablation) and subsequent risk of disease recurrence (**Table 7**).[48,56,61,63,66,68,83,84,88–90,94,95] As would be expected, for any serum Tg level, the risk of recurrence is higher in patients selected for RAI ablation as opposed to low-risk patients who are followed without RAI. Nonetheless, most series have reported a risk of recurrence of approximately 1% to 3% in patients with a postoperative (preablation) stimulated Tg level less than 2 ng/mL. Stimulated Tg values between 2 and 10 ng/mL have a 2% to 8% risk of recurrence range, whereas

Table 7
Risk of recurrent/persistent disease based on postsurgical (pre-RAI ablation) Tg values

	Persistent/Recurrence Rates Patients Submitted to TT and RAI (%)	Persistent/Recurrence Rates Patients Treated With TT Without RAI (%)
Stimulated postoperative Tg value (ng/mL)		
<0.2		≤1
<1.0	<1–3	≤1
<1.5	8.5	
<2.0	1.6–3.7	
<3.2	7	
<5.0		<1
<10.0	1.8–7.4	
>10.0	20–78.5	
>30.0	43.3	
>50.0	96.6	
Nonstimulated postoperative Tg value (ng/mL)		
<0.2	<1	
<2.0		<1

Data from Refs.[48,56,61,63,66,68,83,84,86,88–90,94,95,100]

stimulated Tg values greater than 10 ng/mL are associated with more than 20% risk of recurrent/persistent disease.

Based on this information, we propose the following response to therapy definitions for patients treated with total thyroidectomy without RAI ablation.

- Excellent response: no clinical, biochemical or structural evidence of disease. This definition includes either a TSH stimulated Tg level less than 2 ng/mL or non-stimulated Tg level less than 0.2 ng/mL in the absence of interfering anti-Tg antibodies.
- Biochemical incomplete response: abnormal Tg or increasing TgAb levels in the absence of localizable disease. An abnormal Tg is defined as a TSH stimulated Tg level greater than 10 ng/mL; or a nonstimulated Tg level greater than 5 ng/mL, (because essentially all suppressed Tg values greater than 5 ng/mL correspond with a stimulated Tg level greater than 10 ng/mL in the absence of interfering TgAb,[96]) or consistently increasing Tg values over time with similar TSH levels.
- Structural incomplete response: persistent or newly identified locoregional or distant metastases with or without abnormal Tg or TgAb.
- Indeterminate response: nonspecific biochemical or structural findings that cannot be confidently classified as either benign or malignant. This category includes patients without definitive structural evidence of disease and with 1 of the following: stable or declining TgAb levels; nonstimulated Tg level between 0.2 and 5 ng/mL or stimulated Tg values between 2 and 10 ng/mL in the absence of interfering TgAb.

Thyroid Lobectomy Alone

Evolving evidence indicates that properly selected patients with DTC treated with lobectomy (unilateral lobectomy ± isthmusectomy) and no RAI have excellent outcomes. ATA low-risk to intermediate-risk patients properly selected for thyroid lobectomy had a recurrence rate in the thyroid remnant of 4.1% to 5.7%, in regional lymph nodes of less than 1% to 8.5%, in distant metastatic sites in 0% to 3.2%, and a mortality of 0% to 2.0%.[48,97–99]

The precise Tg value cutoffs for patients submitted to lobectomy remain to be defined. Nevertheless, for these patients, based on the available data, it is reasonable to consider the nonstimulated Tg value after 3 to 4 weeks after initial surgery as a starting point from which any consistent increasing values of nonstimulated Tg over time should lead to imaging procedures to search for structural evidence of disease. The study from Vaisman and colleagues[99] reported that an increasing suppressed Tg value over time was significantly more likely to be found in patients with structural disease recurrence than in those with NED (80% vs 21.5%). Furthermore, an increasing nonstimulated Tg level had an negative predictive value of 98% and a positive predictive value of 22%, indicating that, despite the lack of specificity for an increasing nonstimulated Tg level, a stable or declining nonstimulated Tg level is a good predictor for NED.[99] Aside from the Tg trend, the nonstimulated Tg cutoff value of 30 ng/mL seems to be a reasonable indicator for evidence of structural disease, because this constitutes about 50% of the amount of Tg that would be expected from a normal thyroid gland (reference range usually 20–60 ng/mL).

Follow-up after lobectomy relies on serial neck US examinations and nonstimulated Tg levels initially at 6-month to 12-month intervals, and then less frequently over time. This approach identifies the small percentage of these patients who manifest structural persistent/recurrent disease that may require additional therapies.[46,91,99]

Based on this information, we propose the following response to therapy definitions for patients treated with thyroid lobectomy without RAI ablation.

- Excellent response: no clinical, biochemical, or structural evidence of disease. This definition includes a stable, nonstimulated Tg level less than 30 ng/mL and negative TgAb.
- Biochemical incomplete response: abnormal Tg levels in the absence of localizable disease. An abnormal Tg level is defined as a consistently increasing nonstimulated Tg or a nonstimulated Tg level greater than 30 ng/mL in the absence of interfering TgAb. Consistently increasing TgAb levels over time are also classified as a biochemical incomplete response to therapy.
- Structural incomplete response: persistent or newly identified locoregional or distant metastases with or without abnormal Tg or TgAb.
- Indeterminate response: nonspecific structural findings that cannot be confidently classified as either benign or malignant. This category includes patients with stable or declining TgAb levels without definitive structural evidence of disease.

SUMMARY

Accurate, real-time risk stratification is the cornerstone of an individualized management approach for thyroid cancer. Although initial risk estimates are critical to decision making early in the course of the disease, ongoing risk stratification is required to appropriately tailor long-term management recommendations, so that the intensity of treatment and follow-up can be continually modified to reflect changing risks over time.

REFERENCES

1. Tuttle RM, Lobeuf R. Follow-up approaches in thyroid cancer thyroid cancer: a risk adapted approach. Endocrinol Metab Clin North Am 2008;37:419–35.

2. Tuttle RM, Leboeuf R, Martorella AJ. Papillary thyroid cancer: monitoring and therapy. Endocrinol Metab Clin North Am 2007;36:753–78.

3. Mazzaferri EL, Kloos RT. Clinical review 128: current approaches to primary therapy for papillary and follicular thyroid cancer. J Clin Endocrinol Metab 2001;86: 1447–63.

4. Shaha AR, Shah JP, Loree TR. Risk group stratification and prognostic factors in papillary carcinoma of thyroid. Ann Surg Oncol 1996;3:534–8.

5. Tuttle RM, Tala H, Shah J, et al. Estimating risk of recurrence in differentiated thyroid cancer after total thyroidectomy and radioactive iodine remnant ablation: using response to therapy variables to modify the initial risk estimates predicted by the new American Thyroid Association Staging System. Thyroid 2010;20: 1341–9.

6. Vaisman F, Momesso D, Bulzico DA, et al. Spontaneous remission in thyroid cancer patients after biochemical incomplete response to initial therapy. Clin Endocrinol 2012;77:132–8.

7. Vaisman F, Tala H, Grewal R, et al. In differentiated thyroid cancer, an incomplete structural response to therapy is associated with significantly worse clinical outcomes than only an incomplete thyroglobulin response. Thyroid 2011;21: 1317–22.

8. Pitoia F, Bueno F, Urciuoli C, et al. Outcome of patients with differentiated thyroid cancer risk stratified according to the American thyroid association and Latin-American thyroid society risk of recurrence classification systems. Thyroid 2013;23(11):1401–7.

9. Castagna MG, Maino F, Cipri C, et al. Delayed risk stratification, to include the response to initial therapy (surgery and radioiodine ablation), has better outcome predictivity in differentiated thyroid cancer patients. Eur J Endocrinol 2011;165:441–6.

10. Carty SE, Doherty GM, Inabnet WB, et al, for the Surgical Affairs Committee of the American Thyroid Association. American Thyroid Association Statement on the essential elements of interdisciplinary communication of perioperative information for patients undergoing thyroid cancer surgery. Thyroid 2012;4:395–9.

11. Tuttle RM, Sabra MM. Selective use of RAI for ablation and adjuvant therapy after total thyroidectomy for differentiated thyroid cancer: a practical approach to clinical decision making. Oral Oncol 2013;49:676–83.

12. Jukkola A, Bloigu R, Ebeling T, et al. Prognostic factors in differentiated thyroid carcinoma and their implications for current staging classification. Endocr Relat Cancer 2004;11:571–9.

13. Simpson WJ, McKinney SE, Carruthers JS, et al. Papillary and follicular thyroid cancer: prognostic factors in 1,578 patients. Am J Med 1987;83:479–88.

14. Baek SK, Jung KY, Kang SM, et al. Clinical factors associated with cervical lymph node recurrence in papillary thyroid carcinoma. Thyroid 2010;20:147–52.

15. Ghossein R, Ganly I, Biagini A, et al. Prognostic factors in papillary microcarcinoma with emphasis on histologic subtyping: a clinicopathologic study of 148 cases. Thyroid 2013;24(2):245–53.

16. Randolph GW, Duh QY, Heller KS, et al. The prognostic significance of nodal metastases form papillary thyroid carcinoma can be stratified based on the size and number of metastatic lymph nodes, as well as the presence of extranodal extension. Thyroid 2012;22:1144–52.

17. Ito Y, Tomoda C, Uruno T, et al. Prognostic significance of extrathyroid extension of papillary thyroid carcinoma: massive but not minimal extension affects the relapse-free survival. World J Surg 2006;30:780–6.

18. Ortiz Sebastian S, Rodriguez Gonzalez M, Parilla Paricio P, et al. Papillary thyroid carcinoma. Prognostic index for survival including the histological variety. Arch Surg 2000;135:272–7.
19. Greene FL, Page DL, Fleming ID, editors. AJCC/UICC cancer staging handbook: TNM classification of malignant tumors. 7th edition. New York: Springer-Verlag; 2009.
20. Hay ID, Bergstralh EJ, Goellner JR, et al. Predicting outcome in papillary thyroid carcinoma: development of a reliable prognostic scoring system in a cohort of 1779 patients surgically treated at one institution during 1940 through 1989. Surgery 1993;6:1050–8.
21. Hay I, Grant CS, Taylor WF, et al. Ipsilateral versus bilateral lobar resection in papillary thyroid carcinoma: a retrospective analysis of surgical outcome novel prognostic scoring system. Surgery 1987;102:1088–95.
22. Cady B, Rossi R. An expanded view of risk-group definition in differentiated thyroid carcinoma. Surgery 1988;104:947–53.
23. Byar DP, Green SB, Dor P, et al. A prognostic index for thyroid carcinoma. A study of the EORTC thyroid cancer cooperative group. Eur J Cancer 1979;15:1033–41.
24. Shaha AR, Loree TR, Shah JP. Intermediate-risk group for differentiated carcinoma of the thyroid. Surgery 1994;116:1036–41.
25. Beenken S, Roye D, Weiss H, et al. Extent of surgery for intermediate-risk well-differentiated thyroid cancer. Am J Surg 2000;179:51–6.
26. De Groot LJ, Kaplan EL, McCormick M, et al. Natural history, treatment, and course of papillary thyroid carcinoma. J Clin Endocrinol Metab 1990;71:414–24.
27. Lerch H, Schober O, Kuwert T, et al. Survival of differentiated thyroid carcinoma studied in 500 patients. J Clin Oncol 1997;15:2067–75.
28. Sherman SI, Brierley JD, Sperling M, et al. Prospective multicenter study of treatment of thyroid carcinoma: initial analysis of staging and outcome. National Thyroid Cancer Treatment Cooperative Study Registry Group. Cancer 1998;83:1012–21.
29. Mazzaferri EL, Jhiang SM. Long-term impact of initial surgical and medical therapy on papillary and follicular thyroid cancer. Am J Med 1994;97:418–28.
30. Noguchi S, Murakami N, Kawamoto H. Classification of papillary cancer of the thyroid based on prognosis. World J Surg 1994;18:552–7.
31. Schemper M, Stare J. Explained variation in survival analysis. Stat Med 1996;15:1999–2012.
32. Brierley JD, Panzarella T, Tsang RW, et al. A comparison of different staging systems predictability of patient outcome. Thyroid carcinoma as an example. Cancer 1997;79:2414–23.
33. Lang BH, Lo CY, Chan WF, et al. Staging systems for follicular thyroid carcinoma: application to 171 consecutive patients treated in a tertiary referral centre. Endocr Relat Cancer 2007;14:29–42.
34. Lang BH, Lo CY, Chan WF, et al. Staging systems for papillary thyroid carcinoma: a review and comparison. Ann Surg 2007;245:366–78.
35. Passler C, Prager G, Scheuba C, et al. Application of staging systems for differentiated thyroid carcinoma in an endemic goiter region with iodine substitution. Ann Surg 2003;2:227–34.
36. Sherman SI. Toward a standard clinicopathologic staging approach for differentiated thyroid carcinoma. Semin Surg Oncol 1999;16:12–5.
37. Voultilainen PE, Siironen P, Franssila KO, et al. AMES, AMCIS and TNM prognostic classifications in papillary carcinoma. Anticancer Res 2003;23:4283–8.
38. Lo CY, Chan WF, Lam KY, et al. Follicular thyroid carcinoma. The role of histology and staging systems in predicting survival. Ann Surg 2005;242:708–15.

39. D'Avanzo A, Treseler P, Kebebew E, et al. Prognostic scoring systems in patients with follicular thyroid cancer: a comparison of different staging systems in predicting the patient outcome. Thyroid 2004;12:453–8.

40. Xing M, Alzahrani AS, Carson KA, et al. Association between BRAF V600E mutation and mortality in patients with papillary thyroid cancer. JAMA 2013;309: 1493–501.

41. Howell GM, Carty SE, Armstrong MJ, et al. Both BRAF V600E mutation and older age (≥65 years) are associated with recurrent papillary thyroid cancer. Ann Surg Oncol 2011;18(13):3566–71.

42. Lim JY, Hong SW, Lee YS, et al. Clinicopathologic implications of the BRAF V600E mutation in papillary thyroid cancer: a subgroups analysis of 3130 cases in a single center. Thyroid 2013;23(11):1423–30.

43. Cooper DS, Doherty GM, Bryan RH, et al. Revised American Thyroid Association management guideline for patients with thyroid nodules and differentiated thyroid cancer. Thyroid 2009;19:1–48, 24.

44. Pacini F, Schlumberger M, Dralle H, et al. European consensus for the management of patients with differentiated thyroid cancer of the follicular epithelium. Eur J Endocrinol 2006;154:787–803.

45. Pitoia F, Ward L, Wohllk N, et al. Recommendations of the Latin American Thyroid Society on diagnosis and management of differentiated thyroid cancer. Arq Bras Endocrinol Metabol 2009;53:884–7.

46. Vaisman F, Shaha A, Fish S, et al. Initial therapy with either thyroid lobectomy or total thyroidectomy without radioactive remnant ablation is associated with very low rates of structural disease recurrence in properly selected patients with differentiated thyroid cancer. Clin Endocrinol 2011;75:112–9.

47. Schvartz C, Bonnetain F, Debakuyo S, et al. Impact on overall survival of radioactive iodine in low-risk differentiated thyroid cancer patients. J Clin Endocrinol Metab 2012;97:1526–35.

48. Durante C, Montesano T, Attard M, et al. Long term surveillance of papillary thyroid cancer patients who do not undergo postoperative radioiodine remnant ablation: is there a role for serum thyroglobulin measurement? J Clin Endocrinol Metab 2012;97:2748–53.

49. Robbins RJ, Wan Q, Grewal RK, et al. Real-time prognosis for metastatic thyroid carcinoma based on 2-[18F]fluoro-2-deoxy-D-glucose-positron emission tomography scanning. J Clin Endocrinol Metab 2006;91(2):498–505.

50. Berger F, Friedrich U, Knesewitsch P, et al. Diagnostic 131I whole-body scintigraphy 1 year after thyroablative therapy in patients with differentiated thyroid cancer. Eur J Nucl Med Mol Imaging 2011;38:451–8.

51. Soyluk O, Boztepe H, Aral F, et al. Papillary thyroid carcinoma patients assessed to be at low or intermediary risk after primary treatment are at greater risk of long term recurrence if they are thyroglobulin antibody positive or do not have distinctly low thyroglobulin at initial assessment. Thyroid 2011;21:1301–8.

52. Brassard M, Borget I, Edet-Sanson A, et al, THYRDIAG Working Group. Long-term follow-up of patients with papillary and follicular thyroid cancer: a prospective study on 715 patients. J Clin Endocrinol Metab 2011;96:1352–9.

53. Pelttari H, Välimäki MJ, Löyttyniemi E, et al. Post-ablative serum thyroglobulin is an independent predictor of recurrence in low-risk differentiated thyroid carcinoma: a 16-year follow-up study. Eur J Endocrinol 2010;163:757–63.

54. Klubo-Gwiezdzinska J, Burman KD, Van Nostrand D, et al. Does an undetectable rhTSH-stimulated Tg level 12 months after initial treatment of thyroid cancer indicate remission? Clin Endocrinol (Oxf) 2011;74:111–7.

55. Crocetti U, Durante C, Attard M, et al. Predictive value of recombinant human TSH stimulation and neck ultrasonography in differentiated thyroid cancer patients. Thyroid 2008;18:1049–53.

56. Giovanella L, Maffioli M, Ceriani L, et al. Unstimulated high sensitive thyroglobulin measurement predicts outcome of differentiated thyroid carcinoma. Clin Chem Lab Med 2009;47:1001–4.

57. Malandrino P, Latina A, Marescalco S, et al. Risk-adapted management of differentiated thyroid cancer assessed by a sensitive measurement of basal serum thyroglobulin. J Clin Endocrinol Metab 2011;96:1703–9.

58. Kloos RT, Mazzaferri EL. A single recombinant human thyrotropin-stimulated serum thyroglobulin measurement predicts differentiated thyroid carcinoma metastases three to five years later. J Clin Endocrinol Metab 2009;90:5047–57.

59. Kloos RT. Thyroid cancer recurrence in patients clinically free of disease with undetectable or very low serum thyroglobulin values. J Clin Endocrinol Metab 2010;95:5241–8.

60. Han JM, Kim WB, Yim JH, et al. Long-term clinical outcome of differentiated thyroid cancer patients with undetectable stimulated thyroglobulin level one year after initial treatment. Thyroid 2012;22:784–90.

61. Rosario PW, Mineiro Filho AF, Prates BS, et al. Postoperative stimulated thyroglobulin of less than 1 ng/ml as a criterion to spare low-risk patients with papillary thyroid cancer from radioactive iodine ablation. Thyroid 2012;22:1140–3.

62. Verburg FA, Stokkel MP, Düren C, et al. No survival difference after successful (131)I ablation between patients with initially low-risk and high-risk differentiated thyroid cancer. Eur J Nucl Med Mol Imaging 2010;37:276–83.

63. Piccardo A, Arecco F, Morbelli S, et al. Low thyroglobulin concentrations after thyroidectomy increase the prognostic value of undetectable thyroglobulin levels on levothyroxine suppressive treatment in low-risk differentiated thyroid cancer. J Endocrinol Invest 2010;33:83–7.

64. Castagna MG, Brilli L, Pilli T, et al. Limited value of repeat recombinant human thyrotropin (rhTSH)-stimulated thyroglobulin testing in differentiated thyroid carcinoma patients with previous negative rhTSH-stimulated thyroglobulin and undetectable basal serum thyroglobulin levels. J Clin Endocrinol Metab 2008;93:76–81.

65. Torlontano M, Attard M, Crocetti U, et al. Follow-up of low risk patients with papillary thyroid cancer: role of neck ultrasonography in detecting lymph node metastases. J Clin Endocrinol Metab 2004;89:3402–7.

66. Nascimento C, Borget I, Al Ghuzlan A, et al. Persistent disease and recurrence in differentiated thyroid cancer patients with undetectable postoperative stimulated thyroglobulin level. Endocr Relat Cancer 2011;18:R29–40.

67. Chindris AM, Diehnl NN, Crook JE, et al. Undetectable sensitive serum thyroglobulin (<0.1 ng/ml) in 163 patients with follicular cell derived thyroid cancer: results of rhTSH stimulation and neck ultrasonography and long-term biochemical and clinical follow-up. J Clin Endocrinol Metab 2012;97:2714–23.

68. Webb RC, Howard RS, Stojadinovic A, et al. The utility of serum thyroglobulin measurement at the time of remnant ablation for predicting disease-free status in patients with differentiated thyroid cancer: a meta-analysis involving 3947 patients. J Clin Endocrinol Metab 2012;97:2754–63.

69. Castagna MG, Tala Jury HP, Cipri C, et al. The use of ultrasensitive thyroglobulin assays reduces but does not abolish the need for TSH stimulation in patients with differentiated thyroid carcinoma. J Endocrinol Invest 2011;34:e219–23.

70. Biko J, Reiners C, Kreissl MC, et al. Favourable course of disease after incomplete remission on (131) I therapy in children with pulmonary metastases of papillary thyroid carcinoma: 10 years follow-up. Eur J Nucl Med Mol Imaging 2011;38:651–5.

71. Baudin E, Do Cao C, Cailleux AF, et al. Positive predictive value of serum thyroglobulin levels, measured during the first year of follow-up after thyroid hormone withdrawal, in thyroid cancer patients. J Clin Endocrinol Metab 2003;88: 1107–11.

72. Pineda JD, Lee T, Ain K, et al. Iodine-131 therapy for thyroid cancer patients with elevated thyroglobulin and negative diagnostic scan. J Clin Endocrinol Metab 1995;80:1488–92.

73. Padovani RP, Robenshtok E, Brokhin M, et al. Even without additional therapy, serum thyroglobulin concentrations often decline for years after total thyroidectomy and radioactive remnant ablation in patients with differentiated thyroid cancer. Thyroid 2012;22:778–83.

74. Valadão MM, Rosário PW, Borges MA, et al. Positive predictive value of detectable stimulated tg during the first year after therapy of thyroid cancer and the value of comparison with Tg-ablation and Tg measured after 24 months. Thyroid 2006;16:1145–9.

75. Wong H, Wong KP, Yau T, et al. Is there a role for unstimulated thyroglobulin velocity in predicting recurrence in papillary thyroid carcinoma patients with detectable thyroglobulin after radioiodine ablation? Ann Surg Oncol 2012;19: 3479–85.

76. Miyauchi A, Kudo T, Miya A, et al. Prognostic impact of serum thyroglobulin doubling-time under thyrotropin suppression in patients with papillary thyroid carcinoma who underwent total thyroidectomy. Thyroid 2011;21:707–16.

77. Schuff KG, Weber SM, Givi B, et al. Efficacy of nodal dissection for treatment of persistent/recurrent papillary thyroid cancer. Laryngoscope 2008;118:768–75.

78. Al-Saif O, Farrar WB, Bloomston M, et al. Long-term efficacy of lymph node reoperation for persistent papillary thyroid cancer. J Clin Endocrinol Metab 2010; 95:2187–94.

79. Yim JH, Kim WB, Kim EY, et al. The outcomes of first reoperation for locoregionally recurrent/persistent papillary thyroid carcinoma in patients who initially underwent total thyroidectomy and remnant ablation. J Clin Endocrinol Metab 2011;96:2049–56.

80. Rondeau G, Fish S, Hann LE, et al. Ultrasonographically detected small thyroid bed nodules identified after total thyroidectomy for differentiated thyroid cancer seldom show clinically significant structural progression. Thyroid 2011;21: 845–53.

81. Robenshtok E, Grewal RK, Fish S, et al. A low post operative non stimulated serum thyroglobulin level does not exclude the presence of radioactive iodine avid metastatic foci in intermediate-risk differentiated thyroid cancer patients. Thyroid 2013;23:436–42.

82. Rosario PW, Guimaraes VC, Maia FF, et al. Thyroglobulin before ablation and correlation with posttreatment scanning. Laryngoscope 2005;115:264–7.

83. Rosario PW, Xavier AC, Calsolari MR. Value of post-operative thyroglobulin and ultrasonography for the indication of ablation and ^{131}I activity in patients with thyroid cancer and low risk of recurrence. Thyroid 2011;21:49–53.

84. Vaisman A, Orlov S, Yip J, et al. Application of post-surgical stimulated thyroglobulin for radioiodine remnant ablation selection in low-risk papillary thyroid carcinoma. Head Neck 2010;32:689–98.

85. Schlumberger M, Catargi B, Borget I, et al, Tumeurs de la Thyroïde Refractaires Network for the Essai Stimulation Ablation Equivalence Trial. Strategies of radio-iodine ablation in patients with low-risk thyroid cancer. N Engl J Med 2012;366: 1663–73.

86. Phan HT, Jager PL, van der Wall JE, et al. The follow-up of patients with differentiated thyroid cancer and undetectable thyroglobulin (Tg) and Tg antibodies during ablation. Eur J Endocrinol 2008;158:77–83.

87. Mallick U, Harmer C, Yap B, et al. Ablation with low-dose radioiodine and thyrotropin alfa in thyroid cancer. N Engl J Med 2012;366:1674–85.

88. Kim TY, Kim WB, Kim ES, et al. Serum thyroglobulin levels at the time of 131I remnant ablation just after thyroidectomy are useful for early prediction of clinical recurrence in low-risk patients with differentiated thyroid carcinoma. J Clin Endocrinol Metab 2005;90:1440–5.

89. Nascimento C, Borget I, Troalen F, et al. Ultrasensitive serum thyroglobulin measurement is useful for the follow-up of patients treated with total thyroidectomy without radioactive iodine ablation. Eur J Endocrinol 2013;16:689–93.

90. Giovanella L, Ceriani L, Suriano S, et al. Thyroglobulin measurement before rsTSH-aided 131I ablation in detecting metastases from differentiated thyroid carcinoma. Clin Endocrinol 2008;69:659–63.

91. Grewal RK, Tuttle RM, Fox J, et al. The effect of posttherapy 131I SPECT/CT on risk classification and management of patients with differentiated thyroid cancer. J Nucl Med 2010;51:1361–7.

92. Giovanella L, Ceriani L, Maffioli M. Postsurgery serum thyroglobulin disappearance kinetic in patients with differentiated thyroid carcinoma. Head Neck 2010; 32:568–71.

93. Feldt-Rasmussen U, Petersen PH, Date J, et al. Serum thyroglobulin in patients undergoing subtotal thyroidectomy for toxic and nontoxic goiter. J Endocrinol Invest 1982;5(3):161–4.

94. Piccardo A, Arecco F, Puntoni M, et al. Focus on high-risk DTC patients: high postoperative serum thyroglobulin level is a strong predictor of disease persistence and is associated to progression-free survival and overall survival. Clin Nucl Med 2013;38:18–24.

95. Toubeau M, Touzery C, Arveux P, et al. Predictive value for disease progression of serum thyroglobulin levels measured in the postoperative period and after (131)I ablation therapy in patients with differentiated thyroid cancer. J Nucl Med 2004;45:988–94.

96. Spencer C, Fatemi S, Singer P, et al. Serum basal thyroglobulin measured by a second-generation assay correlates with the recombinant human thyrotropin-stimulated thyroglobulin response in patients treated for differentiated thyroid cancer. Thyroid 2010;20:587–95.

97. Matsuzu K, Sugino K, Masudo K, et al. Thyroid lobectomy for papillary thyroid cancer: long-term follow-up study of 1,088 cases. World J Surg 2014;38(1):68–79.

98. Nixon IJ, Ganly I, Patel SG, et al. Thyroid lobectomy for treatment of well differentiated intrathyroid malignancy. Surgery 2012;151:571–9.

99. Vaisman F, Momesso D, Bulzico DA, et al. Thyroid lobectomy is associated with excellent clinical outcomes in properly selected differentiated thyroid cancer patients with primary tumors greater than 1 cm. J Thyroid Res 2013;2013:398194.

100. Hall FT, Beasley NJ, Eski SJ, et al. Predictive value of serum thyroglobulin after surgery for thyroid carcinoma. Laryngoscope 2003;113:77–81.

Update on Medullary Thyroid Cancer

Mimi I. Hu, MD, Anita K. Ying, MD, Camilo Jimenez, MD*

KEYWORDS

- Medullary thyroid carcinoma • MEN type 2 • Pathophysiology • Diagnosis
- Treatment

KEY POINTS

- Increased understanding of the pathogenesis of medullary thyroid carcinoma (MTC) has led to improved development of targeted agents in the treatment of MTC.
- Calcitonin (Ct) and carcinoembryonic antigen (CEA) doubling time (DT) and somatic mutations of *RET* are indicators of poor prognosis.
- Cabozantinib and vandetanib are approved for the management of aggressive, progressive MTC.
- Understanding the potential side-effect profile of approved drugs is essential for making the decision regarding which agent to use for patients with progressive MTC.

INTRODUCTION

Malignant tumors are characterized by independent cell growth and their capacity to invade surrounding normal tissues and distant sites. Genes associated with growth, angiogenesis, tumor spread, apoptosis, and differentiation are frequently mutated in cancer. Receptor tyrosine kinases (TKs) comprise a large family of genes with members involved in all of these tumor-related pathways. TK receptors are membrane-spanning proteins that have a large N-terminal extracellular domain containing ligand-binding sites; a transmembrane domain that anchors the receptor to the cell membrane; and an intracellular domain that catalyzes the transfer of phosphate from adenosine-5′-triphosphate to tyrosine residues and hydroxyl groups in target proteins.

MTC is a rare neuroendocrine tumor that accounts for 3% to 5% of all thyroid gland cancers. Despite the rarity of MTC, it is one of the best-characterized solid tumors in

Disclosures: Research support (AstraZeneca) (M.I. Hu); None (A.K. Ying & C. Jimenez).
Department of Endocrine Neoplasia and Hormonal Disorders, The University of Texas MD Anderson Cancer Center, 1515 Holcombe Boulevard, Unit 1461, Houston, TX 77030, USA
* Corresponding author. Department of Endocrine Neoplasia and Hormonal Disorders, The University of Texas MD Anderson Cancer Center, 1400 Pressler Street, Unit 1461, Houston, TX 77030.
E-mail address: cjimenez@mdanderson.org

Endocrinol Metab Clin N Am 43 (2014) 423–442
http://dx.doi.org/10.1016/j.ecl.2014.02.004
0889-8529/14/$ – see front matter © 2014 Elsevier Inc. All rights reserved.

terms of its pathologic, biochemical, and molecular genetic properties. Understanding of this cancer's initiation and progression, clinical manifestations, and treatment is based largely in the discovery of tumor-specific mutations in and the abnormal expression of several TK receptors and pathways.

TK RECEPTORS AND PATHWAYS INVOLVED IN MTC DEVELOPMENT
The RET Receptor

Unlike other thyroid tumors, MTC has a strong familial predisposition.[1] Activating germline mutations in the rearranged during transfection (*RET*) oncogene are present in 25% to 35% of MTCs. In addition, up to 65% of patients with sporadic MTC may have somatic *RET* mutations.[2–4] Thus, *RET* mutations are likely the primary oncogenic event in most MTC cases. *RET* mutations are referred to as gain-of-function mutations because they lead to a constitutively active TK.

The *RET* gene is located on chromosome 10q11.21[5] and consists of 21 exons spanning approximately 55,000 base pairs.[6] *RET* encodes a transmembrane receptor with an extracellular portion that contains 4 calcium-dependent cell-adhesion (cadherin) domains and multiple glycosylation sites and a cysteine-rich region necessary for the tertiary structure of the protein and for receptor dimerization. The intracellular domain contains 2 TK regions that activate intracellular signal transduction pathways. RET activation requires the association of a ligand, such as glial cell line–derived neurotrophic factor (GDNF), neurturin, artemin, or persephin, with a membrane surface coreceptor, glycosylphosphatidylinositol-anchored GDNF–family receptor alpha (GFRα).[7–9] The GDNF–GFRα complex interacts with RET to facilitate its dimerization followed by autophosphorylation of tyrosine residues on the intracellular domains. The activated tyrosine residues serve as docking sites for adaptor proteins, which coordinate cellular signal transduction pathways, such as the mitogen-activated protein kinase (MAPK), phosphatidylinositol 3-kinase pathway (PI3K/AKT), c-Jun N-terminal protein kinases (JNK), and extracellular signal-regulated kinase (ERK) pathways.[10] These molecular pathways, which have important roles in regulating the cell cycle and angiogenesis and in regulating cell proliferation, differentiation, motility, apoptosis, and survival, are abnormally activated in patients who have MTC that is associated with either germline or somatic *RET* mutations. Important therapies for such MTC patients include cabozantinib and vandetanib, which modulate the mutated RET receptor.[11,12] Information on these drugs is discussed later.

Vascular Endothelial Growth Factor Receptors

MTC exhibits abnormal angiogenesis, which is essential for tumor growth and metastasis. Angiogenesis, along with other processes, such as vascular permeability and endothelial cell proliferation, migration, and survival, are regulated through the interaction of vascular endothelial growth factors (VEGFs) A, B, C, and D with VEGF receptors (VEGFRs) 1, 2, and 3.[13,14] The major mediator of MTC angiogenesis is believed to be VEGFR-2[15]; VEGFR-2 is overexpressed in MTC compared with normal tissue and is associated with an increased rate of metastases.[16,17] The interaction of the endothelial and MTC VEGFR-2 with tumoral production of VEGF A, B, C, and/or D promotes the activation of the MAPK and PI3K/AKT pathways, which leads to neoangiogenesis.[18] Thus, blocking VEGFRs inhibits tumor-mediated angiogenesis.

Epidermal Growth Factor Receptor

The epidermal growth factor receptor (EGFR), also known as HER-1/ErbB-1, is frequently overexpressed in MTC.[19] EGFR is a TK receptor associated with the regulation of cell growth and apoptosis; EGFR is 1 of 4 homologous transmembrane receptors. The others are HER-2/ErbB-2, HER-3/ErbB-3, and HER-4/ErbB-4. These receptors mediate the actions of different growth factors, such as epidermal growth factor, transforming growth factor α, and neuregulins.[20] The binding of ligands to these receptors induces the formation of EGFR homo- and heterodimers, the activation of kinase domains, and the phosphorylation of specific tyrosine residues that serve as docking sites for molecules essential to the activation of several cascades, including the MAPK and PI3K pathways.[21]

Several mechanisms can cause the oncogenic activation of EGFR, including excess ligand or receptor expression, activating mutations, inactivation failure, and transactivation through receptor dimerization.[22] One study of 153 primary and metastatic MTC samples revealed that *EGFR* mutations are rare in MTC and that the level of EGFR expression in the metastases was higher than that in the primary tumors.[17] MTC samples with mutations in the *RET* 883 and 918 codons had a significantly lower number of EGFR polysomies and tended to have less EGFR immunopositivity compared with MTC samples with other *RET* mutations.[17] In another study, EGFR inhibition was reduced in MTC cell lines with mutations in the *RET* 918 codon. Therefore, the most aggressive *RET* mutations may be less dependent on EGFR activation than other *RET* mutations are, which explains why EGFR inhibitors are less effective in codon 918–mutated MTC cell lines than in codon 634–mutated cell lines.[23] Although these studies suggest that EGFR activation is related to *RET* activation, the EGFR activation rate in tumors with *RET* mutations is not significantly different from that in those without *RET* mutations. This observation suggests that other molecular mechanisms could lead to the activation of *RET* (ie, increased transcription of *RET* in tumors without *RET* mutations).

Hepatocyte Growth Factor Receptor

The *MET* proto-oncogene encodes the receptor of the hepatocyte growth factor (c-MET).[24] The abnormal activation of this receptor may induce unrestricted cell proliferation, motility, and migration as well as angiogenesis and local and distant invasiveness.[25] Some MTCs express c-MET, and c-MET expression in MTC is associated with multifocality.[26,27] In addition, c-MET mutations have been found in some MTCs.[27] *RET* may induce MET expression.[28]

Fibroblast Growth Factor Receptor 4

The fibroblast growth factor receptor 4 (FGFR4) may be overexpressed in MTC and could enhance tumor growth. The inhibition of FGFR4 is associated with decreased MTC proliferation.[29,30] Thus, this receptor may be a therapeutic target in patients with progressive MTC.

RAS

The *RAS* genes encode 3 distinct but highly homologous 21-kDa proteins: H-RAS, K-RAS, and N-RAS. These proteins transduce messages from cell membrane receptors to intracellular effectors through the MAPK and PI3K/AKT pathways, which control a wide range of effects on cell proliferation, differentiation, and apoptosis. Activating point mutations in *RAS* genes, which have been extensively described in several tumor types,[31–33] constitutively activate multiple downstream effectors. Somatic mutations in the *RAS* genes (mainly *H-RAS* and *K-RAS*) have been found in some MTCs that are not associated with germline or somatic *RET* mutations, suggesting that these mutations are mutually exclusive.[33,34] Tumors associated with *RAS* mutations seem to exhibit a less aggressive phenotype compared with tumors associated with *RET* 918 and 634 codon mutations.[33] In contrast to the role of *RET* gene mutations, how *RAS* mutations lead to MTC development remains unclear.[35]

SYNDROMES
Sporadic MTC

Sporadic MTC, the most common form of MTC, is not associated with germline *RET* proto-oncogene mutations, C-cell hyperplasia, or a family history of MTC and/or pheochromocytoma. Sporadic MTC is usually unicentric, although multifocality can occur in 20% of the time and most commonly occurs at equivalent rates in women and men in the fourth decade of life. An isolated thyroid nodule is the most common manifestation of sporadic MTC.[36] Metastases to local lymph nodes occur frequently in patients with sporadic MTC; 80% of patients with a palpable tumor or a tumor larger than 1 cm have lymph node metastases. Lymph node metastases are frequently not apparent to surgeons, and they may be missed by pathologists unless each node is removed and carefully studied. The most common pattern of lymph node metastasis is to the ipsilateral nodes in areas II–VI of the neck, although metastases to the contralateral nodes may occur in up to 40% of patients with a palpable primary tumor. Another common pattern of metastasis is to the mediastinal lymph nodes.[37,38] Metastases to lymph nodes in the neck and/or mediastinum can infiltrate and compress the airway contributing to the high rates of morbidity and mortality in MTC patients. Distant metastases to the liver, bones, and lung parenchyma frequently occur in patients with MTC. Liver and lung metastases are usually vascular. Clinicians should be aware that even experienced radiologists commonly report a small focus of liver metastasis detected using contrast-enhanced CT as a hemangioma. A dedicated liver CT/MRI may help differentiate these tumors. Bone metastases are typically lytic and can cause severe bone pain, pathologic fractures, cord compression, and, rarely, hypercalcemia.

Among patients with apparently sporadic MTCs, 6% or 7% are subsequently found to have a germline *RET* mutation indicative of hereditary disease. Therefore, all MTC patients should be evaluated for *RET* proto-oncogene germline mutations.[39]

Hereditary MTC

Hereditary MTC, which is associated with activating germline mutations of the *RET* proto-oncogene, is multifocal and present in the context of simple, diffuse, and nodular C-cell hyperplasia, the precursor lesion of hereditary MTC. Hereditary MTC may manifest in various age groups, but unlike sporadic MTC, hereditary MTC commonly occurs in individuals younger than 20 years. Patients frequently have a family history of MTC and/or pheochromocytoma. Similar to sporadic MTC, hereditary MTC can metastasize to neck and mediastinal lymph nodes and to the liver, bones, and lungs, thereby predisposing patients to high rates of morbidity and mortality.[36]

Hereditary MTC manifests as part of multiple endocrine neoplasia type 2 (MEN2), which is transmitted as an autosomal dominant trait and may present as 1 of 2 variants. MEN2A is the most common variant, accounting for approximately 80% of MEN2 cases. MEN2A is characterized by bilateral, multicentric MTC in more than 90% of *RET* carriers, unilateral or more frequently bilateral pheochromocytomas in 50% of carriers, and primary hyperparathyroidism in 10% to 20% of carriers. The presence of pheochromocytomas in patients with MTC who have mutations in the *RET* 634 codon (the most common mutated codon in MEN2A patients) does not indicate a more aggressive MTC phenotype. Such patients do not have a more advanced stage of MTC at diagnosis or a shorter overall survival duration compared with patients without pheochromocytoma.[40] In addition, pheochromocytomas, even in the setting of MTC, are rarely malignant, thus seldom contribute to morbidity or mortality.[1,40–42]

There are 3 MEN2A subvariants. One is MEN2A with Hirschsprung disease; patients with this subvariant develop Hirschsprung disease in childhood. Another subvariant, found in 20 to 30 families, is MEN2A associated with cutaneous lichen amyloidosis. Patients with this subvariant develop a pruritic cutaneous lesion across the upper back, usually during the second or third decade of life. A variant of MEN2A is familial MTC, which is characterized by MTC but no other manifestations of MEN2. In general, familial MTC tends to be the least aggressive form of hereditary MTC.[1]

MEN2B, accounting for approximately 20% of MEN2 cases, is less common than MEN2A but is the most distinctive form of the syndrome. MEN2B is characterized by MTC in 100% of patients and by MTC and pheochromocytoma in 50% of patients. More than 90% of MEN2B patients have mucosal ganglioneuromas in the distal tongue, eyelids, and gastrointestinal (GI) tract, and nearly all have a marfanoid habitus.

MEN2B-associated hereditary MTC, which usually arises from de novo mutations, is generally the most aggressive form of MTC. It is difficult to cure because its phenotype is often unknown. Local lymph node metastases are common during the first decade of life, warranting early detection of the disease, and distant metastases are seen with some regularity during the second decade. Death from metastatic MTC generally occurs during the third or fourth decade of life, though there are examples of families with 3 or more generations of living MTC patients.[1]

INITIAL DIAGNOSTIC EVALUATION

MTC is most commonly diagnosed by fine-needle aspiration (FNA) of a new thyroid nodule, with a sensitivity of 60% to 90%.[43–45] FNA cannot always distinguish MTC based on cytology alone, so immunohistochemical staining for Ct, chromogranin A, or CEA can increase accuracy.[46] Recent small studies have shown improved sensitivity with calcitonin measurement in FNA washout fluid with as high as 100% accuracy.[47,48]

Serum Ct is the primary biochemical marker used for detection, staging, postoperative management, and prognosis for MTC patients. The positive predictive value of basal Ct for MTC is 100% if levels are greater than 100 pg/mL.[49] Preoperative levels are predictive of tumor size and location, so the American Thyroid Association (ATA) guidelines addressing MTC recommend that the extent of radiologic evaluation and operation be based in part on Ct level.[50] Abnormal preoperative CEA levels suggest advanced disease. CEA levels greater than 30 ng/mL are associated with central and ipsilateral lateral lymph node metastases, whereas levels greater than 100 ng/mL signify contralateral lateral lymph node and distant metastasis.[51]

All patients with suspected or confirmed MTC should undergo a comprehensive neck ultrasound. There is an increased risk for lymph node metastasis with multifocal disease in thyroid gland and hereditary MTC.[51] If lymph node disease is present in imaging or Ct greater than 400 pg/mL, then additional imaging with neck and chest CT and liver 3-phase contrast-enhanced CT or contrast-enhanced MRI is indicated. If skeletal metastases are suspected, MRI is preferred imaging modality.

Radiologic Surveillance

Imaging for distant metastasis in the chest, liver, and bone should be performed when suspected based on high levels of Ct or CEA. Standard practice includes chest CT, liver CT or MRI, bone scan, and axial skeleton MRI. Sensitivity of these imaging techniques ranges, however, from 25% to 50%.[52–54] Despite the high sensitivity of Ct to predict the presence of MTC, it is a difficult neoplasm to document with imaging studies. Recent radiologic studies have focused on testing different radiotracers and modalities that could provide more sensitive and efficient imaging for persistently elevated Ct levels.

^{18}F-FDG PET

Fludeoxyglucose F 18 (^{18}F-FDG) positron emission tomography (PET) can detect tumor recurrence with reported patient-based sensitivities ranging from 15% to 78% and lesion-based sensitivities ranging from 28% to 96%.[53–58] An early multicenter clinical trial showed promise for ^{18}F-FDG PET with lesion-based sensitivity of 78% compared with 50%.[59] Subsequent comparative and prospective studies, however, have found much lower sensitivity, especially when the Ct value is less than 1000 pg/mL.[56,60] Skoura and colleagues[60] studied patients with elevated Ct levels but negative or equivocal conventional imaging and found patient sensitivity of 44% with ^{18}F-FDG PET; however, that rose to 87% when evaluation only patients with Ct value over 1000 pg/mL.

Some studies have found that ^{18}F-FDG PET positivity correlates with shorter Ct DTs or a more aggressive MTC.[61,62] The prognostic value of ^{18}F-FDG PET, however, is still controversial.[56] Location of the recurrence seems to affect performance of the imaging modality. ^{18}F-FDG PET has higher sensitivity than conventional CT in lymph node recurrence but worse sensitivity in lung, bone, or liver.[54,55,62]

^{18}F-DOPA and ^{68}Ga-DOTA PET

PET imaging using the radiotracer ^{18}F-dihydroxyphenylalanine (DOPA) has increased sensitivity compared with ^{18}F-FDG. Neuroendocrine tumor cells like MTC can take up and decarboxylate amine precursors, such as DOPA, thus allowing visualization by ^{18}F-DOPA PET imaging.[52] Multiple comparative studies report better sensitivity for ^{18}F-DOPA ranging from 63% to 87%.[54,55,57,63] Currently, ^{18}F-DOPA is not commercially available in the United States.

Several different gallium 68 (^{68}Ga)-labeled somatostatin analogues (DOTA peptides) are being studied, but the diagnostic role in MTC is not clear. The few studies that have compared ^{68}Ga-DOTA PET to ^{18}F-FDG PET in MTC have not found improved sensitivity with the newer tracer.[54,64]

^{18}F-NaF PET

Sodium fluoride F 18 (^{18}F-NaF) PET scanning has sensitivity similar to MRI for imaging bone metastases with the added benefit of whole-body imaging with one scan.[65,66] The uptake of the fluoride ion represents bone mineralization. Schirrmeister and colleagues[65,66] reported added benefit to ^{18}F-NaF PET imaging to bone scan in identifying bone metastases in differentiated thyroid cancers. Although some centers are investigating its use in MTC, no comparative studies have been published.

Somatostatin Receptor Scintigraphy

Octreotide scintigraphy can be useful in detecting neuroendocrine tumors, but somatostatin receptor scintigraphy (SRS) has not shown as high sensitivity in MTC compared with conventional imaging. Sensitivity ranges from 57% to 67%, with decreased sensitivity with low tumor volume. There is also inconsistency in study findings, with Frank-Raue and colleagues[67] showing no detection of liver metastasis by SRS compared with Baudin and colleagues,[68] who found better sensitivity in the liver (50%) compared with the neck (25%). Indium In 111–octreotide SRS in children and adolescents with hereditary MTC has even lower lesional sensitivity at 24.5%.[69]

SRS is not helpful in detecting lesions less than 1 cm and has not been shown to alter therapeutic decisions based on conventional imaging findings.[67,68]

PROGNOSIS

Biochemical markers, clinical characteristics, and somatic mutation status have prognostic value to predict recurrence and survival. The DTs of Ct and CEA are both predictive of recurrence-free and overall survival.[53,70,71] Patients with Ct and CEA DT less than 6 months have worse prognosis and progressive disease, and those with DT over 24 months had excellent prognosis or stable disease.[53,70] The ATA has a calculator to determine both measures, which is most accurate when at least 4 values available over a 2-year period (www.thyroid.org). A recent meta-analysis found the best prognostic value for recurrence and survival was Ct and CEA DT at the 1-year point.[72] Meijer and colleagues[72] found the 5- and 10-year survival rates for patients with Ct DT less than 1 year were 36% and 18%, respectively, compared with 95% and 95% for those with Ct DT longer than 1 year; 5- and 10-year survival rates with CEA DT were 43% and 21%, respectively, compared with 100% and 100%. A subgroup of patients also had favorable Ct DT yet unfavorable CEA DT with poor outcomes, suggesting that during the process of dedifferentiation, there may be less than expected production of Ct.[72,73]

Patients with nodal disease are at greatest risk for persistent or recurrent disease. Nodal disease at diagnosis along with presence of vascular invasion on histologic examination are also independent predictors of distant metastases.[74]

The most common somatic RET in sporadic MTC is M918T.[3,75] RET 918 mutation is present in approximately 35% of sporadic MTC patients and is correlated with lymph node metastasis at diagnosis, persistent disease after surgery, and increased chance of recurrence.[3,76,77] In a multivariate analysis, somatic RET and advanced stage of disease were independent predictors of worse outcome.[3]

The 5-year survival of sporadic and hereditary MTC ranges from 70% to 90% and 10-year survival from 56% to 87%.[78–84] Older age and later stage of disease were independent prognostic variables influencing survival with relative risk of death 7.9 and 18.7, respectively.[80] When there is adjustment for the baseline mortality of the general population, however, extrathyroidal extension (defined as T4) and doubling of Ct within the first year after treatment are the only independent predictors of mortality.[85] Multiple studies have not shown sporadic MTC influenced survival in multivariate analysis, but others have shown that sporadic tumors have a poorer prognosis.[78–80,85]

TREATMENT
Prophylactic Surgical Management in Germline RET-Positive Patients

The most effective method to prevent development of MTC or metastatic disease is to perform prophylactic total thyroidectomy in germline RET-positive patients who have preclinical disease. Since 1993, information collected regarding RET mutations and their respective clinical expression has driven consensus recommendations for evaluation and treatment to prevent morbidity and mortality associated with hereditary MTC. The prediction of aggressiveness of MTC associated with a specific RET mutation can be extrapolated by examination of the earliest age at which MTC has been identified and earliest age presenting with metastases.[86] Based on this knowledge, mutations of RET have been classified using a system of levels A through D by the ATA Guidelines Task Force, depending on the aggressiveness observed in the respectively associated MTCs.[50]

The highest-risk ATA mutations of codons 883 and 918, associated with MEN2B phenotype (level D), predispose to very aggressive MTC and are characterized by the initiation of tumor development and even metastases before the first year of life. Consequently, carriers of these mutations are candidates for a total thyroidectomy as soon as possible and within the first year of life, with central lymph node dissection for clinical metastases. Codon 634 *RET* mutation is the only one categorized as a level C risk with the earliest age of detected MTC reported in a 10 month old and documented earliest lymph node metastases in a 6 year old. The ATA guidelines recommend prophylactic thyroidectomy for an *RET* 634 carrier by age 5 years. Less aggressive risk mutations (level B) include codons 609, 611, 618, 620, 630, and 631. Patients with level B mutations could consider surgery before age 5 years or delay surgery beyond that if there are no concerning features on ultrasound, Ct levels are low, and there is a less aggressive MTC family history. Least aggressive risk mutations (level A) are localized in codons 768, 790, 791, 804, and 891 and typically are associated with lower serum Ct levels and less advanced tumor stage at diagnosis than level B mutations. In certain large kindreds with these mutations, a death has never been caused by MTC; in others, metastases and death attributable to MTC have occurred infrequently. If there has never been a death attributable to MTC in one of these kindreds (and the kindred is of sufficient size and the follow-up encompasses multiple generations), delaying total thyroidectomy with or without central lymph node dissection to a later age with active surveillance may be a reasonable course.

Surgical Management of MTC Presenting with Clinically Apparent Disease

At present, the only curative treatment of MTC, sporadic or hereditary, is complete surgical resection when the disease is confined to the neck. Complete resection of MTC, however, could be difficult due to the high likelihood of regional or distant metastases at diagnosis. Ipsilateral (80%) and contralateral cervical lymph nodes (40%) metastases are often present at initial diagnosis with a high incidence of distant metastatic disease to the liver, bones, and/or lung parenchyma.[87] Patients with cervical adenopathy found at diagnosis have a higher incidence of residual disease after surgical resection (90%) compared with those without cervical adenopathy (38%).[88] Consequently, for surgical purposes, patients with MTC can be classified into 1 of 3 groups: those with localized disease (no evidence of metastases to regional lymph nodes as indicated by sonography, no disease outside of the neck as indicated by CT scans of the chest and abdomen with liver protocol and bone scan, and serum Ct values usually <500 pg/mL), in whom cure is possible; those with metastatic disease limited to the neck, for which cure may be possible; and those with metastatic disease outside of the neck, for which there is no chance for surgical cure.

The appropriate surgical procedure for a patient with localized MTC is a total thyroidectomy with central (levels VI and VII) compartmental dissection.[50] Lateral neck (levels II to V) lymph node dissections are considered when there are image or biopsy-positive compartments. In the setting of extensive distant metastases or advanced local features, surgical goals are more palliative with care to minimize complications.

A question that arises in this group of patients is how thoroughly distant metastatic disease should be looked for. Guidance may be provided by a combination of measuring the serum Ct and CEA levels and reviewing high-quality sonography of the neck. If there is nodal disease noted on ultrasound or serum Ct concentration exceeds 400 pg/mL, it is recommended to perform chest CT and 3-phase contrast-enhanced liver CT or MRI abdomen.[50] The challenge is to differentiate between patients in whom surgical cure is possible and those with distant metastasis in whom extensive neck surgery, in most cases, does not affect long-term outcomes. In patients for whom surgical cure is not possible, the goals change. In this situation, it is appropriate to perform a total thyroidectomy with surgical resection of identifiable disease to protect the aerodigestive tract or recurrent laryngeal nerve from future compromise.

Patients with clear evidence of distant metastasis are more straightforward to identify. These patients may have substantial elevations of serum Ct (>5000 pg/mL), have metastatic disease easily identifiable on imaging studies, and frequently have diarrhea and flushing. In these patients, total thyroidectomy with removal of identifiable disease to protect the airway is indicated. When there are lymph nodes with metastasis in the upper mediastinum or perihilar area that are likely to affect the airway, consideration should be given to a mediastinal lymph node dissection.

Persistent Elevation of Serum Calcitonin and Carcinoembryonic Antigen After Surgery

After initial thyroidectomy and central lymph node dissection, it is necessary to allow 3 to 4 months to elapse before concluding that an elevated serum Ct or CEA concentration is related to the presence of residual MTC and not to the postoperative inflammatory effects on Ct synthesis or a failure of circulating Ct and CEA to clear because of their prolonged half-lives (approximately 30 hours for Ct).[8] Patients with undetectable Ct should have annual measurements of serum Ct and CEA.

Frequently, patients with MTC undergo a total thyroidectomy with limited or no lymph node dissection. In these patients and in patients treated with total thyroidectomy and bilateral lateral neck lymph node dissection, persistent elevation of Ct and CEA is likely associated with residual disease in the cervical lymph nodes. Because patients have undergone a total thyroidectomy, the decision to perform a neck lymph node dissection should be based on a realistic estimate of the probability of surgical cure. In patients with serum Ct concentrations of less than 100 pg/mL, it is unusual to find any detectable radiographic abnormalities in the neck, and long-term clinical surveillance with periodic sonography of the neck is then indicated. In patients with higher Ct values without radiographic evidence of macroscopic disease, close follow-up with periodic imaging (sonography of the neck, chest radiographs, and CT scans of the chest and abdomen) is necessary. In most circumstances, reoperation of the neck does not normalize serum Ct concentrations. Additionally, the risk of hypoparathyroidism is much higher than that observed if the neck dissection is performed during the initial surgical intervention.

Patients with serum Ct concentrations higher than 5000 pg/mL after total thyroidectomy and lymph node dissection generally have metastatic disease outside of the neck. These areas should be evaluated with imaging techniques (discussed previously). Depending on a patient's symptoms, possible locoregional complications of invasive disease and pace of disease progression, areas of distant metastatic disease may be followed with active surveillance or treated with targeted modalities or systemic chemotherapy, which are discussed in the following sections.

Active Surveillance for Progression of Metastatic MTC

Because patients with regional or distant metastatic disease can demonstrate variable behavior from indolent to rapidly progressive disease (discussed previously), active surveillance for pace of disease change is needed after thyroidectomy with routine testing of Ct and CEA levels and appropriate radiologic imaging.[89]

The optimal timing intervals for surveillance have not been recommended by any published guidelines, but the authors typically recommend evaluating tumor markers every 3 months for the first 6 months after thyroidectomy with tumor-relevant imaging as needed. Thereafter, follow-up is performed every 6 months for the first 2 years after diagnosis to establish an estimation of the serum Ct and CEA DTs and to monitor for possible short-term changes of distant sites of disease.

Locoregional Targeted Treatments of Metastases or Paraneoplastic Syndromes

Patients with persistent or recurrent metastatic disease that may lead to locoregional compromise should be referred for adjunctive, palliative treatment. Situations, such as potential invasiveness into tracheoesophageal tissue, impending neurologic damage from brain metastases or spinal lesions, or pain from destructive bone lesions, necessitate radiotherapy. Although radiotherapy seems effective in preventing and controlling complications associated with MTC activity in the neck and mediastinum, there is no evidence that such therapy has an effect on improving survival.[90,91] Radiofrequency ablation and transarterial chemoembolization of hepatic metastases have also been shown to have effectiveness in locoregional control.[92]

Bone metastases from solid tumors may be targeted by antiresorptive therapy with parenteral bisphosphonates or denosumab. There is limited published evidence that there is benefit in treating patients with MTC-related metastatic bone disease with either of these agents; however, a published study of patients with differentiated thyroid cancer with bone metastases found that zoledronic acid was effective in decreasing skeletal-related events (SREs) or prolonging the time to develop an SRE.[93,94] According to published ATA guidelines, there is no recommendation for or against the use of bisphosphonates for MTC-related bone metastases. The most recent National Comprehensive Cancer Network (NCCN) guidelines for MTC does recommend consideration of bisphosphonates or denosumab for metastatic bone disease, with particular care to monitor for post-treatment hypocalcemia, which is important in patients at risk for hypoparathyroidism and vitamin D deficiency.[95] In the context of hypercalcemia induced by bone osteolysis, intravenous bisphosphonate or subcutaneous denosumab can control this complication and improve the associated symptoms.

Diarrhea associated with MTC is common (approximately 30%) and a clinically significant paraneoplastic syndrome in many patients, leading to weight loss, dehydration, skin irritation, and poor quality of life. It is often associated with advanced, metastatic disease and frequently seen in patients with hepatic metastases. The diarrhea can be hypersecretory and/or related to increased GI motility. Treatment includes the use of antimotility drugs (loperamide, diphenoxylate/atropine, or tincture of opium) as first-line agents. Somatostatin analogs may have some benefit based on small, nonrandomized studies.[96,97] Surgical debulking or transarterial hepatic chemoembolization may be considered in these patients.[92]

Ectopic Cushing syndrome is a rare endocrine complication of MTC (less than 1%) associated with excessive tumoral production of adrenocorticotropic hormone or its precursor peptides. When this complication is associated with a localized tumor, curative resection of the tumor cures this paraneoplastic syndrome. In the context of ectopic Cushing syndrome secondary to broadly metastatic disease, bilateral adrenalectomy after adequate adrenal inhibition with ketoconazole or metyrapone, followed by adrenal replacement therapy with glucocorticoids and mineralocorticoids, may be necessary.

Systemic Chemotherapy—Tyrosine Kinase Inhibitors

Chemotherapy based on dacarbazine has been associated with a reduction in tumor size in approximately 25% of patients treated with this agent in combination with a variety of other agents (eg, cyclophosphamide, vincristine, and 5-fluorouracil).[98] Complete remission has not been observed, however, and there is no obvious demonstrated survival benefit. Given the potential toxicity profile of cytotoxic chemotherapeutic agents, the recent NCCN guidelines (version 2.2013) for MTC recommends dacarbazine-based chemotherapy for patients with progressive, advanced MTC after considering TK inhibitor (TKI) (discussed later) or referral to a clinical trial.[95] Treatment with somatostatin analogues or radioiodinated metaiodobenzylguanidine has demonstrated limited responses in small case series.[99–101]

Over the past decade of preclinical and clinical studies of various therapeutic agents for metastatic MTC, the most impressive and exciting data have arisen from the evaluation of responses to small molecule TKIs that compete with the ATP-binding site of the catalytic domain of a TK. Occupation of this site by the TKI inhibits autophosphorylation and activation of the TK domain of protumoral transmembrane receptors (eg, VEGFR-2, RET, c-KIT, and EGFR) and prevents further activation of intracellular signaling pathways, which are integral to cell activation, division, migration, and survival. A TKI can be specific to one or many homologous TKs. Although numerous TKIs have been investigated in MTC patients in various phases of clinical trials, 2 agents recently have been approved for the treatment of advanced, progressive, or symptomatic MTC: vandetanib (approved in the United States in April 2011 and in Europe in February 2012) and cabozantinib (approved in the United States in November 2012) (**Fig. 1**).[102] Consideration of sunitinib or sorafenib is recommended by the NCCN if a patient cannot receive or has progressed with vandetanib or cabozantinib or has no access to a clinical trial.

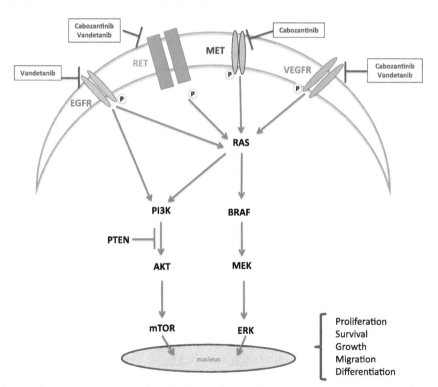

Fig. 1. The MTC receptors and molecular pathways that are targeted by vandetanib and cabozantinib.

Vandetanib is a multi-TKI of RET (IC_{50} 100 nM), VEGFR-2 (IC_{50} 40 nM), and EGFR (IC_{50} 500 nM).[103] Two phase II clinical trials evaluated hereditary MTC patients using 2 different dosing regimens: 100 mg daily and 300 mg daily.[104,105] Wells and colleagues[12] demonstrated that the 300-mg daily dose led to a 20% partial response (PR) and 53% of the patients had stable disease. Responses did not seem to correlate with the underlying *RET* mutation. These encouraging findings led to the ZETA study, which was a large, multicenter, randomized-controlled phase III trial for patients with MTC (hereditary and nonhereditary) and measurable disease by the Response Evaluation Criteria in Solid Tumors (RECIST) (n = 331).[106] Patients were randomized in a 2:1 ratio to vandetanib or placebo between December 2006 and November 2007, with the ability to crossover to active drug if placebo-treated patients demonstrated progression while on study. At the time of publication of the results, vandetanib led to a statistically significant prolonged progression-free survival (PFS) compared with placebo: estimated 30.5 months in the vandetanib group versus 19.3 months in the placebo group. The overall response rate was 45% in the vandetanib group versus 13% in the placebo group. These results led to the approval of the drug by the United States Food and Drug Administration (FDA) in April 2011.

Cabozantinib is a multikinase inhibitor of RET (IC_{50} 4.5 nM), VEGFR-2 (IC_{50} 0.035 nM), and c-MET (IC_{50} 1.8).[103] The authors' experience with cabozantinib in MTC started with a phase I clinical trial for patients with solid tumors, which became enriched for MTC patients once favorable responses were seen.[107] Of the 37 patients with MTC enrolled in this trial, all of whom had progressive disease prior to study entry, 29% had a PR with a combined benefit (PR plus stable disease) seen in 68% of the patients. Due to these encouraging findings, a multicenter, randomized controlled phase III trial (EXAM trial) was conducted where patients with MTC were randomized to cabozantinib or placebo in a 2:1 distribution (n = 330).[11] There are some important differences to highlight in this trial compared with the ZETA study. One is that patients in the EXAM trial had to demonstrate progression by RECIST within 14 months prior to study entry, whereas the ZETA study included patients who had stable disease at baseline. The other is that the study design of the EXAM trial did not allow crossing over to active drug treatment if a patient on placebo demonstrates progression due to the primary objective of measuring PFS. The median PFS was significantly longer in the cabozantinib-treated patients (11.2 months) compared with the placebo group (4.0 months), with a PR of 28% for cabozantinib but 0% in placebo-treated patients. Responses were observed regardless of *RET* mutation status and correlations of radiologic response were made with changes in Ct and CEA levels from baseline. Findings from this study led to the approval of cabozantinib in the United States by the FDA in November 2012 for patients with progressive MTC.

Treatment with TKIs is associated with multiple side effects, which can be dose limiting. Common toxicities with TKIs include the following: dermatologic (palmar-plantar erythrodysesthesia, photosensitivity), mucocutaneous (stomatitis and taste changes), cardiovascular (hypertension), GI (diarrhea, nausea, and anorexia), systemic (fatigue), and uncontrolled hypothyroidism. In relation to vandetanib, the most common side effects ($\geq$20%) included (in descending frequency) diarrhea, rash, nausea, hypertension, fatigue, headache, and diminished appetite.[12] QTc prolongation was observed in 14% patients (any grade) treated with vandetanib and an 8% incidence of grade 3 or above (by Common Terminology Criteria for Adverse Events), although there were no reports of torsades de pointes. Thus, there is a black box warning on the package insert for vandetanib specifying the necessity to monitor ECGs routinely when treated with this agent, avoid medications which are known to prolong the QT interval, correct electrolyte abnormalities (hypocalcemia, hypokalemia, and hypomagnesemia), and correct hypothyroidism. Cabozantinib was associated with the following common side effects (≥20%, in descending frequency): diarrhea, palmar-plantar erythrodysesthesia, weight loss, diminished appetite, nausea, fatigue, taste change, hair color changes, hypertension, stomatitis, constipation, hemorrhage, vomiting, mucosal inflammation, asthenia, and dysphonia.[11] Grade 3 or above adverse events of greater than or equal to 5% involved diarrhea, palmar-plantar erythrodysesthesia, fatigue, hypertension, and asthenia. VEGF-related inhibition with cabozantinib is associated with hemorrhage, venous thrombosis, GI perforation, and fistula formation (adverse events grade 3 or above of 1%–3.7%). Due to these findings, there is a black box warning on the package insert for cabozantinib for the risks of GI perforation, fistula, and hemorrhage. Given the side effect profiles of each of these drugs and the variable propensity for specific side effects, careful recommendation of systemic chemotherapy for MTC patients must be patient centered with consideration of the underlying risk for serious side effects, such as QT prolongation or hemorrhage/fistula/perforation. There is an ongoing trial evaluating 2 different doses of vandetanib (150 mg or 300 mg daily doses). A study looking at 2 different doses cabozantinib is planned (140 mg daily or a lower dose). These 2 postmarketing studies would enlighten as to whether a lower dose can maintain effectiveness with fewer adverse effects.

At this time, there are no formal guidelines on when to recommend systemic therapy or which drug to use. In the authors' experience, patients with the following should be considered for treatment with vandetanib or cabozantinib: progressive disease as determined by RECIST within 14 months, symptomatic disease despite best supportive care or localized therapy, local or impending compromise of neighboring structures not amenable for targeted treatment, or select cases with MTC-related problems not controlled with standard treatments (diarrhea and Cushing syndrome).

Beyond the TKIs, other systemic treatments may have future promise. Vaccine-based and radioisotope immunotherapy in MTC have been studied or are still under investigation; these have not been established as yet to be of clinical benefit.[108–111] There is an ongoing, multicenter, phase II trial with an MTOR inhibitor, everolimus, for metastatic thyroid cancer of all histologies; the results have not been presented to date. Another phase II trial with everolimus, however, in patients with thyroid cancer of any histology reported that of the 8 patients with MTC, all had stable disease as the best response.[112]

SUMMARY

The recognition that activating mutations in the *RET* proto-oncogene cause a substantial number of hereditary and sporadic MTCs has facilitated the identification of specific syndromes and genotype-phenotype correlations. These genotype-phenotype correlations predict the clinical behavior and prognosis of MTC, delineating the characteristics of its follow-up. Furthermore, this knowledge has led to one of the most perfect forms of cancer prevention as a total thyroidectomy is offered to patients with predisposition for MTC. Unfortunately, many patients with hereditary and sporadic MTC still present with noncurable disease. Nevertheless, the characterization of receptors and molecular pathways responsible for MTC development has allowed the discovery of molecular targeted therapies that cause reduction of tumor size, disease stabilization, and symptomatic improvement. Clinical trials are now guiding clinicians on how to treat patients with MTC. There is much research needed, however, to understand which patients would most benefit from drug therapy given the side-effect profiles of current available agents and the lack of survival benefit from the clinical data available to date. On the brighter side, the past decade of basic science and clinical research has led to great advancements in the understanding of the pathogenesis of MTC and reaching the ultimate goal of discovering a cure.

REFERENCES

1. Jimenez C, Gagel RF. Genetic testing in endocrinology: lessons learned from experience with multiple endocrine neoplasia type 2 (MEN2). Growth Horm IGF Res 2004;14(Suppl A):S150–7.
2. Dvorakova S, Vaclavikova E, Sykorova V, et al. Somatic mutations in the RET proto-oncogene in sporadic medullary thyroid carcinomas. Mol Cell Endocrinol 2008;284(1–2):21–7.
3. Elisei R, Cosci B, Romei C, et al. Prognostic significance of somatic RET oncogene mutations in sporadic medullary thyroid cancer: a 10-year follow-up study. J Clin Endocrinol Metab 2008;93(3):682–7.
4. Moura MM, Cavaco BM, Pinto AE, et al. Correlation of RET somatic mutations with clinicopathological features in sporadic medullary thyroid carcinomas. Br J Cancer 2009;100(11):1777–83.
5. Gardner E, Papi L, Easton DF, et al. Genetic linkage studies map the multiple endocrine neoplasia type 2 loci to a small interval on chromosome 10q11.2. Hum Mol Genet 1993;2(3):241–6.
6. Pasini B, Hofstra RM, Yin L, et al. The physical map of the human RET proto-oncogene. Oncogene 1995;11(9):1737–43.
7. Anders J, Kjar S, Ibanez CF. Molecular modeling of the extracellular domain of the RET receptor tyrosine kinase reveals multiple cadherin-like domains and a calcium-binding site. J Biol Chem 2001;276(38):35808–17.
8. Tsui-Pierchala BA, Milbrandt J, Johnson EM Jr. NGF utilizes c-Ret via a novel GFL-independent, inter-RTK signaling mechanism to maintain the trophic status of mature sympathetic neurons. Neuron 2002;33(2):261–73.
9. Airaksinen MS, Saarma M. The GDNF family: signalling, biological functions and therapeutic value. Nat Rev Neurosci 2002;3(5):383–94.
10. Ichihara M, Murakumo Y, Takahashi M. RET and neuroendocrine tumors. Cancer Lett 2004;204(2):197–211.
11. Elisei R, Schlumberger MJ, Muller SP, et al. Cabozantinib in progressive medullary thyroid cancer. J Clin Oncol 2013;31(29):3639–46.
12. Wells SA Jr, Robinson BG, Gagel RF, et al. Vandetanib in patients with locally advanced or metastatic medullary thyroid cancer: a randomized, double-blind phase III trial. J Clin Oncol 2012;30(2):134–41.
13. Terman BI, Dougher-Vermazen M, Carrion ME, et al. Identification of the KDR tyrosine kinase as a receptor for vascular endothelial cell growth factor. Biochem Biophys Res Commun 1992;187(3):1579–86.
14. Shibuya M, Claesson-Welsh L. Signal transduction by VEGF receptors in regulation of angiogenesis and lymphangiogenesis. Exp Cell Res 2006;312(5):549–60.
15. Kerbel RS. Tumor angiogenesis. N Engl J Med 2008;358(19):2039–49.
16. Capp C, Wajner SM, Siqueira DR, et al. Increased expression of vascular endothelial growth factor and its receptors, VEGFR-1 and VEGFR-2, in medullary thyroid carcinoma. Thyroid 2010;20(8):863–71.
17. Rodriguez-Antona C, Pallares J, Montero-Conde C, et al. Overexpression and activation of EGFR and VEGFR2 in medullary thyroid carcinomas is related to metastasis. Endocr Relat Cancer 2010;17(1):7–16.

18. Gomez K, Varghese J, Jimenez C. Medullary thyroid carcinoma: molecular signaling pathways and emerging therapies. J Thyroid Res 2011;2011: 815826.
19. Mitsiades CS, Kotoula V, Poulaki V, et al. Epidermal growth factor receptor as a therapeutic target in human thyroid carcinoma: mutational and functional analysis. J Clin Endocrinol Metab 2006;91(9):3662–6.
20. Jorissen RN, Walker F, Pouliot N, et al. Epidermal growth factor receptor: mechanisms of activation and signalling. Exp Cell Res 2003;284(1):31–53.
21. Holbro T, Civenni G, Hynes NE. The ErbB receptors and their role in cancer progression. Exp Cell Res 2003;284(1):99–110.
22. Vlahovic G, Crawford J. Activation of tyrosine kinases in cancer. Oncologist 2003;8(6):531–8.
23. Croyle M, Akeno N, Knauf JA, et al. RET/PTC-induced cell growth is mediated in part by epidermal growth factor receptor (EGFR) activation: evidence for molecular and functional interactions between RET and EGFR. Cancer Res 2008; 68(11):4183–91.
24. Bottaro DP, Rubin JS, Faletto DL, et al. Identification of the hepatocyte growth factor receptor as the c-met proto-oncogene product. Science 1991;251(4995): 802–4.
25. Corso S, Migliore C, Ghiso E, et al. Silencing the MET oncogene leads to regression of experimental tumors and metastases. Oncogene 2008;27(5):684–93.
26. Papotti M, Olivero M, Volante M, et al. Expression of Hepatocyte Growth Factor (HGF) and its Receptor (MET) in Medullary Carcinoma of the Thyroid. Endocr Pathol 2000;11(1):19–30.
27. Wasenius VM, Hemmer S, Karjalainen-Lindsberg ML, et al. MET receptor tyrosine kinase sequence alterations in differentiated thyroid carcinoma. Am J Surg Pathol 2005;29(4):544–9.
28. Ivan M, Bond JA, Prat M, et al. Activated ras and ret oncogenes induce overexpression of c-met (hepatocyte growth factor receptor) in human thyroid epithelial cells. Oncogene 1997;14(20):2417–23.
29. Ezzat S, Huang P, Dackiw A, et al. Dual inhibition of RET and FGFR4 restrains medullary thyroid cancer cell growth. Clin Cancer Res 2005;11(3):1336–41.
30. St Bernard R, Zheng L, Liu W, et al. Fibroblast growth factor receptors as molecular targets in thyroid carcinoma. Endocrinology 2005;146(3):1145–53.
31. Bos JL. RAS oncogenes in human cancer: a review. Cancer Res 1989;49(17): 4682–9.
32. Pylayeva-Gupta Y, Grabocka E, Bar-Sagi D. RAS oncogenes: weaving a tumorigenic web. Nat Rev Cancer 2011;11(11):761–74.
33. Ciampi R, Mian C, Fugazzola L, et al. Evidence of a low prevalence of RAS mutations in a large medullary thyroid cancer series. Thyroid 2013;23(1): 50–7.
34. Agrawal N, Jiao Y, Sausen M, et al. Exomic sequencing of medullary thyroid cancer reveals dominant and mutually exclusive oncogenic mutations in RET and RAS. J Clin Endocrinol Metab 2013;98(2):E364–9.
35. Giunti S, Antonelli A, Amorosi A, et al. Cellular signaling pathway alterations and potential targeted therapies for medullary thyroid carcinoma. Int J Endocrinol 2013;2013:803171.
36. Jimenez C, Hu MI, Gagel RF. Management of medullary thyroid carcinoma. Endocrinol Metab Clin North Am 2008;37(2):481–96, x–xi.
37. Moley JF, Wells SA. Compartment-mediated dissection for papillary thyroid cancer. Langenbecks Arch Surg 1999;384(1):9–15.

38. Moley JF, Lairmore TC, Doherty GM, et al. Preservation of the recurrent laryngeal nerves in thyroid and parathyroid reoperations. Surgery 1999;126(4):673–7 [discussion: 677–9].

39. Wohllk N, Cote GJ, Bugalho MM, et al. Relevance of RET proto-oncogene mutations in sporadic medullary thyroid carcinoma. J Clin Endocrinol Metab 1996;81(10):3740–5.

40. Thosani S, Ayala-Ramirez M, Palmer L, et al. The characterization of pheochromocytoma and its impact on overall survival in multiple endocrine neoplasia type 2. J Clin Endocrinol Metab 2013;98(11):E1813–9.

41. Ayala-Ramirez M, Feng L, Johnson MM, et al. Clinical risk factors for malignancy and overall survival in patients with pheochromocytomas and sympathetic paragangliomas: primary tumor size and primary tumor location as prognostic indicators. J Clin Endocrinol Metab 2011;96(3):717–25.

42. Jimenez C, Cote G, Arnold A, et al. Review: should patients with apparently sporadic pheochromocytomas or paragangliomas be screened for hereditary syndromes? J Clin Endocrinol Metab 2006;91(8):2851–8.

43. Chang TC, Wu SL, Hsiao YL. Medullary thyroid carcinoma: pitfalls in diagnosis by fine needle aspiration cytology and relationship of cytomorphology to RET proto-oncogene mutations. Acta Cytol 2005;49(5):477–82.

44. Papaparaskeva K, Nagel H, Droese M. Cytologic diagnosis of medullary carcinoma of the thyroid gland. Diagn Cytopathol 2000;22(6):351–8.

45. Bugalho MJ, Santos JR, Sobrinho L. Preoperative diagnosis of medullary thyroid carcinoma: fine needle aspiration cytology as compared with serum calcitonin measurement. J Surg Oncol 2005;91(1):56–60.

46. Chen H, Sippel RS, O'Dorisio MS, et al. The North American Neuroendocrine Tumor Society consensus guideline for the diagnosis and management of neuroendocrine tumors: pheochromocytoma, paraganglioma, and medullary thyroid cancer. Pancreas 2010;39(6):775–83.

47. Boi F, Maurelli I, Pinna G, et al. Calcitonin measurement in wash-out fluid from fine needle aspiration of neck masses in patients with primary and metastatic medullary thyroid carcinoma. J Clin Endocrinol Metab 2007;92(6):2115–8.

48. Kudo T, Miyauchi A, Ito Y, et al. Diagnosis of medullary thyroid carcinoma by calcitonin measurement in fine-needle aspiration biopsy specimens. Thyroid 2007;17(7):635–8.

49. Costante G, Meringolo D, Durante C, et al. Predictive value of serum calcitonin levels for preoperative diagnosis of medullary thyroid carcinoma in a cohort of 5817 consecutive patients with thyroid nodules. J Clin Endocrinol Metab 2007;92(2):450–5.

50. Kloos RT, Eng C, Evans DB, et al. Medullary thyroid cancer: management guidelines of the American Thyroid Association. Thyroid 2009;19(6):565–612.

51. Machens A, Ukkat J, Hauptmann S, et al. Abnormal carcinoembryonic antigen levels and medullary thyroid cancer progression: a multivariate analysis. Arch Surg 2007;142(3):289–93 [discussion: 294].

52. Ambrosini V, Marzola MC, Rubello D, et al. (68)Ga-somatostatin analogues PET and (18)F-DOPA PET in medullary thyroid carcinoma. Eur J Nucl Med Mol Imaging 2010;37(1):46–8.

53. Laure Giraudet A, Al Ghulzan A, Auperin A, et al. Progression of medullary thyroid carcinoma: assessment with calcitonin and carcinoembryonic antigen doubling times. Eur J Endocrinol 2008;158(2):239–46.

54. Treglia G, Castaldi P, Villani MF, et al. Comparison of 18F-DOPA, 18F-FDG and 68Ga-somatostatin analogue PET/CT in patients with recurrent medullary thyroid carcinoma. Eur J Nucl Med Mol Imaging 2012;39(4):569–80.

55. Beheshti M, Pocher S, Vali R, et al. The value of 18F-DOPA PET-CT in patients with medullary thyroid carcinoma: comparison with 18F-FDG PET-CT. Eur Radiol 2009;19(6):1425–34.
56. Ong SC, Schoder H, Patel SG, et al. Diagnostic accuracy of 18F-FDG PET in restaging patients with medullary thyroid carcinoma and elevated calcitonin levels. J Nucl Med 2007;48(4):501–7.
57. Verbeek HH, Plukker JT, Koopmans KP, et al. Clinical relevance of 18F-FDG PET and 18F-DOPA PET in recurrent medullary thyroid carcinoma. J Nucl Med 2012; 53(12):1863–71.
58. Wong KK, Laird AM, Moubayed A, et al. How has the management of medullary thyroid carcinoma changed with the advent of 18F-FDG and non-18F-FDG PET radiopharmaceuticals. Nucl Med Commun 2012;33(7):679–88.
59. Diehl M, Risse JH, Brandt-Mainz K, et al. Fluorine-18 fluorodeoxyglucose positron emission tomography in medullary thyroid cancer: results of a multicentre study. Eur J Nucl Med 2001;28(11):1671–6.
60. Skoura E, Datseris IE, Rondogianni P, et al. Correlation between calcitonin levels and [(18)F]FDG-PET/CT in the detection of recurrence in patients with sporadic and hereditary medullary thyroid cancer. ISRN Endocrinol 2012; 2012:375231.
61. Bogsrud TV, Karantanis D, Nathan MA, et al. The prognostic value of 2-deoxy-2-[18F]fluoro-D-glucose positron emission tomography in patients with suspected residual or recurrent medullary thyroid carcinoma. Mol Imag Biol 2010;12(5): 547–53.
62. Oudoux A, Salaun PY, Bournaud C, et al. Sensitivity and prognostic value of positron emission tomography with F-18-fluorodeoxyglucose and sensitivity of immunoscintigraphy in patients with medullary thyroid carcinoma treated with anticarcinoembryonic antigen-targeted radioimmunotherapy. J Clin Endocrinol Metab 2007;92(12):4590–7.
63. Hoegerle S, Altehoefer C, Ghanem N, et al. 18F-DOPA positron emission tomography for tumour detection in patients with medullary thyroid carcinoma and elevated calcitonin levels. Eur J Nucl Med 2001;28(1):64–71.
64. Conry BG, Papathanasiou ND, Prakash V, et al. Comparison of (68)Ga-DOTATATE and (18)F-fluorodeoxyglucose PET/CT in the detection of recurrent medullary thyroid carcinoma. Eur J Nucl Med Mol Imaging 2010;37(1):49–57.
65. Schirrmeister H, Guhlmann A, Elsner K, et al. Sensitivity in detecting osseous lesions depends on anatomic localization: planar bone scintigraphy versus 18F PET. J Nucl Med 1999;40(10):1623–9.
66. Schirrmeister H, Guhlmann A, Kotzerke J, et al. Early detection and accurate description of extent of metastatic bone disease in breast cancer with fluoride ion and positron emission tomography. J Clin Oncol 1999;17(8):2381–9.
67. Frank-Raue K, Bihl H, Dorr U, et al. Somatostatin receptor imaging in persistent medullary thyroid carcinoma. Clin Endocrinol 1995;42(1):31–7.
68. Baudin E, Lumbroso J, Schlumberger M, et al. Comparison of octreotide scintigraphy and conventional imaging in medullary thyroid carcinoma. J Nucl Med 1996;37(6):912–6.
69. Lodish M, Dagalakis U, Chen CC, et al. (111)In-octreotide scintigraphy for identification of metastatic medullary thyroid carcinoma in children and adolescents. J Clin Endocrinol Metab 2012;97(2):E207–12.
70. Barbet J, Campion L, Kraeber-Bodere F, et al. Prognostic impact of serum calcitonin and carcinoembryonic antigen doubling-times in patients with medullary thyroid carcinoma. J Clin Endocrinol Metab 2005;90(11):6077–84.

71. Miyauchi A, Onishi T, Morimoto S, et al. Relation of doubling time of plasma calcitonin levels to prognosis and recurrence of medullary thyroid carcinoma. Ann Surg 1984;199(4):461–6.

72. Meijer JA, le Cessie S, van den Hout WB, et al. Calcitonin and carcinoembryonic antigen doubling times as prognostic factors in medullary thyroid carcinoma: a structured meta-analysis. Clin Endocrinol 2010;72(4):534–42.

73. Wang TS, Ocal IT, Sosa JA, et al. Medullary thyroid carcinoma without marked elevation of calcitonin: a diagnostic and surveillance dilemma. Thyroid 2008; 18(8):889–94.

74. Pazaitou-Panayiotou K, Chrisoulidou A, Mandanas S, et al. Predictive factors that influence the course of medullary thyroid carcinoma. Int J Clin Oncol 2013. [Epub ahead of print].

75. Taccaliti A, Silvetti F, Palmonella G, et al. Genetic alterations in medullary thyroid cancer: diagnostic and prognostic markers. Curr Genomics 2011;12(8):618–25.

76. Romei C, Elisei R, Pinchera A, et al. Somatic mutations of the ret protooncogene in sporadic medullary thyroid carcinoma are not restricted to exon 16 and are associated with tumor recurrence. J Clin Endocrinol Metab 1996;81(4):1619–22.

77. Schilling T, Burck J, Sinn HP, et al. Prognostic value of codon 918 (ATG–>ACG) RET proto-oncogene mutations in sporadic medullary thyroid carcinoma. Int J Cancer 2001;95(1):62–6.

78. Abraham DT, Low TH, Messina M, et al. Medullary thyroid carcinoma: long-term outcomes of surgical treatment. Ann Surg Oncol 2011;18(1):219–25.

79. Cupisti K, Wolf A, Raffel A, et al. Long-term clinical and biochemical follow-up in medullary thyroid carcinoma: a single institution's experience over 20 years. Ann Surg 2007;246(5):815–21.

80. Pelizzo MR, Boschin IM, Bernante P, et al. Natural history, diagnosis, treatment and outcome of medullary thyroid cancer: 37 years experience on 157 patients. Eur J Surg Oncol 2007;33(4):493–7.

81. Brierley J, Tsang R, Simpson WJ, et al. Medullary thyroid cancer: analyses of survival and prognostic factors and the role of radiation therapy in local control. Thyroid 1996;6(4):305–10.

82. Hyer SL, Vini L, A'Hern R, et al. Medullary thyroid cancer: multivariate analysis of prognostic factors influencing survival. Eur J Surg Oncol 2000;26(7):686–90.

83. Kebebew E, Ituarte PH, Siperstein AE, et al. Medullary thyroid carcinoma: clinical characteristics, treatment, prognostic factors, and a comparison of staging systems. Cancer 2000;88(5):1139–48.

84. Saad MF, Ordonez NG, Rashid RK, et al. Medullary carcinoma of the thyroid. A study of the clinical features and prognostic factors in 161 patients. Medicine 1984;63(6):319–42.

85. de Groot JW, Plukker JT, Wolffenbuttel BH, et al. Determinants of life expectancy in medullary thyroid cancer: age does not matter. Clin Endocrinol 2006;65(6): 729–36.

86. Waguespack SG, Rich TA, Perrier ND, et al. Management of medullary thyroid carcinoma and MEN2 syndromes in childhood. Nat Rev Endocrinol 2011; 7(10):596–607.

87. Moley JF, DeBenedetti MK. Patterns of nodal metastases in palpable medullary thyroid carcinoma: recommendations for extent of node dissection. Ann Surg 1999;229(6):880–7 [discussion: 887–8].

88. Machens A, Schneyer U, Holzhausen HJ, et al. Prospects of remission in medullary thyroid carcinoma according to basal calcitonin level. J Clin Endocrinol Metab 2005;90(4):2029–34.

89. Roman S, Lin R, Sosa JA. Prognosis of medullary thyroid carcinoma: demographic, clinical, and pathologic predictors of survival in 1252 cases. Cancer 2006;107(9):2134–42.
90. Giuliani M, Brierley J. Indications for the use of external beam radiation in thyroid cancer. Curr Opin Oncol 2013;26(1):45–50.
91. Yen TW, Shapiro SE, Gagel RF, et al. Medullary thyroid carcinoma: results of a standardized surgical approach in a contemporary series of 80 consecutive patients. Surgery 2003;134(6):890–9 [discussion: 899–901].
92. Fromigue J, De Baere T, Baudin E, et al. Chemoembolization for liver metastases from medullary thyroid carcinoma. J Clin Endocrinol Metab 2006;91(7):2496–9.
93. Orita Y, Sugitani I, Toda K, et al. Zoledronic acid in the treatment of bone metastases from differentiated thyroid carcinoma. Thyroid 2011;21(1):31–5.
94. Vitale G, Fonderico F, Martignetti A, et al. Pamidronate improves the quality of life and induces clinical remission of bone metastases in patients with thyroid cancer. Br J Cancer 2001;84(12):1586–90.
95. Available at: https://www.nccn.org/professionals/physician_gls/pdf/thyroid.pdf. Accessed November 24, 2013.
96. Mahler C, Verhelst J, de Longueville M, et al. Long-term treatment of metastatic medullary thyroid carcinoma with the somatostatin analogue octreotide. Clin Endocrinol 1990;33(2):261–9.
97. Vainas I, Koussis C, Pazaitou-Panayiotou K, et al. Somatostatin receptor expression in vivo and response to somatostatin analog therapy with or without other antineoplastic treatments in advanced medullary thyroid carcinoma. J Exp Clin Cancer Res 2004;23(4):549–59.
98. Vitale G, Caraglia M, Ciccarelli A, et al. Current approaches and perspectives in the therapy of medullary thyroid carcinoma. Cancer 2001;91(9):1797–808.
99. Castellani MR, Seregni E, Maccauro M, et al. MIBG for diagnosis and therapy of medullary thyroid carcinoma: is there still a role? Q J Nucl Med Mol Imaging 2008;52(4):430–40.
100. Diez JJ, Iglesias P. Somatostatin analogs in the treatment of medullary thyroid carcinoma. J Endocrinol Invest 2002;25(9):773–8.
101. Monsieurs M, Brans B, Bacher K, et al. Patient dosimetry for 131I-MIBG therapy for neuroendocrine tumours based on 123I-MIBG scans. Eur J Nucl Med Mol Imaging 2002;29(12):1581–7.
102. Lalami Y, Awada A. Recurrent thyroid cancer: a molecular-based therapeutic breakthrough. Curr Opin Oncol 2011;23(3):235–40.
103. Sherman SI. Advances in chemotherapy of differentiated epithelial and medullary thyroid cancers. J Clin Endocrinol Metab 2009;94(5):1493–9.
104. Robinson BG, Paz-Ares L, Krebs A, et al. Vandetanib (100 mg) in patients with locally advanced or metastatic hereditary medullary thyroid cancer. J Clin Endocrinol Metab 2010;95(6):2664–71.
105. Wells SA Jr, Gosnell JE, Gagel RF, et al. Vandetanib for the treatment of patients with locally advanced or metastatic hereditary medullary thyroid cancer. J Clin Oncol 2010;28(5):767–72.
106. Available at: http://www.recist.com. Accessed November 25, 2013.
107. Kurzrock R, Sherman SI, Ball DW, et al. Activity of XL184 (Cabozantinib), an oral tyrosine kinase inhibitor, in patients with medullary thyroid cancer. J Clin Oncol 2011;29(19):2660–6.
108. Bachleitner-Hofmann T, Friedl J, Hassler M, et al. Pilot trial of autologous dendritic cells loaded with tumor lysate(s) from allogeneic tumor cell lines in patients with metastatic medullary thyroid carcinoma. Oncol Rep 2009;21(6):1585–92.

109. Papewalis C, Wuttke M, Jacobs B, et al. Dendritic cell vaccination induces tumor epitope-specific Th1 immune response in medullary thyroid carcinoma. Horm Metab Res 2008;40(2):108–16.
110. Salaun PY, Campion L, Bournaud C, et al. Phase II trial of anticarcinoembryonic antigen pretargeted radioimmunotherapy in progressive metastatic medullary thyroid carcinoma: biomarker response and survival improvement. J Nucl Med 2012;53(8):1185–92.
111. Stift A, Sachet M, Yagubian R, et al. Dendritic cell vaccination in medullary thyroid carcinoma. Clin Cancer Res 2004;10(9):2944–53.
112. Lim SM, Chang H, Yoon MJ, et al. A multicenter, phase II trial of everolimus in locally advanced or metastatic thyroid cancer of all histologic subtypes. Ann Oncol 2013;24(12):3089–94.

Surgery for Thyroid Cancer

Glenda G. Callender, MD[a], Tobias Carling, MD, PhD[a],
Emily Christison-Lagay, MD[b], Robert Udelsman, MD, MBA[a,c,*]

KEYWORDS

- Thyroid cancer surgery • Central neck dissection • Modified radical neck dissection
- Pediatric thyroid cancer

KEY POINTS

- Surgery is the treatment of choice for most patients with thyroid cancer.
- Surgical experience is directly related to favorable outcomes.
- Several aspects of thyroid cancer surgery are controversial and expert judgment is required.

INTRODUCTION

The incidence of thyroid cancer is rising rapidly. In women, the incidence of thyroid cancer is rising more rapidly than that of any other malignancy. According to the National Cancer Institute Surveillance, Epidemiology and End Results database, approximately 60,220 people in the United States were diagnosed with thyroid cancer in 2013 and 1850 people died from their disease.[1,2] Papillary thyroid carcinoma (PTC) is the most common endocrine malignancy, and the rising incidence of thyroid cancer in the United States is largely related to the rising incidence of PTC. In 1990, the annual incidence rate of PTC was 5.50 per 100,000 people per year, and by 2010, the annual incidence had reached 13.83 per 100,000 people per year.[3–6] Although much of the rising incidence of PTC is accounted for by an increased rate of detection of papillary thyroid microcarcinoma (PTMC; PTC ≤1 cm) related to medical surveillance and more sensitive diagnostic studies, particularly ultrasound, there is evidence that increased diagnosis cannot completely explain the observed increase in the incidence of PTC.[3,4] The incidence rates of the other histologic subtypes of thyroid cancer (follicular thyroid carcinoma [FTC], medullary thyroid carcinoma [MTC], and anaplastic thyroid carcinoma [ATC]) have increased modestly over the past four decades.[3,4]

Disclosure Statement: The Authors have nothing to disclose.
[a] Section of Endocrine Surgery, Department of Surgery, Yale University School of Medicine, New Haven, CT, USA; [b] Section of Pediatric Surgery, Department of Surgery, Yale University School of Medicine, New Haven, CT, USA; [c] Yale-New Haven Hospital, Yale University School of Medicine, 330 Cedar Street, FMB 102, PO Box 208062, New Haven, CT 06520–8062, USA
* Corresponding author. Yale-New Haven Hospital, Yale University School of Medicine, 330 Cedar Street, FMB 102, PO Box 208062, New Haven, CT 06520–8062.
E-mail address: robert.udelsman@yale.edu

Endocrinol Metab Clin N Am 43 (2014) 443–458
http://dx.doi.org/10.1016/j.ecl.2014.02.011
0889-8529/14/$ – see front matter © 2014 Elsevier Inc. All rights reserved.

The rising incidence of thyroid cancer is accompanied by an increased need for physicians and surgeons with a thorough understanding of the management of thyroid cancer. Although the extent of surgery for thyroid cancer remains controversial, patients with thyroid cancer usually require more extensive resections than do patients with benign thyroid disease. A study of 5860 thyroidectomies in Maryland from 1991 to 1996 demonstrated that, when operating for thyroid cancer, high-volume thyroid surgeons (>100 cases over the 6-year period) experienced complication rates at least two-thirds lower than those of low-volume surgeons (one to nine cases over the 6-year period), and lower hospital lengths of stay and lower costs.[7] It is inappropriate for surgeons to be mere "technicians" in the care of patients with thyroid cancer; the surgeon must understand how to translate emerging data and new technology into optimal care for the patient with thyroid cancer.

This article focuses on the surgical management of thyroid cancer in adult and pediatric patients. Because this issue of *Endocrinology Clinics of North America* is comprehensive, we have purposefully excluded lengthy discussions of thyroid nodules and molecular markers, alternative surgical approaches to the thyroid gland, and MTC, because these are covered in detail elsewhere in the issue.

INDICATIONS

Surgery for thyroid cancer is typically performed for one of the following reasons: (1) diagnostic resection of a thyroid lobe containing a nodule suspected to be a thyroid cancer, (2) treatment of a known thyroid cancer, (3) prophylaxis in patients who screen positive for a genetic mutation that places them at high risk for development of thyroid cancer, or (4) to treat recurrent thyroid cancer.

Thyroid cancer typically presents as a solitary thyroid nodule discovered because of symptoms, a palpable mass, or imaging performed for another reason. According to American Thyroid Association management guidelines published in 2009, ultrasound-guided fine-needle aspiration (FNA) biopsy is recommended for all thyroid nodules greater than or equal to 1 cm, unless the sonographic appearance is completely characteristic of a benign nodule (eg, a pure cystic or spongiform nodule); FNA biopsy should also be considered for subcentimeter thyroid nodules with a suspicious appearance (eg, solid, hypoechoic, with calcifications) and factors that put the individual at increased risk of thyroid cancer because of personal or family history or prior radiation exposure.[8]

The interpretation of thyroid cytopathology has historically been difficult and fraught with wide interobserver variability. In 2009, the Bethesda classification system of thyroid cytopathology was published, and its widespread adoption has helped standardize thyroid FNA reporting. The Bethesda system requires that cytologists assign thyroid cytology to one of six categories based on the adequacy of the sample and the risk of malignancy (**Table 1**).[9] This standardized approach removes much of the vague language of cytology reports that existed previously, and the information ultimately assists clinicians in determining appropriate management. However, it is important that institutions not rely solely on published categorical malignancy rates, but rather, determine their own rates. For example, published rates of malignancy in the diagnostic category "suspicious for PTC" range from 50% to 75%, suggesting that diagnostic thyroid lobectomy may be appropriate initial management; however, in our institution, this category is associated with PTC in more than 90%, and therefore, a formal oncologic operation is usually selected.

Molecular markers are increasingly used to improve the diagnostic accuracy of thyroid nodule FNA biopsy. The BRAF V600E mutation is the most commonly used

Table 1
Bethesda classification system for thyroid cytopathology

Category	Risk of Malignancy	Recommended Initial Management
1. Nondiagnostic/unsatisfactory	1%–4%	Repeat FNA
2. Benign	0%–3%	Clinical follow-up
3. Follicular lesion (atypia) of uncertain significance	5%–15%	Repeat FNA, clinical follow-up, or diagnostic thyroid lobectomy[a]
4. Follicular neoplasm	20%–30%	Diagnostic thyroid lobectomy
5. Suspicious for malignancy	60%–75%	Diagnostic thyroid lobectomy with frozen section and formal thyroid cancer operation if frozen section positive; or up-front formal thyroid cancer operation[a]
6. Malignant	97%–99%	Formal thyroid cancer operation

Abbreviation: FNA, fine-needle aspiration.
[a] Depending on institutional rates of malignancy; BRAF and other molecular markers may be useful in interpretation of risk of malignancy in these categories.
From Cibas ES, Ali SZ. The Bethesda System for reporting thyroid cytopathology. Am J Clin Pathol 2009;132:660; with permission.

mutation marker. It is present in 40% to 70% of PTCs, and has a positive predictive value of nearly 100%; however, its negative predictive value is low, and therefore it cannot be reliably used to rule out cancer in an indeterminate FNA.[10] This topic is addressed in detail elsewhere in this issue.

PREOPERATIVE SURGICAL EVALUATION

The patient history should include symptoms of mass effect, such as globus sensation, difficulty swallowing or breathing, pressure in the neck when lying supine or when turning the head, and stridor. Voice changes or hoarseness could signal involvement of the recurrent laryngeal nerve. Symptoms of thyrotoxicosis or hypothyroidism should be elicited. Patients with MTC should be asked about symptoms of hypercalcitoninemia, including flushing and diarrhea, indicating advanced disease. They should also be asked about symptoms suggestive of a pheochromocytoma. Patients should be asked specifically about all prior surgery, especially procedures in the central and lateral neck, and a history of radiation to the head or neck.

It is important to investigate a personal or family history of thyroid cancer and other cancers. In tertiary centers, approximately 25% of cases of MTC result from germline *RET* protooncogene mutations and the consequent inherited autosomal-dominant syndromes (multiple endocrine neoplasia [MEN] 2A, MEN2B, or familial MTC; an expanded discussion of MTC can be found elsewhere in this issue).[11–13] Nonmedullary thyroid cancers (PTC and FTC) are familial in up to 5% of cases, although a specific mutation has not been identified.[14] Several other inherited cancer syndromes include nonmedullary thyroid cancers. Cowden syndrome results from autosomal-dominant mutations in the *PTEN* suppressor gene and is characterized by hamartomas and an increased risk of breast, endometrial, thyroid, colorectal, and kidney cancers. In Cowden syndrome, up to 70% of patients have benign thyroid nodules, and approximately 10% develop thyroid cancers, which are usually FTC or (less commonly) the follicular variant of PTC.[15] Familial adenomatous polyposis is an autosomal-dominant syndrome that results from mutations in the *APC* gene, and leads to adenomatous polyps carpeting the colon, with nearly 100% incidence of colon cancer if prophylactic colectomy is not performed. Approximately 2% of patients with familial adenomatous polyposis develop thyroid cancer, which is almost invariably the cribiform morular variant of PTC.[16] Carney complex is a rare autosomal-dominant syndrome associated with mutations in the PRKAR1A gene. Patients develop characteristic spotty skin pigmentation, myxomas, schwannomas, primary pigmented nodular adrenocortical disease, and thyroid cancer (FTC or PTC in up to 10% of patients).[17]

Physical examination must include a general assessment of the patient and focused palpation of the thyroid, with particular attention to the characteristics of palpable nodules. Benign nodules are usually smooth and mobile. Cancers are often hard and irregular. Advanced, locally invasive cancers may be fixed to neck structures. The inability to palpate the inferior aspect of the thyroid gland suggests the presence of a substernal goiter and additional imaging with non–intravenous-contrast computed tomography may be warranted to evaluate the extent. Palpation of the lymph node basins of the neck may detect nodes that are grossly involved with metastatic disease. Auscultation over the carotid arteries to detect a carotid bruit is important, because thyroidectomy requires lateral retraction of the carotid arteries, a maneuver that can lead to intraoperative stroke in patients with carotid atherosclerotic disease.

Preoperative evaluation of the vocal cords may be performed using indirect (mirror) or direct (flexible fiberoptic or rigid) laryngoscopy. Preoperative laryngoscopy is essential in a patient whose voice is impaired, or in a patient with a normal voice, but who has previously undergone neck or mediastinal surgery that increases the risk of laryngeal nerve injury or who has thyroid cancer with suspected extrathyroidal extension.[18] However, in a patient with a normal voice, and in whom there is no reason to suspect an immobile vocal cord, formal laryngoscopy seems to add little to the surgeon's evaluation.[19] Nonetheless, in our practice, preoperative (and postoperative) laryngoscopy is routine. We find that it adds little time to the physical examination, represents minimal risk or discomfort to the patient, and has the potential to provide useful information.

Preoperative diagnostic studies in all patients undergoing thyroid surgery must include bloodwork to verify that the patient is euthyroid (ie, FT4 and thyroid-stimulating hormone) and a serum calcium level to screen for concomitant parathyroid disease that should be addressed during thyroidectomy. In a patient with MTC, preoperative genetic testing for RET protooncogene mutations is essential. Failure to diagnose a pheochromocytoma preoperatively (eg, by measuring plasma free metanephrines and normetanephrines) in a patient with syndromic MTC may lead to life-threatening consequences; in addition, the intraoperative management of the parathyroid glands may differ for a patient with syndromic disease.[20,21]

Patients with known thyroid cancer should undergo preoperative staging of the lateral neck lymph node basins by ultrasound mapping. The sensitivity of ultrasound to detect metastatic thyroid cancer in lateral cervical lymph nodes is 90% to 100%.[22] Abnormal lymph nodes should be evaluated by FNA biopsy; biopsy-proved disease in the lateral neck is an indication for modified radical neck dissection.

SURGERY FOR DIFFERENTIATED THYROID CANCER

Surgery is the primary treatment of patients with differentiated thyroid cancer (PTC and FTC). The goals of surgery are to (1) remove locoregional disease (primary tumor and involved regional lymph nodes); (2) facilitate accurate staging; (3) minimize risk of locoregional disease recurrence and metastasis; (4) minimize morbidity; (5) facilitate postoperative treatment with radioactive iodine (RAI), if appropriate; and (6) allow for accurate long-term surveillance for recurrence.[8] Standard treatment of most patients with PTC and FTC is total or near-total thyroidectomy, with dissection of involved lymph node basins.[8]

The optimal extent of thyroidectomy for patients with PTC is controversial. For patients with primary tumors greater than 1 cm, total or near-total thyroidectomy is indicated; in a study of more than 50,000 patients, this approach reduced recurrence and improved survival in patients with PTC greater than 1 cm.[8,23] However, for patients with single, small tumors less than or equal to 1 cm (PTMC), thyroid lobectomy may be considered.[8] Because of the overall excellent prognosis of patients with PTMC, most studies do not demonstrate increased survival rates after total thyroidectomy compared with thyroid lobectomy.[24] However, recurrence rates are higher after lobectomy than total thyroidectomy, even after adjustment for extent of disease.[23,25] Total thyroidectomy also allows postoperative use of RAI scanning to screen for metastatic disease and thyroglobulin use as a tumor marker to detect recurrence. Because of the excellent overall prognosis of patients with PTC, most studies comparing treatment strategies for PTC are underpowered: several thousand patients would be required in each arm to definitively determine that there is no difference between groups.[26] In addition, recent data from Japan demonstrate that observation may be an acceptable option for selected patients with subcentimeter cytologically proved PTC in the absence of worrisome features.[27]

Therapeutic central neck dissection should be performed for clinically involved central neck lymph nodes (**Fig. 1**).[8] Because PTC is metastatic to regional lymph nodes in 20% to 90% of patients at the time of diagnosis, prophylactic central neck dissection

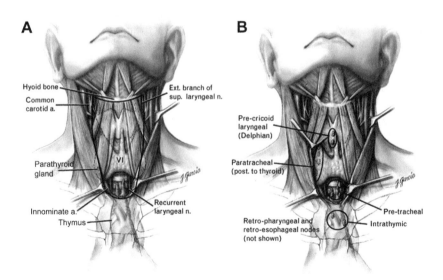

Fig. 1. Anatomy of the central neck (level VI). (*A*) The boundaries of the central neck extend to the medial carotid artery bilaterally, from the hyoid bone to the sternal notch/brachiocephalic vessels. (*B*) A central neck lymph node dissection includes the precricoid laryngeal (Delphian), pretracheal, paratracheal, intrathymic, retropharyngeal, and retroesophageal lymph nodes. (*From* Carty SE, Cooper DS, Doherty GM, et al. Consensus statement on the terminology and classification of central neck dissection for thyroid cancer. Thyroid 2009;19:1156–7; with permission.)

may be considered for patients without clinically involved central neck lymph nodes, especially with larger tumors.[8] Ultrasound is not a good modality for detecting central neck lymph node metastasis, identifying disease preoperatively in only approximately half of patients who ultimately have histopathology-proved involved lymph nodes.[28–30] Thus, central neck disease is usually not diagnosed by preoperative FNA biopsy and central neck dissection is performed either based on clinical suspicion or for prophylactic reasons.

The role of prophylactic central neck dissection in PTC is controversial. There are no randomized data to guide management; an adequately powered randomized trial is unrealistic because of the large number of patients and long follow-up time that would be required to detect a meaningful difference in survival.[26] Existing retrospective data are also underpowered. However, arguments in favor of prophylactic central neck dissection include the following (**Table 2**): (1) metastasis to central neck lymph nodes cannot be reliably detected preoperatively or intraoperatively; (2) central neck dissection improves accuracy in staging, upstaging a substantial proportion of patients from Nx to N1a disease, which may be the only indication for RAI in a subset of patients; (3) central neck dissection results in decreased postoperative serum thyroglobulin levels, allowing greater sensitivity of thyroglobulin to detect recurrence; (4) central neck dissection leads to reduced recurrence rates (and possibly reduced mortality rates); (5) reduced recurrence rates decrease the need for reoperation in the central neck with the associated morbidity; and (6) in the hands of a high-volume endocrine surgeon, central neck dissection can be performed with essentially the same morbidity as thyroidectomy alone.[31,32] Arguments against routine prophylactic central neck dissection include (1) potential for increased rates of hypoparathyroidism and recurrent laryngeal nerve injury, (2) absence of level 1 data that central neck dissection leads to lower recurrence and mortality rates, and (3) most thyroidectomies in the United States (76%) are not performed by high-volume surgeons.[31,33] Therefore, the patient's overall prognosis (based on age and size of the primary tumor), the findings on careful inspection of the central neck lymph nodes at the time of surgery, and the experience of the surgeon all play into the risk-benefit ratio of routine prophylactic central neck dissection for PTC.

Table 2
Arguments for and against prophylactic central neck dissection for papillary thyroid carcinoma

For	Against
May lead to lower recurrence and mortality rates	No level 1 data that recurrence and mortality rates are lower
Can be performed with essentially the same morbidity as thyroidectomy alone in experienced hands	Most thyroidectomies in the United States are not performed by a high-volume surgeon
Preoperative and intraoperative detection of central neck lymph node metastasis is not reliable	May lead to higher rates of hypoparathyroidism and recurrent laryngeal nerve injury
Improves accuracy in staging Decreases postoperative thyroglobulin levels Decreases need for reoperation in the central neck	

From Carling T, Long WD 3rd, Udelsman R. Controversy surrounding the role for routine central lymph node dissection for differentiated thyroid cancer. Curr Opin Oncol 2010;22:32; with permission.

Modified radical neck dissection should be performed for biopsy-proved metastatic disease in the lateral neck (**Fig. 2**).[8] In contrast to the radical neck dissection originally described by George Crile in 1906 for the treatment of head and neck squamous cell carcinoma, modified radical neck dissection preserves the sternocleidomastoid muscle, internal jugular vein, and spinal accessory nerve (functional neck dissection) with much less morbidity.[34] Nonetheless, potential complications include hematoma, seroma, wound infection, chylous leak, pneumothorax, and nerve injury (spinal accessory, marginal mandibular, hypoglossal, vagus, phrenic, sympathetic trunk, brachial plexus, and cutaneous cervical plexus).[35]

FTC differs from PTC in that the diagnosis cannot be reliably made by preoperative FNA biopsy, and FTC does not have the same propensity for lymph node metastasis, but does frequently metastasize distally. Surgery is usually performed for FNA findings of follicular lesion of undetermined significance or follicular neoplasm. Diagnostic thyroid lobectomy is appropriate in many cases, with completion thyroidectomy if final pathology reveals cancer. Frozen section is of little use for the intraoperative diagnosis

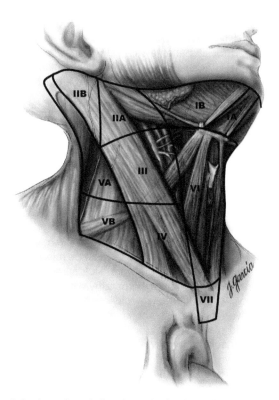

Fig. 2. Anatomy of the lateral neck (levels II–V). The boundary between the central and lateral neck is the medial aspect of the carotid artery. The spinal accessory nerve delineates the boundary between levels IIA and IIB. The boundary between levels IIA and III occurs at the level of the hyoid bone. The boundary between levels III and IV and levels VA and VB occurs at the level of the cricoid cartilage. (*Reprinted from* Mary Ann Liebert Publishers, with permission; and *From* Carty SE, Cooper DS, Doherty GM, et al. Consensus statement on the terminology and classification of central neck dissection for thyroid cancer. Thyroid 2009;19:1155; with permission.)

of FTC; a randomized prospective evaluation demonstrated that frozen section for follicular neoplasms was not informative in 96.4% of patients.[36] Because of the increased risk of cancer in follicular or Hürthle cell neoplasms greater than 4 cm, up-front total thyroidectomy is indicated.[37–39]

SURGERY FOR MTC

Surgery is the primary treatment of MTC. MTC originates from the calcitonin-producing C cells in the thyroid, which do not take up iodine. Thus, unlike differentiated thyroid cancer, RAI is ineffective for the treatment of residual disease. Surgical treatment of locoregional MTC is therefore often more aggressive than surgical treatment of differentiated thyroid cancer. Approximately 25% of cases of MTC are syndromic, resulting from a RET protooncogene mutation inherited in an autosomal-dominant fashion. Three syndromes are observed: (1) MEN2A, characterized by MTC in 100%, pheochromocytoma in 40%, and primary hyperparathyroidism in up to 30%; (2) MEN2B, characterized by aggressive, early onset MTC in 100%, pheochromocytoma in 40%, and characteristic physical features (marfanoid habitus, mucosal neuromas, ganglioneuromatosis of the gastrointestinal tract, and megacolon); and (3) familial MTC, which is likely a variant of MEN2A in which only MTC is seen.[40–42] The surgical management of syndromic disease differs from sporadic disease; RET protooncogene mutation testing is recommended for all patients with MTC before surgical intervention.[43] In general, patients with MTC should be evaluated biochemically for the presence of pheochromocytoma or primary hyperparathyroidism before thyroid surgery even if the RET analysis is negative.

Surgery for MTC is performed in two distinct contexts: to treat clinically evident disease (therapeutic) or to prevent MTC development in a patient identified to carry a RET protooncogene mutation (prophylactic). Prophylactic thyroidectomy is discussed in the pediatric section of this article. Sporadic or syndromic clinically evident MTC is treated with (therapeutic) thyroidectomy and bilateral central neck dissection; modified radical neck dissection is performed for biopsy-proved lateral neck disease or in cases in which metastatic disease to the lateral compartment is likely (eg, larger primary tumors, extensive central neck disease, a patient with MEN2B who did not undergo prophylactic thyroidectomy).[43]

Syndromic patients are at risk for other tumors that affect decision-making in the surgical treatment of MTC. Pheochromocytoma must be ruled out before thyroid surgery, and if present, should be resected before neck surgery. Patients with MEN2A who have clinical evidence of primary hyperparathyroidism should undergo concurrent parathyroidectomy. At the time of thyroidectomy, enlarged parathyroid glands are usually resected, even in a patient who is eucalcemic. Most endocrine surgeons leave normal parathyroid glands in situ; very few centers recommend total parathyroidectomy with autotransplantation at the time of initial surgery to reduce the risk that primary hyperparathyroidism will develop in residual cervical parathyroid tissue, requiring reoperation.[20] In sporadic patients, parathyroid glands that are inadvertently devascularized may be autotransplanted to neck muscles; however, in patients with MEN2A, normal parathyroid glands that are inadvertently devascularized should be autotransplanted into the forearm musculature, before they are at risk of developing primary hyperparathyroidism.[21,43]

SURGERY FOR ATC

Undifferentiated (anaplastic) thyroid carcinoma (ATC) is a rare, highly lethal tumor that accounts for approximately 1% of thyroid cancers, but results in approximately half of all deaths attributed to thyroid cancer annually in the United States.[44] Disease is usually advanced at presentation, and the mainstay of therapy is chemotherapy and radiation in most patients. Surgery is reserved for select situations: (1) open biopsy if FNA cannot differentiate ATC from thyroid lymphoma, (2) tracheostomy to secure an airway in patients with rapidly progressive local disease, and (3) complete tumor resection in the limited number of patients who are discovered to have ATC confined to the thyroid.[45] Several studies have evaluated tumor debulking followed by chemotherapy and radiation versus chemotherapy and radiation alone, with conflicting results: in general, unless complete microscopic tumor resection can be achieved, there is no survival benefit and incomplete resectional surgery is not recommended.[46–49]

REOPERATIVE THYROID SURGERY

Disease recurrence occurs in 10% to 30% of patients with differentiated thyroid cancer after initial surgical treatment of curative intent.[50] Approximately 80% of recurrences are locoregional (thyroid bed or central or lateral neck lymph nodes).[51,52] Surgical resection in cases of recurrence is associated with an increased risk of complications, particularly temporary or permanent hypoparathyroidism.[53] Although PTC usually displays an indolent course, the combination of high-quality ultrasound, increasingly sensitive assays for the detection of serum thyroglobulin, zealous physicians, and anxious patients has resulted in identification of PTC recurrence of ever-smaller clinical significance. The morbidity of reoperation must be balanced against the overall low morbidity of recurrent PTC in most cases.

A report of 70 patients who underwent surgery for recurrent PTC revealed that in approximately 10%, surgery failed to identify and remove the disease recurrence and only 27% experienced undetectable postoperative thyroglobulin.[54] Thus, surgery may not be the ideal management strategy for all patients. Other options for recurrent PTC include RAI, percutaneous ethanol injection, and radiofrequency ablation.[55–58] In some cases, particularly in recurrences less than 1 cm, careful observation alone may suffice.[59]

MINIMALLY INVASIVE THYROID SURGERY

Many surgical procedures, including thyroidectomy, have become less invasive. Several novel approaches have been developed in the quest for a cosmetically superior incision. In a thin patient with a small thyroid, conventional "open" thyroidectomy is possible with reduction of the incision length to 3 to 4 cm. Miccoli and coworkers developed the video-assisted endoscopic technique for thyroidectomy, which is performed through a 1.5- to 2-cm incision in the neck, and is the most widely adopted minimally invasive technique.[60,61] Transaxillary, transbreast, and postauricular incisions have been used with a variety of endoscopic and robotic techniques to avoid an incision on the neck.[62–72] No skin incision is required for "natural orifice" transoral thyroidectomy, first performed by Wilhelm and Metzig in 2009.[73]

Minimally invasive techniques that use extracervical incisions seem to carry additional morbidity not seen in conventional thyroid surgery. These include esophageal, tracheal, and brachial plexus injuries; skin necrosis; and spread of a fractured specimen along the approach route.[74] Because of the complication profile, cost, increased technology requirement, and training needed to perform thyroidectomy using these approaches, they have not been widely adopted in the United States. Alternative approaches to the thyroid gland are discussed in detail elsewhere in this issue.

PEDIATRIC THYROID SURGERY

Pediatric thyroid disease affects approximately 3% to 4% of school-aged children with diffuse gland hypertrophy comprising approximately half of all cases, followed by Hashimoto's thyroiditis, Graves' disease, and benign nodules.[75] Malignant tumors are rare but are diagnosed with increasing frequency and comprise approximately 2% of patients with newly diagnosed thyroid cancer.[76] The National Cancer Institute Surveillance, Epidemiology and End Results registry demonstrated the incidence of pediatric thyroid cancer per 100,000 population to be increasing at a rate of 1.1% yearly between 1973 and 2004.[77] This has also been observed in population-based studies in Great Britain in which a 275% increase in thyroid cancer in boys and a 68% increase in girls aged 0 to 14 was recently reported over approximately the same time period.[78] PTC comprises approximately 80% to 85% of all pediatric thyroid cancers, FTC approximately 10%, and MTC 5%.[79] As survival rates after treatment of other pediatric malignancies have improved, thyroid cancer is increasingly recognized as a secondary malignancy.[80,81] This incidence increases linearly with doses of radiation up to 30 Gy but declines at higher doses, likely secondary to the cytotoxic effects of radiation.[82] The rate of secondary malignancies continues to increase with age.[81,82]

Thyroid cancer should be considered in all pediatric patients in whom a nodule is discovered either on physical examination or diagnostic imaging, and a formal thyroid ultrasound should be performed. Studies have exhibited a wide variance in the reported prevalence of cancer in pediatric patients with thyroid nodules from 9.2% to 50% with an average prevalence of 26% in 1134 patients aggregated over 16 studies, significantly greater than the estimated 10% to 14% prevalence of cancer in thyroid nodules in adults.[83] As in adults, ultrasound-guided FNA biopsy is the gold standard for preoperative diagnosis of thyroid nodules in the pediatric population. A recent meta-analysis of 12 pediatric studies of FNA reported a sensitivity of 82% and a specificity of 91%, yielding a diagnostic accuracy of 83.6%, a positive predictive value of 55.3%, and a negative predictive value of 98.2%.[84]

There is no consensus on the optimal surgical management of well-differentiated thyroid cancer (WDTC; PTC and FTC) in the pediatric population, reflecting an absence of prospective randomized trials to evaluate various surgical approaches. Proponents of lobectomy cite a lack of survival benefit for total thyroidectomy and an increased rate of complication with long-term hypocalcemia reported in 2% and permanent recurrent laryngeal nerve injury in 1% of patients.[77,85] Countering this argument is evidence for a lower recurrence rate after total or near-total thyroidectomy, and the observation that at least 40% of WDTC in children is multifocal.[76,86] Moreover, total thyroidectomy allows for the administration of postoperative RAI to be directed to sites of microscopic metastatic disease and for the use of serum thyroglobulin measurement as a sensitive marker of disease recurrence.

The role of prophylactic central lymphadenectomy is also controversial in the pediatric population. Residual disease after initial operation has been demonstrated to correlate with recurrence.[87] Upfront bilateral central neck dissection has been reported to decrease the rate of a second operation from 20.6% to 7.2%; however, the morbidity of bilateral central neck dissection must be balanced against the indolent nature of WDTC.[88]

MTC comprises approximately 5% of all pediatric thyroid cancers. MTC is inherited in an autosomal-dominant fashion in approximately 20% to 25% of cases.[89] Syndromic MTC is associated with germline mutations in the *RET* protooncogene; affected individuals develop primary C-cell hyperplasia that progresses to invasive MTC.[90] Genotype-phenotype correlations based on the specific *RET* mutation give rise to risk levels for the development of aggressive MTC. The American Thyroid Association has published guidelines based on genotype with regards to the timing of surgery in children with inherited MTC.[43] It is now recommended that all patients with MTC and first-degree relatives of patients with MEN2 undergo early screening to identify a possible *RET* mutation.[43] Affected individuals should undergo neck ultrasound and measurement of serum calcitonin. For patients with the highest-risk mutations (MEN2B), these tests should be carried out shortly after birth, with prophylactic total thyroidectomy and bilateral central neck dissection performed in infancy. Patients with a mutation leading to MEN2A or familial MTC should undergo screening between the ages of 3 and 5 years. Patients with MEN2A who carry higher risk mutations (codon 634) should undergo prophylactic thyroidectomy before age 5 with bilateral central neck dissection if calcitonin is elevated or nodules greater than 5 mm are visible on ultrasound. Patients with lower-risk mutations may be monitored with serial ultrasound and serum calcitonin levels, with thyroidectomy delayed until they are older and surgery is safer. Stage of disease at diagnosis remains the best predictor of survival from MTC. Pediatric patients with localized disease experience survival rates in excess of 90%, whereas regional and distant disease is associated with survival rates of 78% and 40%, respectively.[91]

SUMMARY

Surgery for thyroid cancer involves complex decision-making and technical expertise, both of which correlate with surgeon experience. Reoperative surgery in the central or lateral neck can be difficult and can involve increased risk to the patient; therefore, it is important to perform an optimal initial operation in every patient with thyroid cancer. Thyroid surgery, and particularly thyroid cancer surgery, should be performed in a high-volume endocrine surgery center.

REFERENCES

1. Cancer Research UK. Cancer incidence for common cancers. Available at: http://www.cancerresearchuk.org/cancer-info/cancerstats/incidence/common cancers/#Trends. Accessed January 10, 2014.
2. National Cancer Institute Surveillance Epidemiology and End Results. Thyroid fact sheet. Available at: http://seer.cancer.gov/statfacts/html/thyro.html. Accessed August 16, 2013.
3. Enewold L, Zhu K, Ron E, et al. Rising thyroid cancer incidence in the United States by demographic and tumor characteristics, 1980-2005. Cancer Epidemiol Biomarkers Prev 2009;18:784–91.
4. Udelsman R, Zhang Y. The epidemic of thyroid cancer in the United States: the role of endocrinologists and ultrasounds. Thyroid 2014;24:472–9.
5. Chen AY, Jemal A, Ward EM. Increasing incidence of differentiated thyroid cancer in the United States, 1988-2005. Cancer 2009;115:3801–7.
6. Pacini F. Management of papillary thyroid microcarcinoma: primum non nocere! J Clin Endocrinol Metab 2013;98:1391–3.
7. Sosa JA, Bowman JM, Tielsch JM, et al. The importance of surgeon experience for clinical and economic outcomes from thyroidectomy. Ann Surg 1998;228:320–30.
8. Cooper DS, Doherty GM, Haugen BR, et al. Revised American Thyroid Association management guidelines for patients with thyroid nodules and differentiated thyroid cancer. Thyroid 2009;19:1167–214.

9. Cibas ES, Ali SZ. The Bethesda system for reporting thyroid cytopathology. Am J Clin Pathol 2009;132:658–65.

10. Nikiforov YE, Nikiforov YE, Steward DL, et al. Molecular testing for mutations in improving the fine-needle aspiration diagnosis of thyroid nodules. J Clin Endocrinol Metab 2009;94:2092–8.

11. Kebebew E, Ituarte PH, Siperstein AE, et al. Medullary thyroid carcinoma: clinical characteristics, treatment, prognostic factors, and a comparison of staging systems. Cancer 2000;88:1139–48.

12. Bergholm U, Bergstrom R, Ekbom A. Long-term follow-up of patients with medullary carcinoma of the thyroid. Cancer 1997;79:132–8.

13. Hemminki K, Dong C. Population-based study of familial medullary thyroid cancer. Fam Cancer 2001;1:45–9.

14. Charkes ND. On the prevalence of familial nonmedullary thyroid cancer. Thyroid 1998;8:857–8.

15. Eng C. Will the real Cowden syndrome please stand up? Revised diagnostic criteria. J Med Genet 2000;37:828–30.

16. Perrier ND, van Heerden JA, Goellner JR, et al. Thyroid cancer in patients with familial adenomatous polyposis. World J Surg 1998;22:738–42.

17. Carney JA, Gordon H, Carpenter PC, et al. The complex of myxomas, spotty pigmentation, and endocrine overactivity. Medicine 1985;6:270–83.

18. Chandrasekhar SS, Randolph GW, Seidman MD, et al. Clinical practice guideline: improving voice outcomes after thyroid surgery. Otolaryngol Head Neck Surg 2013;148:S1–37.

19. Jarhult J, Lindestad PA, Nordenstrom J, et al. Routine examination of the vocal cords before and after thyroid and parathyroid surgery. Br J Surg 1991;78:1116–7.

20. Skinner MA, Norton JA, Moley JF, et al. Heterotopic autotransplantation of parathyroid tissue in children undergoing total thyroidectomy. J Pediatr Surg 1997;32:510–3.

21. Kouvaraki M, Perrier N, Shapiro S, et al. Surgical treatment of multiple endocrine neoplasia type 2 (MEN-2). In: Pollock R, Curley S, Ross M, et al, editors. Advanced therapy in surgical oncology. Hamilton (ON): BC Decker Inc; 2008. p. 465–73.

22. Moley JF, DeBenedetti MK. Patterns of nodal metastases in palpable medullary thyroid carcinoma: recommendations for extent of node dissection. Ann Surg 1999;229:880–7.

23. Bilimoria KY, Bentrem DJ, Ko CY, et al. Extent of surgery affects survival for papillary thyroid cancer. Ann Surg 2007;246:375–81.

24. Nixon IJ, Ganly I, Patel SG, et al. Thyroid lobectomy for treatment of well differentiated intrathyroid malignancy. Surgery 2012;151:571–9.

25. Hay ID. Papillary thyroid carcinoma. Endocrinol Metab Clin North Am 1990;19:545–76.

26. Carling T, Carty SE, Ciarleglio MM, et al. American Thyroid Association design and feasibility of a prospective randomized controlled trial of prophylactic central lymph node dissection for papillary thyroid carcinoma. Thyroid 2012;22:237–44.

27. Ito Y, Miyauchi A, Inoue H, et al. An observational trial for papillary thyroid microcarcinoma in Japanese patients. World J Surg 2010;34:28–35.

28. Kouvaraki MA, Shapiro SE, Fornage BD, et al. Role of preoperative ultrasonography in the surgical management of patients with thyroid cancer. Surgery 2003;134:946–54.

29. Solorzano CC, Carneiro DM, Ramirez M, et al. Surgeon-performed ultrasound in the management of thyroid malignancy. Am Surg 2004;70:576–80.

30. Leboulleux S, Girard E, Rose M, et al. Ultrasound criteria of malignancy for cervical lymph nodes in patients followed up for differentiated thyroid cancer. J Clin Endocrinol Metab 2007;92:3590–4.

31. Carling T, Long WD 3rd, Udelsman R. Controversy surrounding the role for routine central lymph node dissection for differentiated thyroid cancer. Curr Opin Oncol 2010;22:30–4.

32. Bonnet S, Hartl D, Leboulleux S, et al. Prophylactic lymph node dissection for papillary thyroid cancer less than 2 cm: implications for radioiodine treatment. J Clin Endocrinol Metab 2009;94:1162–7.

33. Roman S, Boudourakis L, Sosa JA. Health services research in endocrine surgery. Curr Opin Oncol 2008;20:47–51.

34. Crile G. Excision of cancer of the head and neck. JAMA 1906;47:1786–9.

35. Ito Y, Higashiyama T, Takamura Y, et al. Risk factors for recurrence to the lymph node in papillary thyroid carcinoma patients without preoperatively detectable lateral node metastasis: validity of prophylactic modified radical neck dissection. World J Surg 2007;31:2085–91.

36. Udelsman R, Westra WH, Donovan PI, et al. Randomized prospective evaluation of frozen-section analysis for follicular neoplasms of the thyroid. Ann Surg 2001; 233:716–22.

37. Tuttle RM, Lemar H, Burch HB. Clinical features associated with an increased risk of thyroid malignancy inpatients with follicular neoplasia by fine-needle aspiration. Thyroid 1998;8:377–83.

38. Goldstein RE, Netterville JL, Burkey B, et al. Implications of follicular neoplasms, atypia, and lesions suspicious for malignancy diagnosed by fine-needle aspiration of thyroid nodules. Ann Surg 2002;235:656–62.

39. Chen H, Nicol TL, Zeiger MA, et al. Hürthle cell neoplasms of the thyroid: are there factors predictive of malignancy? Ann Surg 1998;227:542–6.

40. Howe JR, Norton JA, Wells SJ. Prevalence of pheochromocytoma and hyperparathyroidism in multiple endocrine neoplasia type 2A: results of long-term follow-up. Surgery 1993;114:1070–7.

41. Mulligan LM, Eng C, Healey CS, et al. Specific mutations of the RET proto-oncogene are related to disease phenotype in MEN2A and FMTC. Nat Genet 1994;6:70–4.

42. Machens A, Holzhausen HJ, Thanh PN, et al. Malignant progression from C-cell hyperplasia to medullary thyroid carcinoma in 167 carriers of RET germline mutations. Surgery 2003;134:425–31.

43. Kloos RT, Eng C, Evans DB, et al. Medullary thyroid cancer: management guidelines of the American Thyroid Association. Thyroid 2009;19:565–612.

44. Gilliland FD, Hunt WC, Morris DM, et al. Prognostic factors for thyroid carcinoma. A population-based study of 15,698 cases from the Surveillance, Epidemiology and End Results (SEER) program 1973-1991. Cancer 1997;79:564–73.

45. Pasieka JL. Anaplastic thyroid cancer. Curr Opin Oncol 2003;15:78–83.

46. Tennvall J, Lundell G, Wahlberg P, et al. Anaplastic thyroid carcinoma: three protocols combining doxorubicin, hyperfractionated radiotherapy and surgery. Br J Cancer 2002;86:1848–53.

47. Sugino K, Ito K, Mimura T, et al. The important role of operations in the management of anaplastic thyroid carcinoma. Surgery 2002;131:245–8.

48. McIver B, Hay ID, Giuffrida DF, et al. Anaplastic thyroid carcinoma: a 50-year experience at a single institution. Surgery 2001;130:1028–34.

49. Passler C, Scheuba C, Prager G, et al. Anaplastic (undifferentiated) thyroid carcinoma (ATC). A retrospective analysis. Langenbecks Arch Surg 1999;384: 284–93.

50. Mazzaferri EL, Jhiang SM. Long-term impact of initial surgical and medical therapy on papillary and follicular thyroid cancer. Am J Med 1994;97:418–28.

51. Dinneen SF, Valikmaki MJ, Bergstralh EJ, et al. Distant metastases in papillary thyroid carcinoma: 100 cases observed at one institution during 5 decades. J Clin Endocrinol Metab 1995;80:2041–5.

52. Samaan NA, Schultz PN, Haynie TP, et al. Pulmonary metastasis of differentiated thyroid carcinoma: treatment results in 101 patients. J Clin Endocrinol Metab 1985;60:376–80.

53. Tufano RP, Bishop J, Wu G. Reoperative central compartment dissection for patients with recurrent/persistent papillary thyroid cancer: efficacy, safety, and the association of the BRAF mutation. Laryngoscope 2012;122: 1634–40.

54. Al-Saif O, Farrar WB, Bloomston M, et al. Long-term efficiency of lymph node reoperation for persistent papillary thyroid cancer. J Clin Endocrinol Metab 2010; 95:2187–94.

55. Maxon HR, Thomas SR, Hertzberg VS, et al. Relation between effective radiation dose and outcome of radioiodine therapy for thyroid cancer. N Engl J Med 1983; 309:937–41.

56. Lewis BD, Hay ID, Charboneau JW, et al. Percutaneous ethanol injection for treatment of cervical lymph node metastases in patients with papillary thyroid carcinoma. Am J Roentgenol 2002;178:699–704.

57. Lim CY, Yun JS, Lee J, et al. Percutaneous ethanol injection therapy for locally recurrent papillary thyroid carcinoma. Thyroid 2007;17:347–50.

58. Monchik JM, Donatini G, Iannuccilli J, et al. Radiofrequency ablation and percutaneous ethanol injection treatment for recurrent local and distant well-differentiated thyroid carcinoma. Ann Surg 2006;244:296–304.

59. Udelsman R. Treatment of persistent or recurrent papillary carcinoma of the thyroid—the good, the bad, and the unknown. J Clin Endocrinol Metab 2010;95: 2061–3.

60. Miccoli P, Berti P, Conte M, et al. Minimally invasive surgery for thyroid small nodules: preliminary report. J Endocrinol Invest 1999;22:849–51.

61. Miccoli P, Berti P, Bendinelli C, et al. Minimally invasive video-assisted surgery of the thyroid: a preliminary report. Langenbecks Arch Surg 2000;385:261–4.

62. Shimizu K, Akira S, Jasmi AY, et al. Video-assisted neck surgery: endoscopic resection of thyroid tumors with a very minimal neck wound. J Am Coll Surg 1999;188:697–703.

63. Yamamoto M, Sasaki A, Asahi H, et al. Endoscopic subtotal thyroidectomy for patients with Graves' disease. Surg Today 2001;31:1–4.

64. Ohgami M, Ishii S, Arisawa Y, et al. Scarless endoscopic thyroidectomy: breast approach for better cosmesis. Surg Laparosc Endosc Percutan Tech 2000;10:1–4.

65. Ishii S, Ohgami M, Arisawa Y. Endoscopic thyroidectomy with anterior chest wall approach. Surg Endosc 1998;12:611.

66. Ikeda Y, Takami H, Sasaki Y, et al. Endoscopic neck surgery by the axillary approach. J Am Coll Surg 2000;191:336–40.

67. Ryu HR, Kang SW, Lee SH, et al. Feasibility and safety of a new robotic thyroidectomy through a gasless transaxillary single-incision approach. J Am Coll Surg 2010;211:e13–9.

68. Kang SW, Lee SC, Lee SH, et al. Robotic thyroid surgery using a gasless, trans-axillary approach and the da Vinci S system: the operative outcomes of 338 consecutive patients. Surgery 2009;146:1048–55.

69. Lee KE, Rao J, Youn YK. Endoscopic thyroidectomy with the da Vinci robot system using the bilateral axillary breast approach (BABA) technique: our initial experience. Surg Laparosc Endosc Percutan Tech 2009;19:e71–5.

70. Choe JH, Kim SW, Chung KW, et al. Endoscopic thyroidectomy using a new bilateral axillo-breast approach. World J Surg 2007;31:601–6.

71. Strik MW, Anders S, Barth M, et al. Total videoendoscopic thyroid resection by the axillobilateral breast approach: operative method and first results. Chirurg 2007;78:1139–44.

72. Shimazu K, Shiba E, Tamaki Y, et al. Endoscopic thyroid surgery through the axillo-bilateral-breast approach. Surg Laparosc Endosc Percutan Tech 2003; 13:196–201.

73. Wilhelm T, Metzig A. Endoscopic minimally invasive thyroidectomy (eMIT): a prospective proof-of-concept study in humans. World J Surg 2011;35:543–51.

74. Clerici T. Minimally invasive techniques in thyroid surgery. In: Oertli D, Udelsman R, editors. Surgery of the thyroid and parathyroid glands. Berlin: Springer-Verlag; 2012. p. 175–86.

75. Rallison ML, Dobyns BM, Meikle AW, et al. Natural history of thyroid abnormalities: prevalence, incidence, and regression of thyroid diseases in adolescents and young adults. Am J Med 1991;91:363–70.

76. Dinauer CA, Breuer C, Rivkees SA. Differentiated thyroid cancer in children: diagnosis and management. Curr Opin Oncol 2008;20:59–65.

77. Hogan AR, Zhuge Y, Perez EA, et al. Pediatric thyroid carcinoma: incidence and outcomes in 1753 patients. J Surg Res 2009;156:167–72.

78. McNally RJQ, Blakey K, James PW, et al. Increasing incidence of thyroid cancer in Great Britain, 1976-2005: age-period-cohort analysis. Eur J Epidemiol 2012; 27:615–22.

79. Zimmerman D. Thyroid carcinoma in children and adolescents: diagnostic implications of analysis of the tumor genome. Curr Opin Pediatr 2013;25:528–31.

80. Maule M, Scelo G, Pastore G, et al. Risk of second malignant neoplasms after childhood leukemia and lymphoma: an international study. J Natl Cancer Inst 2007;99:790–800.

81. Sigurdson AJ, Ronckers CM, Mertens AC, et al. Primary thyroid cancer after a first tumour in childhood (the Childhood Cancer Survivor Study): a nested case-control study. Lancet 2005;365:2014–23.

82. Davies SM. Subsequent malignant neoplasms in survivors of childhood cancer: Childhood Cancer Survivor Study (CCSS) studies. Pediatr Blood Cancer 2007; 48:727–30.

83. Niedziela M. Pathogenesis, diagnosis and management of thyroid nodules in children. Endocr Relat Cancer 2006;86:427–53.

84. Stevens C, Lee JK, Sadatsafavi M, et al. Pediatric thyroid fine-needle aspiration cytology: a meta-analysis. J Pediatr Surg 2009;44:2184–91.

85. LaQuaglia MP, Black T, Holcomb GW, et al. Differentiated thyroid cancer: clinical characteristics, treatment, and outcomes in patients under 21 years of age who present with distant metastases. A report from the surgical discipline committee of the children's cancer group. J Pediatr Surg 2000;35:955–60.

86. Rachmiel M, Charron M, Gupta A, et al. Evidence based review of treatment and follow-up of pediatric patients with differentiated thyroid carcinoma. J Pediatr Endocrinol Metab 2006;19:1377–93.

87. Newman KD, Black T, Heller G, et al. Differentiated thyroid cancer: determinants of disease progression in patients <21 years of age at diagnosis. A report from the surgical discipline committee of the children's cancer group. Ann Surg 1998; 227:533–41.
88. Demidchik I, Kontratovich VA. Repeat surgery for recurrent thyroid cancer in children. Vopr Onkol 2003;49:366–9.
89. Pelizzo MR, Boschin IM, Bernante P, et al. Natural history, diagnosis, treatment and outcome of medullary thyroid cancer: 37 years of experience on 157 patients. Eur J Surg Oncol 2007;33:493–7.
90. Wells SA Jr, Pacini F, Robinson BG, et al. Multiple endocrine neoplasia type 2 and familial medullary thyroid carcinoma: an update. J Clin Endocrinol Metab 2013;98:3149–64.
91. Roman S, Lin R, Sosa JA. Prognosis of medullary thyroid carcinoma: demographic, clinical, and pathologic predictors of survival in 1252 cases. Cancer 2006;107:2134–42.

Alternative Approaches to the Thyroid Gland

William S. Duke, MD, David J. Terris, MD*

KEYWORDS

- Thyroid surgery • Endoscopic • Robotic • Minimally invasive

KEY POINTS

- There are 2 separate mechanisms for reducing the cosmetic burden of thyroid surgery: minimally invasive anterior cervical approaches and remote access approaches.
- Minimally invasive cervical approaches use small incisions on the anterior neck to directly access the thyroid compartment and require limited dissection to remove the thyroid gland.
- Remote access approaches should not be considered minimally invasive; while the incisions are generally well hidden in these techniques, the extent of dissection required and the subsequent prolonged recovery of these approaches is much greater than that of minimally invasive anterior cervical approaches.

INTRODUCTION

The traditional thyroidectomy technique produces a long scar on the neck that is difficult to conceal. While this approach is still warranted in selected cases, many patients may be candidates for innovative procedures designed to customize the incision size, location, and extent of dissection to the individual thyroid pathology being treated. These procedures, which began to emerge in the 1990s, were driven by patient-centered efforts to improve the cosmetic impact of thyroid surgery.

As these novel approaches germinated, 2 divergent avenues of innovation were pursued. Along one pathway, minimally invasive anterior cervical approaches were developed, which sought to reduce the extent of dissection and decrease the length of the cervical scar while still offering direct access to the thyroid. On the other pathway, numerous other techniques were developed that completely remove the thyroidectomy scar from the visible neck. These remote access approaches comprise a heterogeneous group of procedures that use endoscopic or robotic assistance to access the thyroid gland from extracervical incision sites.

Disclosure: None (W.S. Duke); Directed thyroid courses sponsored by Johnson & Johnson (D.J. Terris).

Department of Otolaryngology, GRU Thyroid Center, Georgia Regents University, 1120 Fifteenth Street, BP-4109, Augusta, GA 30912-4060, USA

* Corresponding author.

E-mail address: dterris@gru.edu

Endocrinol Metab Clin N Am 43 (2014) 459–474

http://dx.doi.org/10.1016/j.ecl.2014.02.009

BACKGROUND AND HISTORY

More than a century after becoming a formalized and internationally accepted procedure, thyroid surgery was still being performed as described by Emil Theodor Kocher in the nineteenth century.[1] This traditional approach involves making a large 7- to 10-cm transverse cervical incision, elevating subplatysmal flaps, and widely exposing the contents of the thyroid compartment, using surgical drains and inpatient postoperative care. As endoscopic and minimally invasive techniques became more widespread, interest turned to the application of these approaches to neck surgery, where postoperative scars tend to be more conspicuous. Gagner[2] described the first endoscopic cervical surgery in 1996, performing a subtotal parathyroidectomy using multiple ports and CO_2 insufflation. Although the procedure took 5 hours, generated mild hypercarbia and significant subcutaneous emphysema, and required a 4-day hospital admission, "the cosmetic result was excellent."[3] Although this experience clearly demonstrated obstacles that would need to be addressed when developing alternative approaches to the central region of the neck, the potential to decrease the cosmetic impact of a traditional thyroidectomy scar quickly attracted the attention of both patients and surgeons.

Efforts to improve the cosmetic outcome after thyroid surgery simultaneously evolved along 2 separate pathways. Some teams pursued and refined minimally invasive anterior cervical approaches, such as the minimally invasive video-assisted thyroidectomy (MIVAT)[4,5] and the minimally invasive nonendoscopic thyroidectomy (MINET).[6] These approaches were designed to decrease the length of the cervical scar, reduce the extent of dissection required, and improve the postoperative recovery experience. Other teams sought to remove the scar from the visible portion of the anterior neck completely. These remote access approaches primarily emerged in Asian practices, wherein patients are at an increased risk of hypertrophic scarring and place a premium on the cosmetic appearance of the neck.[7,8]

The earliest attempts at alternative approaches to the thyroid compartment relied on CO_2 insufflation to aid with dissection and maintenance of the operative pocket, and most of them were performed using endoscopic visualization.[4,9–11] After Gagner's[3] initially difficult experience with CO_2 insufflation was confirmed in a subsequent report,[12] surgeons began to develop gasless techniques that could maintain the operative space without the use of CO_2. The minimally invasive anterior cervical approaches came to rely on blunt retraction of the soft tissue,[5,13] whereas the remote access techniques frequently use either percutaneous suspension techniques[14–16] or specialized retractors[17] to maintain the operative space.

DEFINING ALTERNATIVE APPROACHES

Fundamentally, any method of accessing the thyroid gland that deviates from the traditional Kocher thyroidectomy approach may be considered "alternative." A distinction should be clearly made, however, between minimally invasive anterior cervical approaches and remote access approaches (**Table 1**).

Minimally invasive alternative anterior cervical approaches such as MINET and MIVAT use small incisions camouflaged in natural neck creases to access the thyroid compartment. The incision is significantly smaller than that of a conventional thyroidectomy and the extent of dissection is reduced. This feature results in less postoperative pain for the patient and obviates postoperative drainage. In many cases, these procedures are performed on an outpatient basis.[18] These approaches, therefore, are truly minimally invasive, not just involving a minimal incision.

Table 1
Alternative thyroidectomy approaches based on incision location

Category	Incision Site	Approach
Minimally invasive anterior cervical	Anterior region of the neck	• MIVAT • MINET
Remote access	Chest or breast	• CO_2-assisted endoscopic • Gasless endoscopic • Gasless robotic
	Axillary	• CO_2-assisted endoscopic • Gasless endoscopic • Gasless robotic
	Combined	• ABBA • BABA endoscopic
	Postauricular	• RFT
	Oral cavity	• NOTES

Abbreviations: ABBA, axillobilateral breast approach; BABA, bilateral axillo-breast approach; MINET, minimally invasive non-endoscopic thyroidectomy; MIVAT, minimally invasive video-assisted thyroidectomy; NOTES, natural orifice transluminal endoscopic surgery; RFT, robotic facelift thyroidectomy.

In contrast, a remote access approach to the thyroid removes the surgical scar from the visible neck completely. These techniques transfer the site of entry to a more distant, concealed location and use dissection along natural tissue planes to access the central neck compartment. Remote access procedures generally rely on endoscopic or robotic equipment to facilitate visualization and manipulation of the tissue. These procedures require more dissection than that required in a traditional thyroidectomy, put additional structures at risk that are not normally vulnerable during anterior cervical approaches, and frequently necessitate drainage and postoperative hospital admission.[10,11,17,19–21] As such, these procedures neither are minimally invasive nor should they be considered scarless.

ADVANTAGES AND DISADVANTAGES OF ALTERNATIVE APPROACHES

Long-term complications and mortality related to traditional thyroid surgery are uncommon[22,23] and may be even lower in minimally invasive video-assisted anterior cervical approaches.[24,25] MIVAT and MINET afford the surgeon rapid access to the thyroid compartment along a familiar route of dissection. In experienced hands, these approaches are associated with equivalent or shorter operative times, less blood loss, less postoperative pain, and improved cosmetic outcomes than conventional thyroid surgery.[24,26]

Despite these advantages, MINET and MIVAT may not be appropriate for many patients requiring thyroid surgery. Dissection through minimally invasive incisions may be difficult or unsafe in patients with large goiters, substernal extension, or thyroiditis. Patients with invasive carcinomas or lateral neck lymph node metastases should be treated with a more conventional approach. Although the cosmetic results are generally favorable, patients still may be left with a visible anterior cervical scar. Finally, the MIVAT approach requires an additional assistant to operate the endoscope.

Some patients find the prospect of any anterior neck scar unacceptable. For these individuals, remote access procedures, which remove the postoperative scar from a visible location on the anterior part of the neck and replace it with an incision hidden in a less conspicuous location, may be appealing.

Owing to the heterogeneity of this group of procedures, very few generalizations can be made about remote access approaches as a whole. It is unclear if these procedures are consistently less painful or result in a faster recovery time than conventional thyroid surgery, as the potentially smaller incisions may be offset by the more extensive dissection required.[27–29] These procedures generally take longer to perform than anterior cervical approaches, although this parameter may highly depend on the individual technique and the experience of the surgeon.[28–30] What is consistently demonstrated, however, is that remote access thyroid surgery uses more medical resources and is more expensive than conventional thyroid surgery, especially if a prolonged inpatient stay is required.[27,31–33] Although these procedures may reimburse favorably in some Asian markets, there is currently no reimbursement incentive to offset the increased surgical costs in the United States and other Western markets.[32,33]

APPROACHES
Minimally Invasive Anterior Cervical

MIVAT
The procedure begins by marking a 15- to 20-mm incision in a low cervical skin crease while the patient is awake and upright in the holding area. This step helps ensure that the incision is concealed in the most vertically favorable position on the neck. The incision is made in the previously marked skin crease and carried down through the platysma, exposing the sternohyoid and sternothyroid muscles. No subplatysmal flaps are elevated. The strap muscles are separated vertically in the midline and retracted laterally, off the anterior and lateral aspects of the thyroid.

A 5-mm 30° laparoscope is introduced into the wound. The avascular space between the inferior constrictor muscle and the medial aspect of the superior pole is bluntly dissected, thereby isolating the superior vascular pedicle. Although initially described using vessel clips, Harmonic-ACE shears (ACE23P, Ethicon Endo-Surgery, Inc, Cincinnati, OH, USA) are now used to divide the superior pole vessels close to the thyroid capsule (**Fig. 1**). The superior parathyroid gland is identified and preserved. The middle thyroid vein is then divided, and the inferior pole is mobilized. The inferior vascular pedicle is divided, and the inferior parathyroid gland is identified and dissected away from the thyroid.

The lobe is then exteriorized with liberal use of hemostat clamps placed directly on the gland itself, especially the superior pole (**Fig. 2**). The lobe is retracted medially and ventrally, and the recurrent laryngeal nerve (RLN) is identified and traced until it courses under the inferior constrictor muscle. The Harmonic device is used to ligate vessels and divide the tissue during this dissection. The isthmus is then divided and the lobe is removed.

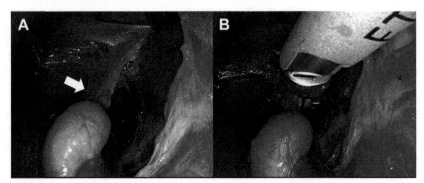

Fig. 1. (*A, B*) Bundle ligation of the superior vascular pedicle (*arrow*) with an advanced energy device during MIVAT.

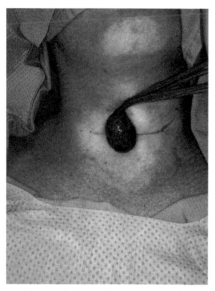

Fig. 2. Delivery of the thyroid lobe through the MIVAT incision.

The contralateral lobe is removed in a similar manner, if required. The surgical field is irrigated, and Surgicel (Ethicon, Inc, Somerville, NJ, USA) is placed into the thyroid bed. The strap muscles are reapproximated in the midline with a single figure-of-eight 3-0 Vicryl suture (Ethicon, Inc). This single fixation point decreases the risk of postoperative airway obstruction by allowing any fluid accumulation to easily escape the thyroid compartment. The subcutaneous tissues are closed with buried interrupted 4-0 Vicryl sutures, and the skin edges are sealed with tissue adhesive and a horizontal $1/4$-inch Steri-Strip (3M Corporation, St. Paul, MN, USA) (**Fig. 3**). No drain is

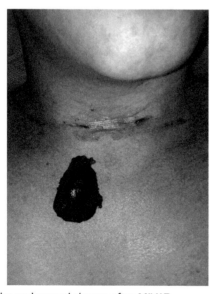

Fig. 3. Right thyroid lobe and wound closure after MIVAT.

used, and the procedure is accomplished on an outpatient basis. **Fig. 4** shows the healing incision.

Originally reported for the treatment of small-volume benign thyroid disease, cytologically indeterminate nodules, and low-risk differentiated thyroid cancer (DTC), the indications for MIVAT have recently been expanded to include select patients with thyroiditis and intermediate-risk DTC[34] and elective central neck dissection has shown to be safe and feasible when combined with this approach.[35] Although they vary by report, potential contraindications include patients with nodules larger than 35 mm, an estimated thyroid volume greater than 25 cm[3], malignancies larger than 20 mm, and the presence or suspicion of metastatic lymph nodes.[34]

In an early multiinstitutional trial of 336 patients, the mean operative time with MIVAT was 69.4 minutes for a hemithyroidectomy and 87.4 minutes for a total thyroidectomy.[36] Complications included hemorrhage in 0.9% of cases, temporary RLN weakness in 2.1% of cases, permanent RLN weakness in 0.3% of cases, temporary hypocalcemia in 2.7% of cases, permanent hypocalcemia in 0.6% of cases, and a conversion rate of 4.5%.[36] This safety profile was validated in a large North American MIVAT study of 228 patients,[25] and Terris and Seybt[37] described several important modifications (detailed above) designed not only to aid with MIVAT procedures but also to be incorporated into any anterior cervical approach. An important potential limitation of this procedure is that 2 surgical assistants are required: one to maintain the operative field with retractors and one to maneuver the endoscope.

MINET

Almost concurrent with the development of MIVAT, a MINET technique was reported from groups in South Korea[26] and the United States.[38] This approach sought to minimize the tissue trauma associated with conventional thyroidectomy while providing an alternative to endoscopic neck surgery.

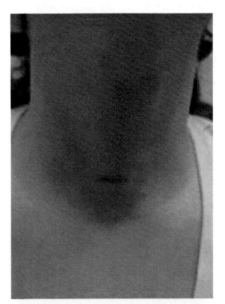

Fig. 4. MIVAT incision 2 weeks after surgery. (*From* Terris DJ, Angelos P, Steward DL, et al. Minimally invasive video-assisted thyroidectomy. A multi-institutional North American experience. Arch Otolaryngol Head Neck Surg 2008;134(1):83; with permission.)

This approach uses a 3- to 5-cm incision marked in a low cervical skin crease to access the thyroid compartment. Dissection is identical to that in the MIVAT technique, except that the slightly larger skin incision is repositioned with retractors as necessary to maintain an optimal view of the operative field, obviating endoscopic assistance. In addition to complete removal of the thyroid, central neck dissection may be performed using this exposure.[26] Closure is the same as for minimally invasive nonendoscopic surgery. No drain is used, and the procedure is accomplished on an outpatient basis.

MINET has been shown to be a safe and effective procedure in properly selected patients. A retrospective comparison of 466 patients undergoing MINET with 437 patients undergoing conventional thyroidectomy demonstrated MINET to have a decreased operative time, less blood loss, a shorter hospital stay, decreased drain utilization, and less postoperative pain with no difference in complication rates.[26]

Remote Access Endoscopic

Chest/breast approaches
Ohgami and colleagues[10] described the first truly remote access thyroidectomy in 2000 when they reported a series of CO_2-assisted endoscopic hemithyroidectomies. The thyroid compartment is accessed through incisions at the parasternal border of one breast and along the superior margins of both areolas. Endoscopic dissection proceeds superiorly over the strap muscles, and the thyroid lobe on the side of the lesion is exposed and removed.

Although Ohgami and colleagues[10] did not describe their patient selection criteria, they reported removing thyroid nodules ranging from 3 to 7 cm. The mean operative time for this series was nearly 4 hours. Using a low insufflation pressure of 6 mm Hg, they experienced minimal cervical emphysema and no other complications related to CO_2 insufflation.

Numerous variations of the anterior chest and breast approach have been described since the initial description of the procedure, including isolated anterior chest wall approaches[15] as well as bilateral[39] and unilateral[40] transareolar approaches. Typical indications for these approaches now include unilateral benign lesions less than 3 cm or papillary microcarcinomas in patients with no concerning lymphadenopathy and no prior history of neck surgery or radiation.[16,39,40]

Despite the lack of cervical scars with these approaches, they do involve incisions on the breast or anterior chest. The anterior chest incisions are subject to hypertrophic scarring,[19] and breast scars, however inconspicuous, may be an unappealing alternative in North American patients.[41,42] These approaches may also be limited by a narrow operative field and restriction of movement by the rigid endoscopic equipment.[19] These factors prompted the development of other remote access techniques.

Axillary approaches
The first viable remote access alternative to the anterior chest and breast approaches was the endoscopic axillary approach, pioneered by Ikeda and colleagues.[11] The patient is positioned supine on the operating table, and the arm on the side to be dissected is elevated to expose the axilla. An incision is made in the axilla, and dissection proceeds along the pectoralis major muscle until the platysma is encountered. Trocars are placed through the incision, and CO_2 insufflation is used to expand the operative field. Using endoscopic visualization, dissection proceeds between the anterior border of the sternocleidomastoid muscle (SCM) and the strap muscles until the thyroid lobe is identified. The strap muscles are divided to expose the thyroid lobe for excision.

This approach is associated with improved cosmetic outcomes when compared with open surgery; however, it takes significantly longer to perform than a conventional open thyroidectomy.[43] This approach is also still subject to the constraints of CO_2-assisted dissection, namely, relatively narrow operative corridors, the need for rigid specialized endoscopic equipment, and the risks of CO_2-related morbidity. To overcome these limitations, gasless remote access techniques that did not require a closed operative pocket and CO_2 insufflation were developed.[44] This approach was later modified so that dissection occurs between the sternal and clavicular heads of the SCM rather than between the SCM and the sternohyoid muscle.[45]

Several hybrid approaches were also developed that combine both axillary and areolar incisions. These techniques, which include the axillobilateral breast approach[19] and the bilateral axillo-breast approach (BABA)[20] were designed to capitalize on the cosmetic benefit of the axillary approaches while providing additional anterior chest working ports without producing a transverse parasternal scar (**Fig. 5**). Despite their cosmetic appeal, these approaches have been associated with several complications not typically associated with traditional thyroid surgery, including transient neurapraxia of the brachial plexus[46] and pneumothorax.[20]

Transoral approaches

While extracervical approaches to the thyroid succeed in removing the incision from the anterior part of the neck, they generally involve extensive dissection and still result in cutaneous scarring. The rise in natural orifice transluminal endoscopic surgery for pelvic and abdominal procedures led to efforts to incorporate these approaches into thyroid compartment surgery. The feasibility of this approach was demonstrated

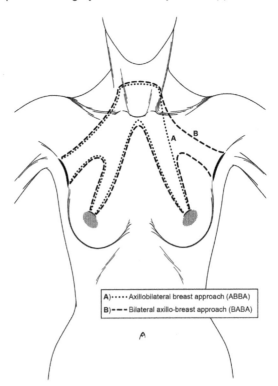

Fig. 5. Comparison of the extent of dissection for the axillobilateral breast approach (ABBA) and the bilateral axillo-breast approach (BABA). (*Courtesy of* Georgia Regents University, Augusta, GA; with permission.)

in cadaver and porcine models,[47,48] but the inaugural clinical implementation of this technique in 8 patients was met with a conversion rate of 38% and a permanent RLN injury rate of 13%.[49] This experience significantly dampened enthusiasm for the technique, with only 1 small series of 8 patients subsequently published.[50]

Remote Access Robotic Procedures

The incorporation of da Vinci surgical robotic technology (Intuitive Surgical, Inc, Sunnyvale, CA, USA) in remote access thyroid surgery has afforded surgeons a 3-dimensional view of the operative field while incorporating surgical instruments whose range of motion exceeds the capabilities of traditional rigid endoscopic equipment. The first use of the surgical robot in thyroid surgery involved a combined robotic and endoscopic transaxillary thyroid lobectomy using CO_2 insufflation.[51] Since that time, surgical robotic technology has been incorporated into a CO_2-assisted BABA,[21] as well as gasless dual incision axillary and chest wall,[17] single incision axillary[52] and facelift[53] approaches (**Fig. 6**). This technology has also been used to perform central and lateral neck dissections in patients with thyroid malignancies.[54] It should be noted that although US Food and Drug Administration approval exists for general surgery procedures, a specific indication for robotic thyroidectomy has not been issued.

Robotic axillary thyroidectomy

The first reports of completely robotic surgery of the thyroid compartment emerged from South Korea in 2009.[17,28,45] An axillary approach was employed combined

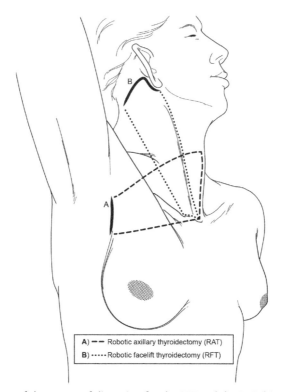

A) − − Robotic axillary thyroidectomy (RAT)
B) ····· Robotic facelift thyroidectomy (RFT)

Fig. 6. Comparison of the extent of dissection for the RFT and the RAT. (*Courtesy of* Georgia Regents University, Augusta, GA; with permission.)

with a gasless dissection facilitated by inserting a specialized retractor (Chung retractor) to elevate the skin and muscle flap.[45] The robotic axillary thyroidectomy (RAT) initially used a secondary parasternal incision on the anterior chest wall (dual incision approach),[28,45] but a single incision in the axilla[52] is now commonly performed. The dissection is the same as described for the endoscopic transaxillary approach, but robotic assistance is used for removal of the thyroid.

There was early enthusiasm that this approach may be widely exportable. However, because of economic considerations and several complications encountered when RAT was initially incorporated into North American practices,[31,33,55–58] this procedure has largely been abandoned in the United States.

Robotic facelift thyroidectomy

The concerns generated by the RAT experience in Western centers, as well as the need for perioperative drains and postoperative hospital admission after this procedure, prompted exploration into alternative robotic approaches to the thyroid compartment. The robotic facelift thyroidectomy (RFT) was developed to address some of these potential disadvantages associated with RAT.[53,59]

Patients must meet specific eligibility criteria to be considered for RFT.[60] As with all remote access techniques, patients should be highly motivated to avoid a visible cervical scar. However, they should also accept the unlikely risk of conversion to an anterior cervical approach. Patients should also be healthy enough to tolerate the extended general anesthesia exposure necessary with this procedure.[53] Patients should not be morbidly obese, although flap elevation in an extremely thin neck must be deliberate to avoid inadvertent skin injury.

The thyroid disease must also conform to selection requirements.[60] The approach vector and current instrumentation only permit unilateral surgery through a single ipsilateral incision. Although cases of staged bilateral completion RFT procedures or total thyroidectomy through 2 incisions have been reported,[53] generally, the thyroid condition to be addressed should be one that is appropriate for unilateral surgery. The largest nodule to be removed should not exceed 4 cm in greatest dimension. There should be no thyroiditis, substernal extension, or concern for malignancy such as pathologic lymphadenopathy or extrathyroidal spread.

The RFT incision begins in the postauricular crease and is carried superiorly, crossing into the occipital hairline (**Fig. 7**). A subplatysmal flap is elevated until the SCM is identified. Dissection proceeds along the SCM as a series of landmarks are encountered, including the great auricular nerve and the external jugular vein. These are preserved as the anteromedial border of the SCM is exposed down to the clavicle.

A muscular triangle bounded by the anterior border of the SCM, the superior border of the omohyoid muscle, and the posterior border of the sternohyoid is defined, and the omohyoid and other strap muscles are elevated ventrally to expose the superior pole of the thyroid gland and the superior vascular pedicle (**Fig. 8**). The modified Chung retractor (Marina Medical, Inc, Sunrise, FL, USA) is positioned to retract the strap muscles ventrally. A Singer hook (Medtronic, Jacksonville, FL, USA) is used to retract the SCM laterally and dorsally, thereby securing the open surgical pocket.

The robot is deployed using a 30° down-facing endoscope. A Harmonic device (Ethicon Endo-Surgery, Inc) is placed in the dominant arm, and a Maryland grasper is used in the nondominant arm.

The superior vascular pedicle is divided with the Harmonic device. The superior thyroid pole is retracted inferiorly and ventrally to expose the inferior constrictor muscle, taking care to avoid injuring the superior laryngeal nerve. The superior parathyroid gland is reflected away from the posterior aspect of the thyroid. The RLN is then

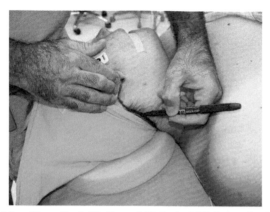

Fig. 7. The RFT incision. (*From* Terris DJ, Singer MC, Seybt MW. Robot facelift thyroidectomy: II. Clinical feasibility and safety. Laryngoscope 2011;121:1637; with permission.)

identified laterally as it courses under the inferior constrictor (**Fig. 9**). The nerve is dissected inferiorly, exposing the ligament of Berry. With the nerve under direct visualization, the ligament is transected with the Harmonic device and the thyroid isthmus is divided. The middle thyroid vein is divided. The inferior parathyroid gland is bluntly dissected away from the thyroid, and the inferior vascular pedicle is divided. All remaining attachments between the thyroid lobe and the surrounding soft tissue are divided, and the specimen is removed. The wound is closed as described above for the MIVAT procedure. No drains are used, and the patient is discharged on the day of surgery. **Fig. 10** shows a patient after the procedure with no visible neck scar.

RFT is a relatively new addition to the remote access armamentarium. More than 60 procedures have been accomplished at the authors' center. In peer-reviewed

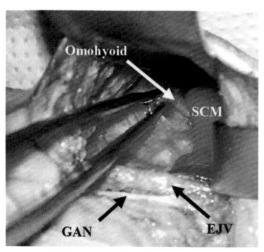

Fig. 8. Dissection pocket in RFT. EJV, external jugular vein; GAN, great auricular nerve. (*From* Terris DJ, Singer MC, Seybt MW. Robot facelift thyroidectomy: II. Clinical feasibility and safety. Laryngoscope 2011;121:1638; with permission.)

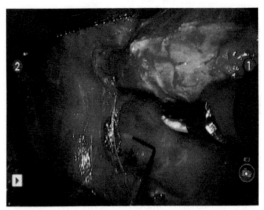

Fig. 9. The recurrent laryngeal nerve is visualized at the tip of the nerve stimulating probe during RFT. (*From* Terris DJ, Singer MC, Seybt MW. Robot facelift thyroidectomy: II. Clinical feasibility and safety. Laryngoscope 2011;121:1639; with permission.)

publications, the procedures were completed on an outpatient basis without drainage in all but the first patient.[53,60,61] There was one incidence of transient vocal fold weakness and 2 seromas, all of which resolved without intervention. There have been no episodes of hypocalcemia and no conversions to an anterior approach. This experience has been repeated in at least 4 centers, with more than 100 procedures accomplished with the same complication profile as described in the original reports.

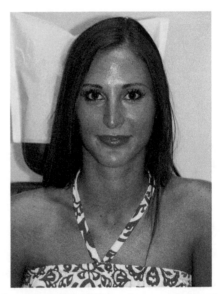

Fig. 10. Frontal view of a patient after RFT showing no anterior cervical scar.

SUMMARY

A commitment to patient-centered and personalized surgery has driven the development of alternative approaches to the thyroid gland. These comprise 2 fundamentally different treatment paradigms. Minimally invasive anterior cervical approaches seek to both lessen the cosmetic impact of thyroid surgery by minimizing the length of the visible incision and improve the postoperative experience for the patient by reducing the extent of dissection required. Remote access techniques completely remove the visible scar from the anterior region of the neck, at the expense of greater dissection and potential jeopardy to structures not normally at risk during thyroid surgery. Although these treatment options may not be appropriate for many individuals requiring thyroid surgery, there are patients who, by nature of medical comorbidities, occupation, lifestyle, or desire, will benefit from these innovative techniques. The surgeon and patient should consider individual risk-benefit analysis to determine if the potential advantages afforded by these techniques are warranted.

REFERENCES

1. Pinchot S, Chen H, Sippel R. Incisions and exposure of the neck for thyroidectomy and parathyroidectomy. Operat Tech Gen Surg 2008;10:63–76.
2. Gagner M. Endoscopic subtotal parathyroidectomy in patients with primary hyperparathyroidism. Br J Surg 1996;83:875.
3. Naitoh T, Gagner M, Garcia-Ruiz A, et al. Endoscopic endocrine surgery in the neck. An initial report of endoscopic subtotal parathyroidectomy. Surg Endosc 1998;12:202–5.
4. Miccoli P, Berti P, Conte M, et al. Minimally invasive surgery for thyroid small nodules: preliminary report. J Endocrinol Invest 1999;22:849–51.
5. Bellantone R, Lombardi CP, Raffaelli M, et al. Minimally invasive, totally gasless video-assisted thyroid lobectomy. Am J Surg 1999;177:342–3.
6. Terris DJ, Seybt MW, Elchoufi M, et al. Cosmetic thyroid surgery: defining the essential principles. Laryngoscope 2007;117:1168–72.
7. McCurdy J. Considerations in Asian cosmetic surgery. Facial Plast Surg Clin North Am 2007;15:387–97.
8. Duh Q. Robot-assisted endoscopic thyroidectomy: has the time come to abandon neck incisions? Ann Surg 2011;253(6):1067–8.
9. Hüscher CS, Chiodinin S, Napolitano C, et al. Endoscopic right thyroid lobectomy. Surg Endosc 1997;11:877.
10. Ohgami M, Ishii S, Arisawa Y, et al. Scarless endoscopic thyroidectomy: breast approach for better cosmesis. Surg Laparosc Endosc Percutan Tech 2000;10:1–4.
11. Ikeda Y, Takami H, Niimi M, et al. Endoscopic thyroidectomy by the axillary approach. Surg Endosc 2001;15:1362–4.
12. Gottlieb A, Sprung J, Zheng XM, et al. Massive subcutaneous emphysema and severe hypercarbia in a patient during endoscopic transcervical parathyroidectomy using carbon dioxide insufflation. Anesth Analg 1997;84:1154–6.
13. Miccoli P, Berti P, Raffaelli M, et al. Minimally invasive video-assisted thyroidectomy. Am J Surg 2001;181:567–70.
14. Shimizu K, Akira S, Tanaka S. Video-assisted neck surgery: endoscopic resection of benign thyroid tumor aiming at scarless surgery on the neck. J Surg Oncol 1998;69:178–80.
15. Kataoka H, Kitano H, Takeuchi E, et al. Total video endoscopic thyroidectomy via the anterior chest approach using the cervical region-lifting method. Biomed Pharmacother 2002;56:68s–71s.

16. Youben F, Bo W, Chunlin Z, et al. Trans-areola single-site endoscopic thyroidectomy: pilot study of 35 cases. Surg Endosc 2012;26:939–47.

17. Kang SW, Lee SC, Lee SH, et al. Robotic thyroid surgery using a gasless, transaxillary approach and the da Vinci S system: the operative outcomes of 338 consecutive patients. Surgery 2009;146:1048–55.

18. Terris DJ, Chin E. Clinical implementation of endoscopic thyroidectomy in selected patients. Laryngoscope 2006;116:1745–8.

19. Shimazu K, Shiba E, Tamaki Y, et al. Endoscopic thyroid surgery through the axillo-bilateral-breast approach. Surg Laparosc Endosc Percutan Tech 2003; 13:196–201.

20. Choe JH, Kim SW, Chung KW, et al. Endoscopic thyroidectomy using a new bilateral axillo-breast approach. World J Surg 2007;31:601–6.

21. Lee KE, Rao J, Youn YK. Endoscopic thyroidectomy with the da Vinci robot system using the bilateral axillary breast approach (BABA) technique. Our initial experience. Surg Laparosc Endosc Percutan Tech 2009;19:e71–5.

22. Rosato L, Avenia N, Bernante P, et al. Complications of thyroid surgery: analysis of a multicentric study on 14,934 patients operated on in Italy over 5 years. World J Surg 2004;28:271–6.

23. Gupta PK, Smith RB, Gupta H, et al. Outcomes after thyroidectomy and parathyroidectomy. Head Neck 2012;34:477–84.

24. Miccoli P, Berti P, Materazzi G, et al. Minimally invasive video-assisted thyroidectomy: five years of experience. J Am Coll Surg 2004;199:243–8.

25. Terris DJ, Angelos P, Steward DL, et al. Minimally invasive video-assisted thyroidectomy. A multi-institutional North American experience. Arch Otolaryngol Head Neck Surg 2008;134:81–4.

26. Park CS, Chung WY, Chang HS. Minimally invasive open thyroidectomy. Surg Today 2001;31:665–9.

27. Tan CT, Cheah WK, Delbridge L. "Scarless" (in the neck) endoscopic thyroidectomy (SET): an evidence-based review of published techniques. World J Surg 2008;32:1349–57.

28. Kang SW, Jeong JJ, Yun JS, et al. Robot-assisted endoscopic surgery for thyroid cancer: experience with the first 100 patients. Surg Endosc 2009;23:2399–406.

29. Jackson NR, Yao L, Tufano RP, et al. Safety of robotic thyroidectomy approaches: meta-analysis and systematic review. Head Neck 2013. http://dx.doi.org/10.1002/hed.23223.

30. Lee J, Yun JH, Nam KH, et al. The learning curve for robotic thyroidectomy: a multicenter study. Ann Surg Oncol 2011;18:226–32.

31. Landry C, Grubbs E, Warneke C, et al. Robot-assisted transaxillary thyroid surgery in the United States: is it comparable to open thyroid lobectomy? Ann Surg Oncol 2012;19:1269–74.

32. Cabot JC, Lee CR, Brunaud L, et al. Robotic and endoscopic transaxillary thyroidectomies may be cost prohibitive when compared to standard cervical thyroidectomy: a cost analysis. Surgery 2012;152:1016–24.

33. Perrier N. Why I have abandoned robot-assisted transaxillary thyroid surgery. Surgery 2012;152:1025–6.

34. Minuto MN, Berti P, Miccoli M, et al. Minimally invasive video-assisted thyroidectomy: an analysis of results and a revision of indications. Surg Endosc 2012;26:818–22.

35. Neidich MJ, Steward DL. Safety and feasibility of elective minimally invasive video-assisted central neck dissection for thyroid carcinoma. Head Neck 2012;34:354–8.

36. Miccoli P, Bellantone R, Mourad M, et al. Minimally invasive video-assisted thyroidectomy: multiinstitutional experience. World J Surg 2002;26:972–5.
37. Terris DJ, Seybt MW. Modifications of Miccoli minimally invasive thyroidectomy for the low-volume surgeon. Am J Otol 2011;32:392–7.
38. Ferzli GS, Sayad P, Abdo Z, et al. Minimally invasive, nonendoscopic thyroid surgery. J Am Coll Surg 2001;192:665–8.
39. Hur SM, Kim SH, Lee SK, et al. New endoscopic thyroidectomy with the bilateral areolar approach: a comparison with the bilateral axillo-breast approach. Surg Laparosc Endosc Percutan Tech 2011;21:e219–24.
40. Youben F, Bomin G, Bo W, et al. Trans-areola single-incision endoscopic thyroidectomy. Surg Laparosc Endosc Percutan Tech 2011;21:e192–6.
41. Yeung GH. Endoscopic thyroid surgery today: a diversity of surgical strategies. Thyroid 2002;12:703–6.
42. Ogden J, Lindridge L. The impact of breast scarring on perceptions of attractiveness. An experimental study. J Health Psychol 2008;13:303–10.
43. Ikeda Y, Takami H, Sasaki Y, et al. Clinical benefits in endoscopic thyroidectomy by the axillary approach. J Am Coll Surg 2003;196:189–95.
44. Yoon JH, Park CH, Chung WO. Gasless endoscopic thyroidectomy via an axillary approach: experience of 30 Cases. Surg Laparosc Endosc Percutan Tech 2006;16:226–31.
45. Kang SW, Jeong JJ, Nam KH, et al. Robot-assisted endoscopic thyroidectomy for thyroid malignancies using a gasless transaxillary approach. J Am Coll Surg 2009;209:e1–7.
46. Bärlehner E, Benhidjeb T. Cervical scarless endoscopic thyroidectomy: axillo-bilateral-breast approach (ABBA). Surg Endosc 2008;22:154–7.
47. Witzel K, von Rahden BH, Kaminski C, et al. Transoral access for endoscopic thyroid resection. Surg Endosc 2008;22:1871–5.
48. Benhidjeb T, Wilhelm T, Harlaar J, et al. Natural orifice surgery on thyroid gland: totally transoral video-assisted thyroidectomy (TOVAT): report of first experimental results of a new surgical method. Surg Endosc 2009;23:1119–20.
49. Wilhelm T, Metzig A. Endoscopic minimally invasive thyroidectomy (eMIT): a prospective proof-of-concept study in humans. World J Surg 2011;35:543–51.
50. Nakajo A, Arima H, Hirata M, et al. Trans-oral video-assisted neck surgery (TOVANS). A new transoral technique of endoscopic thyroidectomy with gasless premandible approach. Surg Endosc 2013;27:1105–10.
51. Lobe T, Wright SK, Irish MS. Novel uses of surgical robotics in head and neck surgery. J Laparoendosc Adv Surg Tech A 2005;15:647–52.
52. Ryu HR, Kang SW, Lee SH, et al. Feasibility and Safety of a New Robotic thyroidectomy through a gasless, transaxillary single-incision approach. J Am Coll Surg 2010;211:e13–9.
53. Terris DJ, Singer MC, Seybt MW. Robot facelift thyroidectomy: II. Clinical feasibility and safety. Laryngoscope 2011;121:1636–41.
54. Kang SW, Park JH, Jeong JS, et al. Prospects of robotic thyroidectomy using a gasless, transaxillary approach for the management of thyroid carcinoma. Surg Laparosc Endosc Percutan Tech 2011;21:223–9.
55. Dionigi G. Robotic thyroidectomy: Seoul is not Varese. Otolaryngol Head Neck Surg 2013;148:178.
56. Kuppersmith R, Holsinger F. Robotic thyroid surgery: an initial experience with North American patients. Laryngoscope 2011;121:521–6.
57. Kandil E, Noureldine S, Yao L, et al. Robotic transaxillary thyroidectomy: an examination of the first one hundred cases. J Am Coll Surg 2012;214:558–66.

58. Inabnet WB. Robotic thyroidectomy: must we drive a luxury sedan to arrive at our destination safely? Thyroid 2012;22:988–90.
59. Terris DJ, Singer MC. Qualitative and quantitative differences between 2 robotic thyroidectomy techniques. Otolaryngol Head Neck Surg 2012;147:20–5.
60. Terris D, Singer MC, Seybt MW. Robotic facelift thyroidectomy: patient selection and technical considerations. Surg Laparosc Endosc Percutan Tech 2011;21(4): 237–42.
61. Terris DJ, Singer MC. Robotic facelift thyroidectomy: facilitating remote access surgery. Head Neck 2012;34:746–7.

Persistent Posttreatment Fatigue in Thyroid Cancer Survivors

A Scoping Review

Anna M. Sawka, MD, PhD, FRCPC[a,b,]*, Asima Naeem, BSc[a],
Jennifer Jones, PhD[c,d], Julia Lowe, MBChB, MMedSci[b,e],
Philip Segal, MD, FRCPC[a,b,f], Jeannette Goguen, MD, MEd, FRCPC[b,g],
Jeremy Gilbert, MD, FRCPC[b,e], Afshan Zahedi, MD, FRCPC[b,f,h],
Catherine Kelly, MD, FRCPC[b,h], Shereen Ezzat, MD, FRCPC[i]

KEYWORDS

- Thyroid cancer • Fatigue • Vitality • Quality of life • Survivorship

KEY POINTS

- There is evidence that long-term fatigue is a common problem among thyroid cancer (TC) survivors.
- It is challenging to make specific recommendations on the treatment of persistent post-treatment fatigue (PPF) in TC survivors, because of a paucity of randomized controlled trials in this population.

Continued

Funding: This work was funded in part by a University of Toronto Department of Medicine Strategic Innovation Fund grant. A.M. Sawka currently holds a Chair in Health Services Research from Cancer Care Ontario, funded by the Ontario Ministry of Health and Long-term Care.
Disclosures: Other than the academic funding listed earlier, the authors have no relevant disclosures to declare.
[a] Division of Endocrinology, Department of Medicine, University Health Network, 200 Elizabeth Street, 12th Floor, Toronto, Ontario M5G 2C4, Canada; [b] Division of Endocrinology, Department of Medicine, University of Toronto, 200 Elizabeth Street, 12 EN-243, Toronto, Ontario M5G 2C4, Canada; [c] Department of Psychiatry, University of Toronto, 250 College Street, 8th Floor, Toronto, Ontario M5T 1R8, Canada; [d] Cancer Survivorship Program, Princess Margaret Hospital, University Health Network, 200 Elizabeth Street, Bcs-045, Toronto, Ontario M5G 2C4, Canada; [e] Division of Endocrinology, Department of Medicine, Sunnybrook Health Sciences Center, 2075 Bayview Avenue, H Wing, Toronto, Ontario M4N 3M5, Canada; [f] Division of Endocrinology, Department of Medicine, Mount Sinai Hospital, 600 University Avenue, Toronto, Ontario M5G 1X5, Canada; [g] Division of Endocrinology, Department of Medicine, St. Michael's Hospital, 61 Queen Street East, 6th Floor, Toronto, Ontario M5C 2T2, Canada; [h] Division of Endocrinology, Department of Medicine, Women's College Hospital, 76 Grenville Street, Toronto, Ontario M5S 1B2, Canada; [i] Endocrine Oncology Site Group, Princess Margaret Hospital, University Health Network, 200 Elizabeth Street, 12NU-1200, Toronto, Ontario M5G 2C4, Canada
* Corresponding author. Toronto General Hospital, 200 Elizabeth Street, 12 EN-212, Toronto, Ontario M5G 2C4, Canada.
E-mail address: Annie.Sawka@uhn.ca

Endocrinol Metab Clin N Am 43 (2014) 475–494
http://dx.doi.org/10.1016/j.ecl.2014.02.007
endo.theclinics.com

Continued

- There is a need for more research in PPF in TC survivors, including studies examining the severity prevalence, modifying factors, natural history, and associated life impact.
- There is a strong need for randomized controlled trials examining treatment of fatigue in TC survivors.

INTRODUCTION

There are currently more than a half a million thyroid cancer (TC) survivors in the United States.[1] Furthermore, TC incidence rates are increasing.[1,2] It is thus important to address any long-term problems in this growing population. Persistent posttreatment fatigue (PPF) is one of the most common problems encountered in general oncology populations,[3–11] with an estimated prevalence of about 19% to 38%.[4] There is no universally accepted definition of PPF (also referred to as cancer-related fatigue) in cancer survivors, but some generally accepted concepts include a multidimensional nature (eg, physical and mental components), symptoms out of proportion to exertion, incomplete relief with rest, and interference with usual functioning.[3,4,7] Cancer-related fatigue may occur as a consequence of malignancy or its treatment,[3,7] or in association with related conditions (eg, psychological distress).[6] The prevalence or severity of PPF in TC survivors is not known.

Our objective was to examine the volume, breadth, and type of research published on PPF in TC survivors. As a secondary objective, we identified some research gaps. The study design was that of a scoping review, with the intention of performing a preliminary search and mapping a broad range of literature on the topic.[12–17]

METHODS

The general method followed was that of a scoping review, which typically involves (1) identifying a broad research question, (2) identifying relevant studies, (3) study selection, (4) abstracting data, (5) summarizing the results (including key themes), and (6) an optional stakeholder consultation phase.[13] A scoping review typically does not include an in-depth critical appraisal of methodological data (found in systematic reviews), nor pooled quantitative data synthesis (found in meta-analyses).[12–17]

Research Questions

Our primary research question was: what is the current scope of published literature, relating to PPF in TC survivors? Our secondary research aim was to identify research gaps in this field.

Inclusion and Exclusion Criteria for Studies

Our focus for this review was TC survivors who had completed primary oncologic treatment such as surgery, with or without radioactive iodine remnant ablation/treatment or external beam radiation treatment. Short-term fatigue associated with current or recent radioactive iodine treatment, surgery, radiation treatment, or systemic oncologic treatment (such as chemotherapy or targeted molecular therapy) was not a focus of this review. For the purpose of this review, we defined PPF as fatigue that is experienced more than 6 months after completion of any combination of such TC treatment(s). Input on a meaningful time frame for measurement of PPF was received from a clinical content expert (SE) as well as an expert in measurement of fatigue in oncology populations (JJ). Short-term fatigue associated with preparation for radioactive iodine treatment or scanning (eg, thyroid hormone withdrawal, or short-term studies comparing thyroid hormone withdrawal with the use of recombinant human thyrotropin) was not a focus of this review. Our target study population was TC survivors (any primary histologic subtype). For inclusion in the review, it was required that more than half the study population meets all inclusion criteria (ie, for studies of mixed populations) or that data on respective subgroups of interest were reported. Furthermore, fatigue measurements more than 6 months after primary treatment were required to be reported in more than half of the study population (ie, for studies reporting a mixture of short-term and long-term fatigue data in 1 outcome analysis). There was no methodological inclusion restriction. Only published English language articles were included, because of resource limitations for translation of articles. We excluded duplicate publications reporting the same outcome measurements in the same TC survivors, at the same time point.

Search for Relevant Studies

The details of our electronic searches are listed in **Table 1**. In summary, we searched the following electronic databases from inception until September, 2013: EMBASE, Ovid MEDLINE, Ovid MEDLINE In-Process and Other Non-Indexed Citations, and PubMed. The search terms incorporated the condition of thyroid carcinoma as well as the general concept of fatigue, with no restrictions on age, language, or methodology. All electronic searches were conducted by a librarian with expertise in electronic database searching. The hand searches were divided between reviewers, and these included reviews of reference lists from team members with content expertise (AMS), potentially relevant cross-references of included articles (AMS), and tables of contents from January 2008 to September 2013 from some key journals (ie, *Thyroid* and *The Journal of Clinical Endocrinology and Metabolism*) (AN).

Study Selection

Two team members (AMS and AN) independently reviewed the citations retrieved from electronic searches for relevance as well as any full-text articles deemed relevant by either reviewer from either the citation review phase or hand searching. A kappa statistic (with 95% confidence intervals [CIs]) was calculated for estimation of agreement between reviewers on (1) citations retrieved from the electronic database search for inclusion in full-text review, and (2) full-text review for inclusion in the study (using Confidence Interval Analysis Software, Version 2.2.0; T.N. Bryant, PhD, of the University of Southampton).[18] Consensus was achieved between reviewers on the final full-text articles for inclusion in the review, after discussion and rereview of the articles in question.

Data Abstraction and Reporting of Results

The flow of information through various phases of the review process was summarized using a flowchart that was adapted from a published template intended for systematic reviews.[19] Data abstraction was independently performed by 2 reviewers (AMS and AN) on standardized data abstraction forms. For studies collecting data at multiple time points, we abstracted only the long-term fatigue data (ie, more than 6 months following completion of TC treatment). Each abstracted data set was checked (by the other reviewer), and a final consensus data set was created. Key aspects of the published research were identified by both reviewers, using

Table 1
Search terms used in the electronic searches[a]

Database	TC Terms	Fatigue-Related Terms
Embase (1974 to September 18, 2013)	Exp thyroid tumor/ Exp thyroid cancer/ Thyroid cancer.tw. Thyroid carcinoma.tw. Thyroid neoplasm.tw.	Exp Fatigue/ Fatigue?.tw. Exhausted.tw. Exhaustion.tw. Tiredness.tw. Lethargy.tw. Lassitude.tw. Languidness.tw. Asthenia/ Vigor.tw.[a] Vitality.tw.[a]
Ovid MEDLINE (1946 to September 18, 2013)	Exp thyroid neoplasms/ Thyroid cancer.tw. Thyroid carcinoma.tw. Thyroid neoplasm.tw.	Exp Fatigue/ Fatigue?.tw. Exhausted.tw. Exhaustion.tw. Tiredness.tw. Lethargy.tw. Lassitude.tw. Languidness.tw. Fatigue syndrome, chronic/ Asthenia/ Vigor.tw.[a] Vitality.tw.[a]
Ovid MEDLINE In-Process and Other Non-Indexed Citations (inception to September 18, 2013)	Same as under Ovid MEDLINE	Same as under Ovid MEDLINE
PubMed[b] (inception to week 2, September, 2013)	Thyroid neoplasms (MeSH terms) Thyroid neoplasms (all fields) "Thyroid cancer" (all fields)	Fatigue (MeSH terms) Fatigue (all fields) Vigor (all fields)[a] Vitality (all fields)[a]

Abbreviations: Exp, explode; MeSH, medical subject headings; tw, text word.

[a] The search terms for TC were combined with those for fatigue-related outcomes. The original electronic search was conducted on September 18, 2013 without the text words for vigor or vitality, and the search was rerun, incorporating these terms on September 26, 2013.

[b] The PubMed search was restricted to exclude references that were also included in Ovid MEDLINE.

the abstracted data sets. Relevant themes from abstracted data sets were then extracted by both reviewers. Abstracted data, including relevant themes, were summarized in tabular and narrative form within the article. For statistical comparisons performed in the primary studies, we assumed that a P value of less than .05 was statistically significant.

Consultation Phase

Our completed article was reviewed by a group of University of Toronto endocrinologists from various academic hospitals. We specifically sought feedback on the key points/research gaps identified in the review. Feedback was received via e-mail, and any necessary edits were made to the article.

RESULTS
Studies Included in the Scoping Review

The process of study selection is shown in **Fig. 1**. Two reviewers independently screened 898 unique citations from the electronic search. In-depth, full-text review was performed by 2 independent reviewers for 43 articles (19 of which originated from the electronic search, and 24 from the hand search).[20–62] We included 24 articles in the review.[20–43] The reasons for exclusion of other full-text articles were that 2 studies had TC population data that overlapped with that of another included publication,[44,45] 8 studies focused on short-term (acute) fatigue,[46,47,51–53,59–61] 7 studies provided insufficient or no extractable raw data on fatigue,[48–50,54,56,58,62] and most of the study population in 2 of the studies were not TC survivors.[55,57] The 2 studies that overlapped already included studies[44,45] were used as a supplement, to clarify any missing or unclear information from the respective included studies.[21,30] One of the citations that had insufficient extractable fatigue data was limited by being a published meeting abstract, and complete details, as would be found in a fully published article, were not available at the time of our review.[48] The kappa scores for agreement between reviewers for various stages of the review process were as follows: (1) electronic database citation review, kappa 0.729 (95% CI, 0.542, 0.916); (2) full-text review 0.580 (95% CI, 0.336, 0.824).

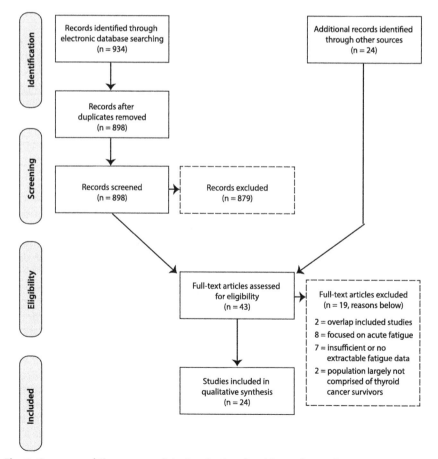

Fig. 1. Summary of the process of study selection for this scoping review.

Description of Studies According to Thematic Content

The studies included in this review, as well as TC survivor and control group characteristics, and instruments used to measure fatigue-related outcomes, are shown in **Table 2**. After abstracting the data, we reviewed the included study characteristics, and agreed on several broad study design themes (categories), as well as relevant subcategories. Studies that provided multiple comparators or multiple outcome analyses are listed in more than one category. The 2 broad categories were: (1) epidemiologic studies, and (2) randomized controlled trials (RCTs) of therapeutic interventions. The epidemiologic analyses were subdivided as follows: (1) 9 studies providing descriptive quantitative data on fatigue in TC survivors at 1 time point (eg, symptom prevalence, fatigue prevalence ranking relative to other symptoms, or measure of fatigue on some form of quantitative measurement instrument), without any non-TC population control comparison[25–27,29,30,35,37,38]; (2) 16 studies providing quantitative comparisons of fatigue-related outcomes between TC populations and non-TC populations, at 1 time point[20,22–24,28,30–34,36,39–43]; and (3) 8 studies providing explanatory data on risk factors or associations for the presence or increasing severity of fatigue-related outcomes at 1 time point.[22,23,28,30–33,42] Three RCTs examined the following types of respective interventions: (1) thyroid hormonal treatment (2 studies; one trial of a combination of synthetic triiodothyronine [T3] with levothyroxine [LT4] substitution for LT4 alone,[21] and another trial of restoration of euthyroidism after prolonged thyroid-stimulating hormone [TSH] suppressive therapy),[24] and (2) supervised exercise.[43]

We could not find various other categories of study designs. For example, we found no long-term prospective studies providing data on the natural history of fatigue in TC survivors at multiple time points beyond 6 months (ie, excluding short-term fatigue measurements in relation to thyroid hormone withdrawal or recombinant human thyrotropin administration for diagnostic surveillance). Furthermore, we found no qualitative studies examining experience descriptions of long-term fatigue, from the perspective of TC survivors. We found no quantitative or qualitative studies examining life impact specifically in relation to severity of PPF (eg, social functioning, missed time from paid work, work productivity, or finances).

Epidemiologic studies

Descriptive fatigue-related data without non-TC control group comparisons This category included descriptive, quantitative data on fatigue in TC survivors at 1 time point (eg, symptom prevalence, fatigue prevalence ranking relative to other symptoms, or measure of fatigue on some form of quantitative measurement instrument), without any non-TC population control group comparison, and consisted of data from 9 studies, including a combined total of 1129 TC survivors.[25–27,29,30,35,37,38,41] In 4 respective clinical samples of TC survivors, fatigue was the most commonly reported physical symptom.[25,29,35,38] The overall prevalence rates of long-term fatigue in clinical populations of TC survivors were reported to be 54.4%[35] and 62.1%[38] in respective studies. Huang and colleagues[29] reported that the prevalence of fatigue in the past month was 41.1% (reported as part of the Quality-of-life Index questionnaire, which was administered 6 to 36 months after TC surgery). Gning and colleagues[25] reported that severe fatigue was experienced by 28.3% of TC survivors, whereas the same percentage of respondents had no fatigue. In a cancer registry–based survey study from the Netherlands, 50% of TC survivors reported experiencing abrupt attacks of fatigue on the Thyroid Cancer Survivors' Association Quality of Life (THYCA-QoL) questionnaire, and this was the third most common complaint, after pain in the joints or muscles (64%) and feeling chilly (52%).[30] In another clinic-based study from Columbia, South America, tiredness, with or without decay or dry skin, was reported as a posttreatment effect in 20% of TC survivors (although the definition of decay was unclear).[27] Four respective studies described a single time point measurement for fatigue-related outcomes from generic quality-of-life instruments, without any control comparison, including 2 studies[26,27] reporting the Vitality subscale of the Short Form 36 (SF-36), another study[37] reporting fatigue symptom data from the European Organization for Research and Treatment of Cancer (EORTC)-QLQ-C30 questionnaire, and a fourth study[41] reporting the Vigor-Vitality and Fatigue-Inertia subscales data from the Profile of Mood States (POMS).

Case-control comparisons of fatigue-related outcomes at 1 time point There was a total of 16 studies,[20,22–24,28,30–34,36,39–43] including a combined total of 2122 TC survivors, that reported 1 or more case-control comparisons of fatigue-related outcome data on TC survivors compared with non-TC controls. For 15 of these studies, the comparator group was a general population or healthy (variably defined) control population.[20,22–24,28,30–32,34,36,39–43] Of the 15 studies (N = 1982 TC survivors) reporting 1 or more case-control comparisons with population or healthy controls, fatigue was reported to be significantly worse in the TC group in 1 or more analyses in 10 of the studies.[20,22,23,28,30–32,41–43] For this descriptive summary, the number of participants in the 2 different outcome studies by Husson and colleagues[30,31] was only counted once. More information, according to type of fatigue-related outcome measured in the study, is detailed later.

There were 7 studies reporting quantitative comparisons of fatigue-related outcomes in TC survivors compared with non-TC population control groups, using dedicated fatigue questionnaires (at 1 time point).[23,24,28,31–33,43] In 6 of the studies, fatigue questionnaire data from TC survivors was compared with general population or healthy control data (variably defined),[23,24,28,31,32,43] whereas in 1 study the comparator group contained individuals treated for autoimmune hypothyroidism.[33] The specific fatigue questionnaires used in these studies included the Brief Fatigue Inventory (1 study[32]), the Chalder Fatigue Scale (2 studies[23,43]), the Fatigue Assessment Scale (1 study[31]), and the Multidimensional Fatigue Inventory-20 (MFI-20) (3 studies[24,28,33]). In 5[23,28,31,32,43] of the 6 studies[23,24,28,31,32,43] comparing fatigue levels in TC survivors with population or healthy controls (variably defined), fatigue levels were statistically significantly worse in the TC group. In 1 of these studies, the prevalence of Fatigue Assessment Scale classification in the fatigued or very fatigued category ranged from 39% to 47% in TC survivors out to more than 15 years after diagnosis, whereas the prevalence was 25% in age-matched and sex-matched population controls (P<.001).[31] In 1 study comparing MFI-20 scores between TC survivors and individuals treated for autoimmune hypothyroidism, fatigue levels were reported to be significantly worse in the latter group (P<.001).[33] However, the autoimmune thyroid group had a significantly shorter mean LT4 treatment period, significantly higher mean TSH measurements, and significantly higher mean body mass index compared with the TC survivors.[33] In this study, the median TSH level was 0.07 mIU/L in the TC survivors, and 1.20 mIU/L in the treated autoimmune hypothyroid group (P<.001 for the difference in TSH).[33]

There were 10 studies that reported quantitative comparisons of fatigue-related outcomes between TC populations and non-TC populations using generic quality-of-life or general symptom questionnaires.[20,22,23,30,34,36,39–42] All of these studies used general population or health control group (variably described) comparator groups.[20,22,23,30,34,36,39–42] The questionnaires and relevant subscales/symptom domains used in these studies included the Vitality subscale of the SF-36 (8 studies[20,22,23,34,39–42]), the Fatigue subscale of the EORTC-QLQ-C30 (1 study[30]),

Table 2
Characteristics of included studies

First Author (Year, Country)	TC Population	Control Population	Fatigue-Related Outcome Measurement Instrument
Botella-Carretero[20] (2003, Spain)	18 women with DTC Mean age 44 y All had suppressed TSH level No active SR	18 healthy, euthyroid women (patients' relatives or hospital employees) Mean age 43 y	SF-36 (Vitality)[63-65] POMS (Vigor-Activity)[66] Visual Analog Mental Scales (Tiredness) Nottingham Health Profile (Energy)[67,68]
Bunevicius[21] (2003, Lithuania)[a,b]	15 women, history TC Mean age 46 y Mean TSH 0.09 mIU/L	Crossover design randomized trial (so same as TC population)	POMS (Vigor-Activity, Fatigue-Inertia)[66]
Crevenna[22] (2003, Austria)	150 DTC survivors, both sexes Mean age 52 y TSH not reported, but free thyroxine normal No active SR	Age-matched and sex-matched reference values	SF-36 (Vitality) (German version)[69]
De Oliveira Chachamovitz[23] (2013, Brazil)	38 DTC survivors, both sexes Mean age 45 y Mean TSH 0.23 mIU/L (inclusion criterion of TSH <0.4 mIU/L) No active SR	54 healthy individuals known to TC group, similar sex to TC group Mean age 43 y Mean TSH 1.70 mIU/L	Chalder Fatigue Scale (Portuguese version)[70-72] SF-36 (Vitality Subscale),[77] Portuguese version
Eustatia-Rutten[24] (2006, Netherlands)[a,b]	For baseline measures for the nonrandomized case-control comparison, total 24 DTC survivors, both sexes Mean age 49 y Median TSH 0.058 mIU/L No active SR For the randomized trial: 12 of the individuals were randomized to be rendered euthyroid	For the nonrandomized case-control comparison: age-related reference Dutch values were used for a comparison with the baseline measures For the randomized trial: half of the TC population (n = 12) was randomized to continue TSH-suppressive therapy	MFI-20[73]

Gning[25] (2009, United States)	60 TC survivors, both sexes Mean age 51 y No active SR in 38%	NA	MD Anderson Symptom Inventory – TC Module (core symptom of fatigue)[74]
Golger[26] (2003, Canada)	181 DTC survivors, both sexes Mean age 43 y Median baseline TSH 0.19 mIU/L No active SR	NA	SF-36 (Vitality)[75,76]
Gomez[27] (2010, Columbia)	75 TC survivors, both sexes Central age range 45–61 y TSH and recurrence status not reported	NA	SF-36 (Vitality)[77] Symptom inquiry
Hoftijzer[28] (2008, Netherlands)	153 DTC survivors, both sexes Mean age 49 y Median TSH 0.1 mIU/L No active SR	Two separate control groups: 1. 113 controls selected by the patients with TC, of comparable age, sex, and socioeconomic status 2. Data pooled from 336 age-matched and gender-matched controls from other Leiden quality-of-life studies	MFI-20[78]
Huang[29] (2004, Taiwan)	146 TC survivors, both sexes Mean age 48 y TSH and current disease status not reported	NA	Quality-of-Life Index[79,80]
Husson[30] (2013, Netherlands)	306 TC survivors, both sexes Mean age 56.4 y TSH and current disease status not reported	800 age-matched and sex-matched cancer-free controls from the Netherlands	THYCA-QOL (fatigue symptom) (only TC group)[81] EORTC-QLQ-C30[82]
Husson[31] (2013, Netherlands)	See row above	530 age-matched and sex-matched controls from the Netherlands	Fatigue Assessment Scale[83]
Lee[32] (2010, South Korea)	316 DTC survivors, both sexes Mean age 46 y Mean TSH 0.49 MIU/L No active SR	Sex-matched and age-matched reference control group data adopted from previously published study of the general Korean population	Brief Fatigue Inventory[84,85]

(continued on next page)

Table 2
(continued)

First Author (Year, Country)	TC Population	Control Population	Fatigue-Related Outcome Measurement Instrument
Louwerens[33] (2012, Netherlands)	140 DTC survivors, both sexes; Mean age 49 y; Mean TSH 0.07 mIU/L; No active SR	138 patients treated for autoimmune hypothyroidism, both sexes; Mean age 48 y; Mean TSH 1.20 mIU/L	MFI-20[86]
Malterling[34] (2010, Sweden)	52 TC survivors, both sexes; Median age 61 y; No TSH data; 6% had active TC	Healthy Swedish population reference data	SF-36 (Vitality)[87-89]
Mendoza[35] (2004,c United States)	54 DTC survivors, both sexes; No TSH data; Although some had history of treated TC recurrence, current active SR status not reported	NA	Symptom inquiry
Peltarri[36] (2009, Finland)	341 DTC survivors, both sexes, with low-risk TC at diagnosis; Mean age 52 y; No TSH measurements	Published reference control group data for the Finnish population from a national health survey	15D Instrument[90]
Roberts[37] (2010, United States)	62 TC survivors, both sexes; Mean age 53 y; No TSH data; No data on active SR	NA	EORTC-QLQ-C30[82]
Roerink[38] (2013, Netherlands)	145 DTC survivors, both sexes; Mean age 40 y; Mean TSH 0.42 mIU/L; Active SR in 6.2%	NA	Distress Thermometer and Problem List (Dutch version)[91,92]
Schroeder[39] (2006, United States)	228 DTC survivors, both sexes; Mean age 47 y; Median baseline TSH 0.08–0.10 mIU/L[49]; 21% had radioactive iodine scan positivity outside the thyroid bed[49]	Published general United States population norms (not reported if any specific age or sex adjustment performed in the analysis)	SF-36 (Vitality)[75,77]

Study	Participants	Comparison	Measure
Shah[40] (2006, Canada)	55% of population had TC, the rest benign thyroid disorder; all had thyroid surgery, both sexes; Mean age 46 y; No TSH data; No data on active SR	Published median SF-36 scores for the United States general population	SF-36 (Vitality)[77]
Tagay[41] (2005, Germany)	100 DTC survivors, both sexes; Mean age 50 y; Median TSH <0.01 mIU/L; No data on active SR	Published German general population data for the SF-36, matched for age; No comparison group for the POMS data	SF-36 (Vitality)[93]; POMS (Vigor-Vitality)[94]
Tan[42] (2007, Singapore)	144 DTC survivors, both sexes; Mean age 48 y; No TSH data; No data on active SR	SF-36 population norms for the Singaporean population, adjusted for age, sex, race, and survey language	SF-36 (Vitality)[76,95–97]
Vigario[43] (2011, Brazil)[a,d]	For the nonrandomized case-control comparison: 36 DTC survivors, both sexes (in case-control comparison); Median age 48 y; Median TSH 0.02 mIU/L; No active SR; For the randomized trial: 19 of these individuals were randomized to a 12-wk exercise program	For the nonrandomized case-control comparison: 48 controls without thyroid disease, of both sexes, were recruited; Median age 51 y; Median TSH 1.56 mIU/L; For the randomized trial, 17 of the individuals in the preceding column were randomized to be physically inactive	Chalder Fatigue Scale[70]

Abbreviations: DTC, differentiated TC; EORTC-QLQ, European Organization for Research and Treatment of Cancer Quality-of-life Questionnaire; MFI-20, Multidimensional Fatigue Inventory 20; NA, not applicable; POMS, Profile of Mood States; SR, structural recurrence; THYCA-QOL, Thyroid Cancer Survivors' Association Quality of Life; TSH, thyroid-stimulating hormone.

a Randomized controlled trial.
b Some blinding in the randomized controlled trial.
c Retrospective chart review.
d No blinding in the randomized controlled trial.
Data from Refs.[20–43]

the Vitality subscale of the 15D questionnaire (1 study[36]), the Fatigue-Inertia and the Vigor-Activity subscales of the POMS, the Energy subscale of the Nottingham Health Profile, and the Fatigue symptom on the Visual Analog Mental Scales (all in 1 study[20]). Three[22,41,42] of the 8 analyses of the Vitality subscale of the SF-36 questionnaire[20,22,23,34,39–42] showed statistically significantly worse vitality scores in TC survivors, compared with controls. The only study that used the Fatigue subscale of the EORTC-QLQ-C30 reported a statistically significant difference in fatigue levels between TC survivors and age-matched and sex-matched cancer-free controls.[30] Also, in 1 analysis of the Energy subscale data from the Nottingham Health Profile, TC survivors had significantly worse levels compared with controls.[20] There were no significant differences between TC survivors and controls in respective analyses on fatigue-related subscales of the POMS,[20] 15D,[36] or the Visual Analog Mental Scales.[20] In summary, of the 10 respective studies[20,22,23,30,34,36,39–42] comparing fatigue-related outcomes between TC survivors and non-TC controls using generic quality-of-life or symptom questionnaires, 5 of the studies[20,22,30,41,42] reported that fatigue was worse in TC survivors, in at least 1 such analysis.

Explanatory studies We identified 8 explanatory studies,[22,23,28,30–33,42] including a total of 1247 TC survivors, that explored risk factors or associations for the presence or increasing severity of fatigue-related outcomes at 1 time point. Crevenna and colleagues[22] reported that, in a multiple regression analysis, time since initial diagnosis was significantly associated with reduced SF-36 Vitality subscale score, but not gender, age, number of concomitant diseases, or partnership status. Furthermore, Hoftijzer and colleagues[28] reported that, using a stepwise univariable linear regression, longer duration of differentiated TC (DTC) cure was associated with statistically significantly less fatigue on the MFI-20 subscales of General Fatigue ($P = .035$), Physical Fatigue ($P = .003$), and Mental Fatigue ($P = .038$). Husson and colleagues[30] reported no statistically significant difference between Fatigue subscale scores of the EORTC-QLQ-C30 between TC survivors at less than 5 years after diagnosis, compared with those 5 to 10 years after diagnosis, and those more than 10 years after diagnosis ($P = .4$), but having one or more comorbidities was associated with more fatigue ($P<.05$). Furthermore, in the same population, Husson and colleagues[31] reported that Fatigue Assessment Scale Questionnaire scores were not significantly different between survivors according to time since diagnosis (ie, <5 years, 5–10 years, 10–15 years, or >15 years), but there was some variability in statistical significance of fatigue associations with age, comorbidity, presence of psychological problems, and marital status, among various multivariable logistic regression models explored.[31] Some variables that were not statistically significantly associated with higher Fatigue Assessment Scale score in any of the multivariable models in this study included sex, clinicopathologic stage of disease, or the presence of any additional TC treatment after TC surgery.[31] De Oliveira Chachamovitz and colleagues[23] reported in respective secondary subgroup analyses of 30 female and 8 male TC survivors whose TSH was less than 0.4 mIU/L (with normal free thyroxine measurements) that levels of fatigue measured by Chalder Fatigue Scale were not significantly different when the mean TSH value was less than 0.1 mIU/L, compared with those when the mean TSH was greater than or equal to 0.1 mIU/L. Furthermore, in this study, Vitality subscale measurements were not significantly different between these two TSH categories in an analysis of 30 women (male vitality data not reported for this subgroup analysis).[23] In a univariate analysis, Lee and colleagues[32] reported no significant difference in Brief Fatigue Inventory scores between TC survivors who were treated with TC surgery alone, compared with those groups treated with TC surgery with various dose activities of radioactive iodine. Tan and colleagues[42] reported that, in a multivariable analysis, reduced Vitality score on the SF-36 questionnaire was statistically significantly predicted by the presence of more than 5 medical appointment days in the past 12 months, but not level of education or employment status. Furthermore, age, race, and the presence of 2 or more TC surgeries did not significantly predict this outcome in univariable analyses in this study.[42] In a univariable analysis, Louwerens and colleagues[33] suggested that the presence of the TSH receptor–Asp727Glu polymorphic allele was associated with significantly more fatigue in DTC survivors on 4 out of 5 subscales of the MFI-20 (ie, General Fatigue, Physical Fatigue, Reduced Activity, and Reduced Motivation) compared with the wild type for the allele. The Asp/Glu polymorphism was present in 10.7% of the DTC survivors in this study.[33] It was hypothesized in this study that the Asp/Glu polymorphism was more sensitive than the wild-type TSH receptor, thereby theoretically increasing neuronal ability to modulate intracellular thyroid hormone levels in patients with the polymorphism.[33] There was reported to be no significant difference in biochemical parameters between genotypes in the patients with DTC in this study.[33]

RCTs of interventions

There were 3 RCTs, examining the effect of interventions on fatigue-related outcomes, in a combined total of 75 TC survivors.[21,24,43] None of these trials had a specific eligibility criterion, requiring participants to have any degree of fatigue before enrollment in the study. Bunevicius and colleagues[21] reported a subgroup analysis in 15 female TC survivors who had been enrolled as part of a larger, single-center, blinded, crossover design RCT,[44] in which the use of the usual LT4 dose was compared with the combination of T3 and LT4 (where 50 μg of the usual LT4 dose was substituted with 12.5 μg of T3) for 5 weeks, and vice versa. The results of the POMS questionnaire subscales were conflicting, showing statistically significant improvements in the Fatigue-Inertia subscale, but no significant difference in the Vigor-Activity subscale of the same questionnaire, for the combination therapy group compared with the LT4 group (secondary subgroup analyses in the RCT).[21] In a single-blinded parallel-design RCT of 6 months' duration, Eustatia-Rutten and colleagues[24] compared the use of the usual LT4 dose (with a target TSH <0.4 mIU/L) with a reduced dose of LT4 with placebo with the intention of achieving euthyroidism (target TSH 0.4–4.8 mIU/L). This RCT included 24 DTC survivors who had been on TSH-suppressive therapy for more than 10 years (mean of 12 years, standard deviation 1 year).[24] Eustatia-Rutten and colleagues[24] compared the baseline and 6-month subscale scores from the Multidimensional Fatigue Index 20 (ie, subscales of General Fatigue, Physical Fatigue, Reduced Activity, Reduced Motivation, and Mental Fatigue) for respective study arms. There was no significant change in all of these fatigue-related subscales in participants who had been maintained on TSH-suppressive therapy, and no significant change in most of the subscales in the euthyroid group, with the exception of statistically significant improvement in the Reduced Motivation subscale ($P = .003$).[24] In a third, unblinded, RCT, Vigário Pdos and colleagues[43] randomized 36 DTC survivors who were on TSH-suppressive therapy (TSH <0.4 mIU/L) to an individually prescribed supervised exercise program (treadmill-based aerobic activity with warm-up and cool-down, for a total 60 minutes, twice a week, for 12 weeks), compared with prescribed physical inactivity (ie, participants instructed to do as little as possible for 12 weeks). Fatigue (measured by the Chalder Fatigue Scale) was significantly reduced in the exercise group, and significantly worsened in the inactivity group, at 3 months.[43]

SUMMARY

In this scoping review, we found that most of the published literature on PPF in TC survivors is epidemiologic in nature, and there is a paucity of RCTs. Most of the epidemiologic literature is focused on cross-sectional comparisons of fatigue-related outcome measurements relative to control populations. Furthermore, the control group comparisons are largely composed of general population or healthy individuals (variably defined). In uncontrolled clinical studies, fatigue seems to be one of the most frequently reported problems. Also, most studies evaluating levels of fatigue in TC survivors compared with the general population or healthy controls suggest that fatigue is worse in the TC group on at least one measurement. However, there is some variability in study findings, which may be partly caused by variability in measurement tools. We found little research examining the prevalence of fatigue according to severity levels. Furthermore, risk or explanatory factors for fatigue were inconsistent among the studies examining this issue. The relationship between fatigue and thyroid hormone biochemical indices was not clear in the limited data for this issue. Some limitations of this review include exclusion of unpublished literature, a modest level of agreement between reviewers for study inclusion at the full-text review stage (largely caused by challenges in interpreting the minimum threshold for data that could be abstracted for inclusion, from studies in which outcomes of interest were not clearly reported), abstraction of limited clinical details, limited methodological appraisal of primary studies, and no quantitative meta-analyses of abstracted data. However, our intention was to provide a broad general overview of the topic in TC populations, rather than a systematic review of specific details of the individual studies, or any pooled statistical analysis. In the process of performing this scoping review, we have determined that there are sufficient data for one or more in-depth systematic reviews in this area, which could provide more detailed, in-depth insights on the results.

There are many research gaps PPF in TC survivors that may be identified from this review. For example, there is a need for more RCTs for the treatment of fatigue in affected TC survivors. There is also a need for more research examining fatigue severity, modifying factors, natural history, and associated life impact in TC survivors. Qualitative research examining the experience of fatigue from TC survivors' perspectives would also be valuable.

The results of this scoping review may be considered in the broader findings of other reviews, summarizing the knowledge and research priorities in cancer-related fatigue,[98] and cancer survivorship.[99] Some research priorities recently identified by experts in cancer-related fatigue that may be relevant to TC include examining the biology and behavioral mechanisms of fatigue (ideally using long-term, prospective cohort studies), clarifying the minimal clinically important differences in the measurement of fatigue (ie, the smallest difference that is perceived to be important by patients), establishing fatigue severity thresholds for participation in intervention RCTs, and conducting dissemination trials of effective management strategies.[98] Moreover, as part of a scoping review of research in cancer survivorship care, Richardson and colleagues[99] suggested that research priorities (including in management of PPF), should incorporate (1) large-scale prospective cohort studies, describing the needs of long-term survivors and predicting those at highest risk; (2) RCTs of specific delivery-ready interventions; and (3) research identifying the most effective and efficient ways to guide organization of care. Such goals have not yet been met in TC survivorship research, and it is likely that this scoping review will generate more questions than answers. Nevertheless, we hope that this work will broaden thoughtful consideration by stakeholders on PPF in a significant subset of TC survivors.

ACKNOWLEDGMENTS

We thank Ms Junhui Zhang, MEd, MLIS, an Information Specialist at the Princess Margaret Hospital, for assistance with the electronic database searches. We also acknowledge the research administrative assistance of Mrs Coreen Marino for retrieving many of the articles for review.

REFERENCES

1. National Cancer Institute – Surveillance Epidemiology and End Results. 2013 SEER stat fact sheets: thyroid. Available at: http://seer.cancer.gov/statfacts/html/thyro.html. Accessed October 3, 2013.
2. Statistics Canada. 2013 Canadian cancer statistics 2013. Available at: http://www.cancer.ca/~/media/cancer.ca/CW/publications/Canadian%20Cancer%20Statistics/canadian-cancer-statistics-2013-EN.pdf. Accessed October 9, 2013.
3. Hofman M, Ryan JL, Figueroa-Mosely CD, et al. Cancer-related fatigue: the scale of the problem. Oncologist 2007;12(Suppl):4–10.
4. Prue G, Rankin J, Allen J, et al. Cancer-related fatigue: a critical appraisal. Eur J Cancer 2006;42:846–63.
5. Donovan KA, McGinty HL, Jacobsen PB. A systematic review of research using diagnostic criteria for cancer-related fatigue. Psychooncology 2012;22:737–44.
6. Oh HS, Seo WS. Systematic review and meta-analysis of correlates of cancer-related fatigue. Worldviews Evid Based Nurs 2011;8(4):191–201.
7. Neefjes EC, van der Vorst MJ, Blauwhoff-Buskermolen S, et al. Aiming for a better understanding and management of cancer-related fatigue. Oncologist 2013; 18(10):1135–43.
8. Curt GA. The impact of fatigue on patients with cancer: overview of FATIGUE 1 and FATIGUE 2. Oncologist 2000;5(Suppl 2):9–12.
9. Baker F, Denniston M, Smith T, et al. Adult cancer survivors: how are they faring? Cancer 2005;104(Suppl 11):2565–76.
10. Lawrence DP, Kupelnick B, Miller K, et al. Evidence report on the occurrence, assessment, and treatment of fatigue in cancer patients. J Natl Cancer Inst Monogr 2004;(32):40–50.
11. Vogelzang NJ, Breitbart W, Cella D, et al. Patient, caregiver, and oncologist perceptions of cancer-related fatigue: results of a tri-part assessment survey. The Fatigue Coalition. Seminars in Hematology 1997;34(3 Suppl 2):4–12.
12. Grant MJ, Booth A. A typology of reviews: an analysis of 14 review types and associated methodologies. Health Info Libr J 2009;26(2):91–108.
13. Arksey H, O'Malley L. Scoping studies: towards a methodological framework. Int J Soc Res Meth 2005;8(1):19–32.
14. Rumrill PD, Fitzgerald SM, Merchant WR. Using scoping literature reviews as a means of understanding and interpreting existing literature. Work 2010;35: 399–404.
15. Davis K, Drey N, Gould D. What are scoping studies? A review of the nursing literature. Int J Nurs Stud 2009;46(10):1386–400.
16. Levac D, Colquhoun H, O'Brien KK. Scoping studies: advancing the methodology. Implement Sci 2010;5:69.
17. Daudt HM, van Mossel C, Scott SJ. Enhancing the scoping study methodology: a large, inter-professional team's experience with Arksey and O'Malley's framework. BMC Med Res Methodol 2013;13:48.

18. Altman DG. Diagnostic tests: comparison of assessors – the kappa statistic. In: Altman DG, Machin D, Bryant TN, et al, editors. Statistics with confidence. 2nd edition. Bristol (United Kingdom): BMJ Books; 2000. p. 116–8.

19. Moher D, Liberati A, Tezlaff J, et al. Preferred reporting items for systematic reviews and meta-analyses: the PRISMA statement. PLoS Medicine 2009;6(7): e1000097.

20. Botella-Carretero JI, Galán JM, Caballero C, et al. Quality of life and psychometric functionality in patients with differentiated thyroid carcinoma. Endocr Relat Cancer 2003;10(4):601–10.

21. Bunevicius R, Prange AJ. Mental improvement after replacement therapy with thyroxine plus triiodothyronine: relationship to cause of hypothyroidism. Int J Neuropsychopharmacol 2000;3(2):167–74.

22. Crevenna R, Zettinig G, Keilani M, et al. Quality of life in patients with non-metastatic differentiated thyroid cancer under thyroxine supplementation therapy. Support Care Cancer 2003;11(9):597–603.

23. de Oliveira Chachamovitz DS, dos Santos Vigário P, Nogueira Cordeiro MF, et al. Quality of life, muscle strength, and fatigue perception in patients on suppressive therapy with levothyroxine for differentiated thyroid carcinoma. Am J Clin Oncol 2013;36(4):354–61.

24. Eustatia-Rutten CF, Corssmit EP, Pereira AM, et al. Quality of life in longterm exogenous subclinical hyperthyroidism and the effects of restoration of euthyroidism, a randomized controlled trial. Clin Endocrinol (Oxf) 2006;64(3):284–91.

25. Gning I, Trask PC, Mendoza TR, et al. Development and initial validation of the thyroid cancer module of the M. D. Anderson Symptom Inventory. Oncology 2009;76(1):59–68.

26. Golger A, Fridman TR, Eski S, et al. Three-week thyroxine withdrawal thyroglobulin stimulation screening test to detect low-risk residual/recurrent well-differentiated thyroid carcinoma. J Endocrinol Invest 2003;26(10):1023–31.

27. Gomez MM, Gutierrez RM, Castellano SA, et al. Psychological well-being and quality of life in patients treated for thyroid cancer after surgery. Terapia Psicologica 2010;28(1):69–84.

28. Hoftijzer HC, Heemstra KA, Corssmit EP, et al. Quality of life in cured patients with differentiated thyroid carcinoma. J Clin Endocrinol Metab 2008;93(1): 200–3.

29. Huang SM, Lee CH, Chien LY, et al. Postoperative quality of life among patients with thyroid cancer. J Adv Nurs 2004;47(5):492–9.

30. Husson O, Haak HR, Buffart LM, et al. Health-related quality of life and disease specific symptoms in long-term thyroid cancer survivors: a study from the population-based PROFILES registry. Acta Oncol 2013;52(2):249–58.

31. Husson O, Nieuwlaat WA, Oranje WA, et al. Fatigue among short- and long-term thyroid cancer survivors: results from the population-based PROFILES registry. Thyroid 2013;23(10):1247–55.

32. Lee JI, Kim SH, Tan AH, et al. Decreased health-related quality of life in disease-free survivors of differentiated thyroid cancer in Korea. Health Qual Life Outcomes 2010;8:101.

33. Louwerens M, Appelhof BC, Verloop H, et al. Fatigue and fatigue-related symptoms in patients treated for different causes of hypothyroidism. Eur J Endocrinol 2012;167(6):809–15.

34. Malterling RR, Andersson RE, Falkmer S, et al. Differentiated thyroid cancer in a Swedish county–long-term results and quality of life. Acta Oncol 2010;49(4): 454–9.

35. Mendoza A, Shaffer B, Karakla D, et al. Quality of life with well-differentiated thyroid cancer: treatment toxicities and their reduction. Thyroid 2004;14(2):133–40.
36. Pelttari H, Sintonen H, Schalin-Jäntti C, et al. Health-related quality of life in long-term follow-up of patients with cured TNM stage I or II differentiated thyroid carcinoma. Clin Endocrinol (Oxf) 2009;70(3):493–7.
37. Roberts KJ, Lepore SJ, Urken ML. Quality of life after thyroid cancer: an assessment of patient needs and preferences for information and support. J Cancer Educ 2008;23(3):186–91.
38. Roerink SH, de Ridder M, Prins J, et al. High level of distress in long-term survivors of thyroid carcinoma: results of rapid screening using the distress thermometer. Acta Oncol 2013;52(1):128–37.
39. Schroeder PR, Haugen BR, Pacini F, et al. A comparison of short-term changes in health-related quality of life in thyroid carcinoma patients undergoing diagnostic evaluation with recombinant human thyrotropin compared with thyroid hormone withdrawal. J Clin Endocrinol Metab 2006;91(3):878–84.
40. Shah MD, Witterick IJ, Eski SJ, et al. Quality of life in patients undergoing thyroid surgery. J Otolaryngol 2006;35(4):209–15.
41. Tagay S, Herpertz S, Langkafel M, et al. Health-related quality of life, anxiety and depression in thyroid cancer patients under short-term hypothyroidism and TSH-suppressive levothyroxine treatment. Eur J Endocrinol 2005;153(6):755–63.
42. Tan LG, Nan L, Thumboo J, et al. Health-related quality of life in thyroid cancer survivors. Laryngoscope 2007;117(3):507–10.
43. Vigário Pdos S, Chachamovitz DS, Cordeiro MF, et al. Effects of physical activity on body composition and fatigue perception in patients on thyrotropin-suppressive therapy for differentiated thyroid carcinoma. Thyroid 2011;21(7):695–700.
44. Bunevicius R, Kazanavicius G, Zalinkevicius R, et al. Effects of thyroxine as compared with thyroxine plus triiodothyronine in patients with hypothyroidism. N Engl J Med 1999;340(6):424–9.
45. Vissers PA, Thong MS, Pouwer F, et al. The impact of comorbidity on health-related quality of life among cancer survivors: analyses of data from the PROFILES registry. J Cancer Surviv 2013;7(4):602–13.
46. Dow KH, Ferrell BR, Anello C. Quality-of-life changes in patients with thyroid cancer after withdrawal of thyroid hormone therapy. Thyroid 1997;7(4):613–9.
47. Gamper EM, Giesinger JM, Oberguggenberger A, et al. Good prognosis, good quality of life? – Longitudinal assessment of quality of life in thyroid cancer patients. Value Health 2011;14:A461 [abstract PCN146].
48. Giusti M, Mortara L, Cecoli F, et al. Evaluation of quality of life (QoL) with the Thy-PRO questionnaire in patients with disease-free differentiated thyroid carcinoma (DTC). Endocr Rev 2012;33 [abstract MON-436]. In: 94th Annual Meeting of the Endocrine Society. Houston, June 23–26, 2012.
49. Haugen BR, Pacini F, Reiners C, et al. A comparison of recombinant human thyrotropin and thyroid hormone withdrawal for the detection of thyroid remnant or cancer. J Clin Endocrinol Metab 1999;84(11):3877–85.
50. Husson O, Haak HR, Oranje WA, et al. Health-related quality of life among thyroid cancer survivors: a systematic review. Clin Endocrinol (Oxf) 2011;75(4):544–54.
51. Karapanou O, Papadopoulos A, Vlassopoulou B, et al. Health status of Greek thyroid cancer patients after radioiodine administration compared to a demographically matched general population sample. Hell J Nucl Med 2012;15(2):98–102.

52. Ladenson PW. Recombinant thyrotropin for detection of recurrent thyroid cancer. Trans Am Clin Climatol Assoc 2002;113:21–30.

53. Ladenson PW, Braverman LE, Mazzaferri EL, et al. Comparison of administration of recombinant human thyrotropin with withdrawal of thyroid hormone for radioactive iodine scanning in patients with thyroid carcinoma. N Engl J Med 1997; 337(13):888–96.

54. Oren A, Benoit MA, Murphy A, et al. Quality of life and anxiety in adolescents with differentiated thyroid cancer. J Clin Endocrinol Metab 2012;97(10): E1933–7.

55. Prinsen H, Bleijenberg G, Heijmen L, et al. The role of physical activity and physical fitness in postcancer fatigue: a randomized controlled trial. Support Care Cancer 2013;21(8):2279–88.

56. Regalbuto C, Maiorana R, Alagona C, et al. Effects of either LT4 monotherapy or LT4/LT3 combined therapy in patients totally thyroidectomized for thyroid cancer. Thyroid 2007;17(4):323–31.

57. Rodriguez T, Lavis VR, Meininger JC, et al. Substitution of liothyronine at a 1:5 ratio for a portion of levothyroxine: effect on fatigue, symptoms of depression, and working memory versus treatment with levothyroxine alone. Endocr Pract 2005;11(4):223–33.

58. Schultz PN, Stava C, Vassilopoulou-Sellin R. Health profiles and quality of life of 518 survivors of thyroid cancer. Head Neck 2003;25(5):349–56.

59. Singer S, Lincke T, Gamper E, et al. Quality of life in patients with thyroid cancer compared with the general population. Thyroid 2012;22(2):117–24.

60. Singer S, Kuhnt S, Zwerenz R, et al. Age- and sex-standardised prevalence rates of fatigue in a large hospital-based sample of cancer patients. Br J Cancer 2011;105:445–51.

61. Tagay S, Herpertz S, Langkafel M, et al. Health-related quality of life, depression and anxiety in thyroid cancer patients. Qual Life Res 2006;15(4):695–703.

62. Taïeb D, Sebag F, Cherenko M, et al. Quality of life changes and clinical outcomes in thyroid cancer patients undergoing radioiodine remnant ablation (RRA) with recombinant human TSH (rhTSH): a randomized controlled study. Clin Endocrinol (Oxf) 2009;71(1):115–23.

63. Alonso J, Regidor E, Barrio G, et al. Population reference values of the Spanish version of the Health Questionnaire SF-36. Medicina Clinica 1998;111(11): 410–6.

64. Bullinger M, Alsonso J, Apolone G, et al. Translating health status questionnaires and evaluating their quality: the IQOLA Project approach. International Quality of Life Assessment. J Clin Epidemiol 1998;51(11):913–23.

65. Garratt AM, Ruta DA, Abdalla MI, et al. The SF36 Health Survey questionnaire: an outcome measure suitable for routine use within the NHS? BMJ 1993; 306(6890):1440–4.

66. McNair DM, Lorr M, Dropleman LF. POMS manual profile of mood states. San Diego (CA): Educational and Industrial Testing Service; 1992.

67. Alonso J, Anto JM, Moreno C. Spanish version of the Nottingham Health Profile: translation and preliminary validity. Am J Public Health 1990;80(6): 744–8.

68. Alonso J, Prieto L, Anto JM. The Spanish version of the Nottingham Health Profile: a review of adaptation and instrument characteristics. Qual Life Res 1994; 3(6):385–93.

69. Bullinger M. Assessment of health related quality of life with the SF-36 Health Survey. Rehabilitation (Stuttg) 1996;35(3):17–27.

70. Cho HJ, Costa E, Chalder T, et al. Cross-cultural validation of the Chalder Fatigue Questionnaire in Brazilian primary care. J Psychosom Res 2007;62:301–4.
71. Samano ES, Goldenstein PT, Ribeiro Lde M, et al. Praying correlates with higher quality of life: results from a survey on complementary/alternative medicine use among a group of Brazilian cancer patients. Sao Paulo Med J 2004;122(2):60–3.
72. Chalder T, Berelowitz G, Pawlikowska T, et al. Development of a fatigue scale. J Psychosom Res 1993;37(2):147–53.
73. Smets EM, Visser MR, Willems-Groot AF, et al. Fatigue and radiotherapy: (B) experience in patients 9 months following treatment. Br J Cancer 1998;78(7):907–12.
74. Cleeland CS, Mendoza TR, Wang XS, et al. Assessing symptom distress in cancer patients: the M. D. Anderson Symptom Inventory. Cancer 2000;89(7):1634–46.
75. Ware JE. SF-36 Health Survey update. Spine 2000;25(24):3130–9.
76. Ware JE, Snow KK, Kosinski M. SF-36 Health Survey: manual and interpretation guide. Lincoln (RI): Quality Metric Incorporated; 1993. p. 2000.
77. Ware JE, Sherbourne CD. The MOS 36-item short-form health survey (SF-36): I. Conceptual framework and item selection. Med Care 1992;30(6):473–83.
78. Smets EM, Garssen B, Bonke B, et al. The Multidimensional Fatigue Inventory (MFI) psychometric qualities of an instrument to assess fatigue. J Psychosom Res 1995;39(3):315–25.
79. Ferrans CE, Powers MJ. Quality of life index: development and psychometric properties. ANS Advances in Nursing Science 1985;8(1):15–24.
80. Liu HE. An exploration of the psychometrics of the quality of life index of Chinese families. J Nurs Res 1993;1(2):127–36.
81. Husson O, Haak HR, Mols F, et al. Development of a disease-specific health-related quality of life questionnaire (THYCA-QoL). Acta Oncol 2013;52(2):447–54.
82. Aaronson NK, Ahmedzai S, Bergman B, et al. The European Organization for Research and Treatment of Cancer QLQ-C30: a quality-of-life instrument for use in international clinical trials in oncology. J Natl Cancer Inst 1993;85(5):365–76.
83. Michielsen HJ, De Vries J, Van Heck GL. Psychometric qualities of a brief self-rated fatigue measure: the Fatigue Assessment Scale. J Psychosom Res 2003;54(4):345–52.
84. Mendoza TR, Wang XS, Cleeland CS, et al. The rapid assessment of fatigue severity in cancer patients: use of the Brief Fatigue Inventory. Cancer 1999;85(5):1186–96.
85. Yun YH, Wang XS, Lee JS, et al. Validation study of the Korean version of the Brief Fatigue Inventory. J Pain Symptom Manage 2005;29(2):165–72.
86. Smets EM, Garrsen B, Cull A, et al. Application of the Multidimensional Fatigue Inventory (MFI-20) in cancer patients receiving radiotherapy. Br J Cancer 1996;73(2):241–5.
87. Sullivan M, Karlsson J, Ware J. The Swedish SF-36 Health Survey I. Evaluation of data quality, scaling assumptions, reliability and construct validity across general populations in Sweden. Soc Sci Med 1995;41(10):1349–58.
88. Persson LO, Karlsson J, Bengtsson C, et al. The Swedish SF-36 Health Survey II. Evaluation of clinical validity: results from population studies of elderly and women in Gothenburg. J Clin Epidemiol 1998;51(11):1095–103.
89. Sullivan M, Karlsson J. The Swedish SF-36 Health Survey III. Evaluation of criterion-based validity: results from normative population. J Clin Epidemiol 1998;51(11):1005–13.

90. Sintonen H. The 15D instrument of health-related quality of life: properties and applications. Ann Intern Med 2001;33:328–36.

91. Gessler S, Low J, Daniells E, et al. Screening for distress in cancer patients: is the distress thermometer a valid measure in the UK and does it measure change over time? A prospective validation study. Psychooncology 2008;17:538–47.

92. Tuinman MA, Gazendam-Donofrio SM, Hoekstra-Weebers JE. Screening and referral for psychosocial distress in oncologic practice: use of the distress thermometer. Cancer 2008;113(4):870–8.

93. Ware JE, Snow KK, Kosinski M. SF-36 Health Survey: manual and interpretation guide. Lincoln (RI): Quality Metric Incorporated; 2002.

94. McNair DM, Lorr M, Dropleman LF. EITS POMS manual for the profile of mood states. San Diego (CA): Educational and Industrial Testing Service; 1971.

95. Thumbo J, Feng PH, Soh CH, et al. Validation of the Chinese SF-36 for quality of life assessment in patients with systemic lupus erythematosus. Lupus 2000;9(9): 708–12.

96. Thumboo J, Fong KY, Machin D, et al. A community-based study of scaling assumption and construct validity of the English (UK) and Chinese (HK) SF-36 in Singapore. Qual Life Res 2001;10(2):175–88.

97. Thumboo J, Chan SP, Machin D, et al. Measuring health-related quality of life in Singapore: normal values for the English and Chinese SF-36 Health Survey. Ann Acad Med Singapore 2002;31(1):366–74.

98. Barsevick AM, Irwin MR, Hinds P, et al. Recommendations for high-priority research on cancer-related fatigue in children and adults. J Natl Cancer Inst 2013;105(19):1432–40.

99. Richardson A, Addington-Hall J, Amir Z, et al. Knowledge, ignorance and priorities for research in key areas of cancer survivorship: findings from a scoping review. Br J Cancer 2011;105(Suppl 1):S82–94.

Management of Graves' Disease
An Overview and Comparison of Clinical Practice Guidelines with Actual Practice Trends

Becky T. Muldoon, MD[a,b], Vinh Q. Mai, DO[a,b],
Henry B. Burch, MD[a,c],*

KEYWORDS

- Hyperthyroidism • Management • Clinical practice guidelines
- Clinical practice survey

KEY POINTS

- Over the last century, much has been learned about the pathogenesis, manifestations, and management of Graves' disease leading to the establishment of evidence-based clinical practice guidelines.
- The joint clinical practice guidelines from the American Thyroid Association and the American Association of Clinical Endocrinologists give recommendations on both the diagnosis and treatment of hyperthyroidism.

Continued

Disclosures: The authors have nothing to disclose.
The views expressed in this article are those of the authors and do not reflect the official policy of the Department of the Army, Navy, the Department of Defense, or the US government. The authors are military service members (or employees of the US government). This work was prepared as part of the authors' official duties. Title 17, US Code - Section 105: Subject matter of copyright: United States Government works provides that "Copyright protection under this title is not available for any work of the United States Government." Title 17 US Code - Section 101: Defines a US government work as a work prepared by a military service member or employee of the US government as part of that person's official duties. The authors certify that all individuals who qualify as authors have been listed; each has participated in the conception and design of this work, the analysis of data (when applicable), the writing of the document, and/or the approval of the submission of this version; the document represents valid work; if the authors used information derived from another source, they obtained all necessary approvals to use it and made appropriate acknowledgments in the document; and each takes public responsibility for it.

[a] Endocrinology Service, Department of Medicine, Walter Reed National Military Medical Center, 8901 Wisconsin Avenue, Building 19, 5th Floor, Bethesda, MD 20889-5600, USA; [b] Department of Medicine, Uniformed Services University of the Health Sciences, 4301 Jones Bridge Road, Bethesda, MD 20814, USA; [c] Endocrinology Division, Uniformed Services University of the Health Sciences, 4301 Jones Bridge Road, Bethesda, MD 20814, USA
* Corresponding author. 8901 Wisconsin Avenue, Building 19, 5th Floor, Room 5053, Bethesda, MD 20889-5600.
E-mail address: henry.burch@us.army.mil

Endocrinol Metab Clin N Am 43 (2014) 495–516
http://dx.doi.org/10.1016/j.ecl.2014.02.001
0889-8529/14/$ – see front matter Published by Elsevier Inc.

endo.theclinics.com

Continued

- A survey of clinical endocrinologists revealed that current practices diverge from these recently published guidelines in multiple areas.
- These differences will need to be assessed serially to determine the impact of the guidelines on future clinical practice and perhaps vice versa.

INTRODUCTION

Hyperthyroidism is a common endocrine disorder, with a lifetime risk of 2% to 5%.[1] The most frequent cause of hyperthyroidism in iodine-sufficient areas is Graves' disease (GD),[2,3] which often affects younger individuals.[4] Biochemically, it is defined as the presence of a suppressed serum thyrotropin-stimulating hormone (TSH) level, and an elevated thyroxine (T4) and/or triiodothyronine (T3) in overt hyperthyroidism, and normal T4 and/or T3 in subclinical hyperthyroidism. GD is associated with short-term symptomatic manifestations, such as palpitations, unintentional weight loss, hair thinning, increased frequency of bowel movements, visual disturbances, and long-term effects, including bone loss and arrhythmias. Recent data have established strong links between hyperthyroidism and increased all-cause mortality (hazard ratio [HR] 1.42), generally from cardiovascular (HR 1.49) and lung causes (HR 1.91).[5] Additionally, patients with GD are at an increased risk for developing thyroid cancer[6]; these tumors behave more aggressively and are associated with decreased survival.[7]

Clinical practice guidelines (CPGs) provide an in-depth analysis of existing evidence by area experts, with the intention of providing guidance to clinicians.[8–10] As has been noted, these are "not inclusive of all proper approaches, or exclusive of others"[9] and are not meant to replace clinical judgment by health care providers in any individual patient's case.

Current clinical practice surveys provide a snapshot of actual clinical management and, therefore, can be used to both gauge the degree of divergence of guidelines from real clinical practice and to assess the ultimate effect of CPGs on practice trends. The current article is intended to provide an overview of GD, with an emphasis on a comparison between recommendations made in the recently published American Thyroid Association (ATA)/American Association of Clinical Endocrinologists' (AACE) hyperthyroidism guidelines[8,11] and actual clinical practice patterns.[12]

PATHOGENESIS

GD has an underlying autoimmune basis, which is multifactorial and polygenic in nature, with variable penetrance.[13,14] Data from epidemiologic family and twin studies attribute its development to an interaction between genetic predisposition and environmental influence. The concordance rate for monozygotic twins has reportedly been as high as 76% compared with 11% for dizygotic twins.[15] Other epidemiologic studies have noted a familial pattern of inheritance related to the expression of anti-thyroid autoantibodies and an increased rate of polymorphisms of the human thyrotropin receptor (hTSH-R) in relatives of patients with GD.[16–19] In addition, GD has been linked to HLA-B8 and HLA-DR3 in the Caucasian population, whereas other ethnic groups were found to have additional allelic contributions, including HLA-B13, DR1, DR3, DR5, and Drw8.[13] Non-HLA associations, particularly the immune regulatory CTLA-4, have been demonstrated as a susceptibility gene for GD,[13,20] whereas hTSH-R polymorphisms may be related to its severity.[20] The hTSH-R gene locus on chromosome 14q31 was found to represent a susceptibility locus for the development of GD.[21] Environmental implications in the etiologic contribution to GD have recently been linked to *Helicobacter pylori* infection (odds ratio [OR] 4.35), and cytotoxin-associated gene A seropositivity increases the risk for autoimmune thyroid disease by 2.24-fold.[22] Other environmental factors that have been implicated in its pathogenesis include dietary iodine intake, smoking, estrogens, certain drugs, stressful life events, irradiation, infection, allergy, and alcohol consumption and selenium deficiency.[23,24]

CLINICAL MANIFESTATIONS

Manifestations of GD are a result of an increased thyroid hormone production, which affects the tissues in multiple organ systems. In addition, there are clinical manifestations potentially associated with autoimmunity against the human thyroid-stimulating hormone receptor (hTSH-R), including Graves' ophthalmopathy (GO), dermopathy, and thyroid acropachy (**Table 1**).

Cardiovascular

The cardiovascular effects of excess thyroid hormone result from the need to meet the demands of increased metabolic activity but thyroid hormone can also affect cardiac contractility directly.[25] T3 acts on cardiac myocytes, which have thyroid hormone nuclear receptors to regulate expression of genes, such as the α-myosin heavy chain and sarcoplasmic reticulum Ca^{2+}-ATPase, both of which are integral to cardiac contractility.[25–27] Thyroid hormone also affects sodium, potassium, and calcium channels of the heart and vascular smooth muscle cells, serving to increase cardiac output by increasing the heart rate while decreasing systemic vascular resistance.[26]

Sinus tachycardia at rest and with activity is the most common cardiac manifestation in hyperthyroidism. Atrial fibrillation occurs in 5% to 15% of thyrotoxic patients, particularly among those with underlying heart disease.[25] Other arrhythmias, such as atrial flutter, ventricular premature contractions, and ventricular tachyarrhythmias, are rare.[25]

The high cardiac workload in thyrotoxicosis increases the risk for congestive heart failure from tachycardia-related left ventricular dysfunction.[26,28] Reversible pulmonary arterial hypertension has also been associated with hyperthyroidism and can lead to right heart failure.[28,29] These thyrotoxic effects on the heart can be associated with increased morbidity and mortality,[30] especially in those with underlying cardiovascular disease and the elderly.[31]

Pulmonary

Dyspnea, especially with exertion, is a common complaint in hyperthyroid patients and is likely a result of diaphragmatic muscle weakness related to hyperthyroid myopathy.[32] Also contributing to thyrotoxic dyspnea is the hypermetabolic state, which leads to increases in basal metabolic rate, oxygen consumption, and carbon dioxide production, prompting an increased ventilatory response to the excess carbon dioxide and hypoxia.[33] Breathing patterns in hyperthyroid patients are shallower and faster and improve with treatment of thyrotoxicosis.[34]

Gastrointestinal

Common gastrointestinal symptoms associated with hyperthyroidism include hyperphagia, increased frequency of defecation, and liver dysfunction. In a study of 3049 overtly hyperthyroid patients, 60.7% had weight loss, which was the most common

Table 1
Prevalence of clinical findings in patients with overt thyrotoxicosis by period

Period of Study	1984–2008	1960–1988	1943–1945
Study Location	Birmingham, United Kingdom	Honolulu	Boston
Number of Patients[a]	3049	880	247
Symptoms			
Weight loss	61%	61%	85%
Heat intolerance	55%	55%	89%
Tremulousness	54%	NR	NR
Palpitations	51%	65%	89%
Nervousness/anxiety	41%	69%	99%
Hyperdefecation	22%	22%	33%
Neck fullness	22%	NR	NR
Eye symptoms	11%	NR	54%
Dyspnea	10%	NR	75%
Weight gain	7%	12%	2%
Fatigue	NR	69%	88%
Diaphoresis	NR	45%	91%
Increased appetite	NR	42%	65%
Physical findings			
Palpable goiter	69%	93%	100%
Eye signs[b]	63%	34%	71%
Tremor	42%	69%	97%
Atrial fibrillation	4%	3%	10%
Moist skin	NR	34%	NR
Tachycardia	NR	80%	100%

Abbreviation: NR, not reported.
[a] Eye symptoms and signs in 1984–2008 study percentage of the subgroup 1189 patients with confirmed Graves' disease.
[b] Eye signs in Nordyke study limited to lid changes.
From Burch HB. Overview of the clinical manifestations of thyrotoxicosis. In: Braverman LE, Cooper DS, editors. Werner & Ingbar's The Thyroid, 10th Edition. Philadelphia: Lippincott, Williams & Wilkins; 2013. p. 435; with permission.

presenting symptom.[35] Shortened transit time from the mouth to the cecum contributes to more frequent defecation and diarrhea.[36] Steatorrhea is also common in thyrotoxicosis; this has been attributed to hyperphagia with increased intake of dietary fat and, therefore, an increased fecal fat excretion.[32,36,37] Although rare, dysphagia, nausea, vomiting, and abdominal pain can be presenting symptoms of hyperthyroidism.[36,37]

Hyperthyroidism can cause hepatic dysfunction and hepatic injury manifested by elevation of aspartate aminotransferase (AST) and alanine aminotransferase (ALT) and also cholestatic injury with elevation in liver alkaline phosphatase (ALP) and γ-glutamyl transpeptidase (GGT). The hepatic injury has been attributed to relative hypoxia in the liver secondary to increased oxygen demand without an appropriate increase in hepatic blood flow.[38] Approximately 60% of hyperthyroid patients of all causes and 76% of patients with untreated GD have at least one liver function test abnormality.[39,40] In hyperthyroid patients, AST elevation is seen in 6% to 27% and ALT elevation in 23% to 37% of untreated patients.[39–41] ALP elevation was seen in 44% to 60% of untreated patients, but GGT elevation was seen in only 14% to 27% signifying ALP is often largely of bone origin, because of high bone turnover in thyrotoxicosis.[38–40] There may be an increase in hepatic transaminases and ALP after initiation of antithyroid drugs (ATDs), and propylthiouracil (PTU) is known to rarely cause liver failure caused by hepatic necrosis. Because of the prevalence of mild transaminasemia in untreated thyrotoxicosis, it is essential to obtain baseline liver function testing before the initiation of ATD therapy in order to avoid an incorrect attribution of this finding to the ATD.[8] When patients with GD being treated with ATDs were compared with untreated patients, there was a similar elevation of AST and ALT, again reinforcing that liver abnormalities first noted after the start of treatment are often not caused by the ATD therapy.[39]

GD has also been found to be associated with other gastrointestinal diseases, such as autoimmune gastritis, ulcerative colitis, Crohn disease, and celiac disease. In a study in which 111 patients with GD were screened for celiac disease with antigliadin and tissue transglutaminase antibodies, the prevalence of celiac disease in those patients was 4.5% compared with 0.9% in matched healthy controls.[42]

Neuropsychiatric

Neuropsychiatric manifestations in thyrotoxicosis range from restlessness, irritability, and agitation to more severe psychiatric symptoms, such as depression, generalized anxiety disorder, and psychosis. Those patients with hyperthyroidism are more likely to have symptoms of depression and anxiety than healthy subjects.[43,44] In a study of 36 newly diagnosed patients with GD, based on *Diagnostic and Statistical Manual of Mental Disorders* (Fourth Edition) criteria, 15 had generalized anxiety disorder, 6 had mood disorder, 6 had obsessive-compulsive disorder, and 2 each had personality disorder and schizophreniform disorder,[45] showing the high prevalence of psychiatric disorders in these patients. Although less common than anxiety and depression, psychosis also has been associated with thyrotoxicosis. During a 20-year period at a single institution, there were 18 patients who required inpatient admission for psychosis with newly diagnosed thyrotoxicosis. These patients had median inpatient stays of 4 weeks, and 7 of these were considered compulsory hospitalizations. Fourteen of these patients had affective psychoses associated with either mania or major depression.[46]

Reproductive

Hyperthyroidism affects reproductive function in both adult males and females. In hyperthyroid men, sex hormone–binding globulin (SHBG) is increased, leading to an increase in circulating levels of testosterone and normal free testosterone levels but lower bioavailable testosterone in some reports.[47] Total and free estradiol (E2) concentrations are elevated; as a result, the free testosterone/free E2 ratio is lower in hyperthyroid adult males compared with normal individuals, which may contribute to the higher incidence of gynecomastia observed in thyrotoxic men.[47]

Sexual dysfunction, such as delayed ejaculation, premature ejaculation, erectile dysfunction, and decreased libido, is common in hyperthyroid men and usually resolves with treatment of the hyperthyroidism. In a multicenter study that included 34 hyperthyroid men, 50% had premature ejaculation; this percentage was reduced to 15% with therapy for thyrotoxicosis, a rate similar to that of normal controls.[48] Mean sperm motility is lower in thyrotoxic men and improves or normalizes with restoration of euthyroidism.[49] Other seminal parameters, such as semen volume, sperm density, and sperm morphology, were not significantly different in hyperthyroidism compared with normal controls.[49]

In thyrotoxic women, abnormal menses occur more commonly than in controls. In an early study, the incidence of oligomenorrhea in women with hyperthyroidism was 58%[50]; but a more recent study showed a lower prevalence of menstrual irregularity, occurring in 21.5% of 214 hyperthyroid patients compared with 8.4% of controls.[51]

Musculoskeletal

In thyrotoxicosis there is an increased bone turnover caused by a shortened bone remodeling cycle, which can lead to osteoporosis and fragility fractures.[52] Compared with normal controls, hyperthyroid patients have an increased risk for fracture and lower bone mineral density, but these changes improve with effective therapy of the thyrotoxicosis.[53]

Ophthalmopathy

GO occurs in more than 25% to 50% of patients with GD depending on the detection method, and 85% of ophthalmopathy patients will manifest eye changes within 18 months of the diagnosis of thyrotoxicosis.[54,55] Symptoms can range from mild dryness to pain, double vision, and even blindness. GO, especially in the more severe forms, results in significant reduction in quality of life as well as both direct and indirect costs related to loss of productivity and prolonged therapy.[56] Bilateral eye involvement occurs in 85% to 95% of cases and is frequently asymmetric. Fortunately, severe ophthalmopathy only occurs in only 3% to 5% of patients with GD.[55]

The pathogenesis of GO is thought to result from the shared expression of a common thyroid-eye antigen, such as the TSH-receptor, which has been found to be present in orbital fibroblasts, adipocytes, and preadipocytes. Stimulation of the TSH receptor by autoantibodies results in increased retro-orbital fat and glycosaminoglycan synthesis and release from retroocular fibroblasts, leading to swollen orbital muscles leading to proptosis, conjunctival injection, and periorbital edema in GO.[57] Eye changes in GD are frequently classified by subjective and objective measures of clinical activity using a clinical activity score (CAS).[55,58] The CAS can also be used to determine progression or regression of disease.[59,60] The 7 static elements of the CAS include pain behind the globe over the last 4 weeks, pain with eye movement over the last 4 weeks, redness of the eyelids, redness of the conjunctiva, eyelid swelling, chemosis, and swollen caruncle. Additional criteria assess change over time and include an increase in proptosis of more than 2 mm, decrease eye movement of 5° or more, and decreased visual acuity of 1 line or more on the Snellen chart over a 3-month interval. The presence of each static element is awarded one point, and a CAS of 3 or more signifies active GO, which is more likely to respond to antiinflammatory therapy. The severity of GO can be graded using a classification scheme developed by the European Group on Graves' Orbitopathy, with categories including mild, moderate to severe, or sight-threatening disease.[61] Those with sight-threatening GO have optic neuropathy and/or corneal breakdown that require immediate intervention. Patients with moderate to severe GO usually have one or more of the following: lid retraction 2 mm or greater, moderate or severe soft tissue involvement, proptosis 3 mm or more greater than normal, and diplopia; the benefits of therapy with immunosuppression or surgery justify the associated risk of intervention. Patients with mild GO have one or more of the following: lid retraction less than 2 mm, mild soft tissue involvement, proptosis less than 3 mm greater than normal, transient or no diplopia, and corneal exposure responsiveness to lubricants. These features have a minor impact on daily life, and the risk of treatment with immunosuppressive agents or surgery outweighs the benefit.

Dermopathy and Acropachy

Thyroid dermopathy (also known as *localized pretibial myxedema*) and acropachy are rare presentations of GD. The pathogenesis of dermopathy and acropachy may also involve the lymphocyte-derived cytokine activation of fibroblasts in the locations that are involved similar to that of ophthalmopathy. Thyroid dermopathy is characterized by localized thickening of the skin, commonly in the pretibial area that is raised, waxy, and erythematous or yellowish brown.[62,63] Acropachy is characterized by digital clubbing with thickening of the skin of the digits and, in its more severe form, periostitis of the distal bones.[62] These dermatologic conditions are associated with GO, and their presence usually indicates a more severe autoimmune disease.[63,64] It is estimated that among patients with GO, 4% to 13% of these patients have dermopathy and that 20% of the patients with dermopathy have acropachy.[64] Based on these data, it can be roughly estimated that for every 1000 patients with GD, 250 will have clinically obvious ophthalmopathy, 10 will have dermopathy, and 2 will have acropachy. Compared with a GD control group without dermopathy or acropachy, the OR of having severe GO (defined by need for orbital decompression) was 3.55 in patients with dermopathy and 20.68 in patients with acropachy.[62]

Mild cases of thyroid dermopathy do not require intervention as they improve spontaneously or in response to corticosteroids used to treat concurrent ophthalmopathy.[64] Local therapies, including the use of topical steroids applied with an occlusion dressing such as plastic wrap, and intralesional corticosteroids have been used in more moderate to severe cases with variable results. Complete remission is difficult to achieve, occurring in less than 25% of cases treated with topical therapy.[63] In addition to local and systemic corticosteroids to prevent and manage thyroid dermopathy, patients with GD should be instructed to stop smoking, lose weight if obese, and avoid skin trauma.[64]

Apathetic Thyrotoxicosis

In elderly patients, the classic hyperthyroid symptoms may not be apparent, which can delay diagnosis and treatment and likely contributes to the higher morbidity and mortality observed in these patients. Compared with younger patients, those older than 61 years have smaller palpable goiters and a lower number of classic symptoms at presentation, with the exception of weight loss and shortness of breath.[35] Patients older than 70 years had decreased sweating, heat intolerance, nervousness, polydipsia, and appetite changes and lesser degrees of hyperactive reflexes and tremor.[65] Rarely, apathetic hyperthyroidism has been described in adolescents and younger adult patients.[66,67]

TREATMENT

Graves' hyperthyroidism can be treated by one of 3 modalities: (1) ATD therapy, (2) radioactive iodine, and (3) thyroidectomy. Although radioactive iodine (RAI) therapy is still the most frequently selected modality to treat GD in the United States, there has been a shift toward a more frequent use of ATDs.[12,68]

Antithyroid Drugs

The 2 ATDs that are available in the United States are methimazole (MMI) and PTU. Carbimazole is used in the United Kingdom and other parts of the world and is a prodrug that is converted to its active form, MMI, after absorption. ATDs are thionamides, which inhibit thyroid hormone synthesis by impairing thyroid peroxidase action, thereby interfering with the iodination and coupling steps in thyroid hormonogenesis. Unlike MMI, PTU also blocks conversion of T4 to T3 in the thyroid and peripheral tissues. ATDs also have immunosuppressive effects, including apoptosis of intrathyroidal lymphocytes, which may contribute to the observed reductions in TSH-receptor antibodies with ATD treatment.[69] Patients who are good candidates for ATDs include those who have a high likelihood of remission (individuals with small goiters and mild thyrotoxicosis), those who have moderate to severe active ophthalmopathy, and those who have contraindications to radioactive iodine or are at high risk for thyroidectomy.[8,11]

Adverse effects associated with both MMI and PTU include hepatitis, jaundice, urticaria, rash, lupuslike syndrome, and agranulocytosis. Agranulocytosis typically occurs within 90 days of starting ATD therapy, frequently occurring rapidly and within 2 weeks of having a normal granulocyte count.[70] The rate of adverse effects with ATDs is about 13%, with the predominant adverse effect of PTU being hepatic involvement (2.7%) and rash with MMI (6%).[71] Commonly, there may be an increase in hepatic transaminases after the initiation of ATDs. However, a rare but severe adverse effect of thionamides is hepatotoxicity and liver failure, especially with PTU. This effect forms the rationale for the monitoring of liver-associated enzyme in patients on this therapy,[12] though the rapid and unpredictable onset of this complication is such that patients should be warned to immediately report signs of hepatic dysfunction, such as abdominal pain or jaundice.[72]

The 2011 ATA/AACE hyperthyroidism CPGs suggested that MMI should be used in virtually every patient selecting ATD therapy, with the exception of women in the first trimester of pregnancy because of the teratogenic effects of MMI, in thyroid storm because PTU can also block conversion of T4 to T3, and in patients with adverse reactions to MMI who should be given PTU other than agranulocytosis but cannot be treated with radioactive iodine or surgery.[8,11] This recommendation reflects recent observed prescribing patterns in PTU.[73] In a study looking at the prescribing practices in the United States from 1991 to 2008, the number of MMI prescriptions increased 9-fold; by the end of the study period, MMI accounted for 77% of thionamide prescriptions.[73]

The long-term relapse rate after a course of ATDs is in the range of 51% to 68% after 12 to 18 months of therapy.[74] Very high levels of thyrotropin receptor antibody (TRAb) titers at diagnosis, and the rate at which these levels decrease at 6 months or time of discontinuation is the best predictor of remission.[75] In addition to a small goiter and mild thyrotoxicosis, other predictors of long-term remission on ATDs include female sex, absence of tobacco use, absence of ophthalmopathy, and treatment duration.[76] If unable to achieve remission with ATDs alone, radioactive iodine treatment or surgery is recommended, though some patients will elect to continue ATDs indefinitely.[77]

Radioactive Iodine

RAI therapy provides a nonsurgical option for definitive therapy for GD and has been used since the 1940s. When administered orally, RAI (utilizing ^{131}I) is taken up by the thyroid under the influence of stimulating TSH-receptor antibodies, incorporated into thyroid hormone, and stored as colloid, where it emits beta particles that cause irreparable damage to the thyrocyte. RAI may be an appropriate option for those who have contraindications or adverse effects with ATDs, those who want definitive treatment of GD without the invasive risks of surgery, or in women who are planning pregnancy more than 4 to 6 months from treatment time.[8,11]

There are various RAI treatment regimens in use, with the 2 most common being fixed-RAI dosing and calculated dosing. With fixed-RAI dosing, a fixed amount of ^{131}I is given as treatment (usually 10–15 mCi) to all patients, whereas calculated dosing is designed to deliver a fixed number of microcuries per gram of thyroid tissue, based on the measured volume of the thyroid gland and then adjusted for the radioiodine uptake. For example, using a dose of 200 μCi/g, a patient with a 50-g goiter and an radioactive iodine uptake (RAIU) of 50% would receive [(50 × 200) ÷ 0.50] = 15,000 μCi or 15 mCi. Studies have shown little difference in outcome between methods, so the most cost-effective method is to give a fixed dose, which is the recommendation of the ATA.[11,78] If ATDs are used to pretreat patients before RAI, such as in elderly patients, those with underlying coronary artery disease, or multiple comorbidities, they should be discontinued 4 to 5 days before treatment to avoid ATD-mediated interference of RAI uptake, ensuring adequate beta-adrenergic blockade during this interim, as abrupt discontinuation of ATDs is the most common inciting event for thyroid storm.[79] ATDs may be resumed 3 to 7 days after RAI administration in selected high-risk patients who would poorly tolerate a transient worsening of thyrotoxicosis after RAI treatment.[80] The goal of RAI for GD is to achieve hypothyroidism rather than euthyroidism, so patients should have thyroid function tests monitored every 2 to 4 weeks after treatment and started on treatment for hypothyroidism when thyroid hormone levels are low. Hypothyroidism is frequently achieved within 2 months; but a full response may not be seen until 6 months, at which time patients with persistent thyrotoxicosis may be retreated.[11]

The most common adverse effect of RAI is new or worsening of GO, occurring in 15% to 33% of patients, especially in smokers. For this reason, RAI treatment is contraindicated in those with active moderate to severe Graves' ophthalmopathy.[8,11] Radiation thyroiditis, characterized by anterior neck pain and worsening thyrotoxicosis, occurs in approximately 1% of patients.[71] Those patients with active mild GO who select RAI therapy, particularly in the presence of risk factors for worsening eye disease, such as tobacco smoking, high TSH-receptor antibody titers, and high T3 levels, should receive adjunctive glucocorticoid prophylaxis, using a regimen of prednisone 0.2 mg/kg/d, tapered over the 6-week period following RAI therapy.[8,11,81]

Thyroid Surgery

Given the efficacy of ATDs and radioactive iodine, surgical management of GD is the least frequently selected modality because of the risks of surgery, including those related to general anesthesia, evoking thyroid storm, bleeding, hypoparathyroidism, and recurrent laryngeal nerve injury. However, in certain subsets of patients it may be the preferred treatment, such as those with a large goiter causing compressive symptoms, those with a low uptake of radioactive iodine, suspicion for cancer, moderate-severe GO, intolerance to ATDs, planned pregnancy in less than 6 months, or patient refusal of radioactive iodine.[11,82]

When surgery is chosen, there is a trend from subtotal to near or total thyroidectomy. Previously, subtotal thyroidectomy with the preservation of sufficient thyroid remnant to maintain euthyroidism was attempted; but only 60% of patients achieved euthyroidism, and 8% had persistent or recurrent hyperthyroidism.[83] In a meta-analysis of 35 clinical trials including 7241 patients who underwent surgical treatment of GD, there were no reports of thyroid storm, mortality rate was zero, and overall complication rate was 3%, indicating that thyroid surgery is not only effective but also generally safe.[83–85]

The ATA's guidelines for the management of hyperthyroidism recommend that potassium iodide solution (KI) be administered preoperatively for thyroidectomy. KI has been shown to decrease thyroid gland vascularity and blood loss as well as decrease thyroidal iodide uptake and release of thyroid hormones to prevent intraoperative thyroid storm.[11,86] ATD treatment with both PTU and MMI, especially when treated for more than 12 months, was also associated with less thyroid vascularity on Doppler and with less intraoperative blood loss.[87] A recently published single-institution study comparing surgical outcomes in 162 patients with GD with 102 patients with a toxic multinodular goiter in which neither group received KI solution showed similar intraoperative blood loss and rates of surgical complications, suggesting that KI may not be necessary.[88]

Adjuvant Treatment

Beta-adrenergic blockers are the most common adjunctive therapy used in the management of GD. Many of the symptoms of hyperthyroidism, including tachycardia, weight loss, tremors, and anxiety, mimic beta-adrenergic excess and are greatly improved by beta-blockers.[89] The beta-blockers propranolol, atenolol, and alprenolol can also decrease conversion of T4 to T3 by the inhibition of deiodinase enzymes.[90,91]

Corticosteroids are used in the treatment of moderate to severe because of their antiinflammatory and immunosuppressive effects. Intravenous (IV) and oral glucocorticoids are both effective in the treatment of Graves' ophthalmopathy, though IV administration is more effective and has a lower rate of side effects than oral dosing.[92,93] With a 12-week IV regimen of glucocorticoids, the response rate is 80%.[92] As noted previously, glucocorticoids are also given prophylactically to prevent worsening or development of after RAI treatment.[94]

Rituximab, an anti-CD20 monoclonal antibody, is being studied for the treatment of GO. As GD is an autoimmune process involving T and B cells, B-cell depletion with rituximab can disrupt the inflammatory cycle and reduce disease.[95] In a pilot open study, rituximab infusion did not affect thyroid hormone levels or thyroid antibodies but did result in significantly reduced clinical activity score in patients with active GO compared with the control group receiving IV glucocorticoids.[96] Two randomized controlled trials examining the safety and effectiveness of rituximab therapy for GO have recently been completed and are awaiting publication, with preliminary reports showing divergent conclusions regarding its effectiveness. Intraorbital injection of rituximab has also been found to significantly reduce clinical activity scores in GO.[97]

Management of Thyrotoxicosis During Pregnancy

GD in pregnancy occurs in 0.1% to 1.0% of pregnancies.[98] It is important for fetal outcome that GD is controlled during pregnancy as thyrotoxicosis is associated with low birth weight, prematurity, eclampsia, and miscarriage.[99] In GD there is also the potential for transfer of maternal thyrotropin receptor–stimulating antibodies to the fetus, which can result in fetal hyperthyroidism, manifested by intrauterine growth retardation, tachycardia, goiter, heart failure, and hydrops.[99] Rarely fetal hypothyroidism may occur because of blocking TSH-receptor antibodies. TSH-receptor antibodies may also be present in high titers in women with a prior history of GD, particularly after treatment with radioactive iodine, so it is recommended that antibody levels are checked between 20 and 24 weeks to assess for the risk of fetal thyroid dysfunction as then the pregnancy will require closer monitoring for fetal thyroid dysfunction.[98]

Diagnostic or therapeutic use of radioactive iodine is contraindicated during pregnancy and breastfeeding as it can damage the fetus and infant's thyroid gland. ATDs are the mainstay of GD treatment during pregnancy. PTU and MMI have comparable efficacy in terms of the treatment of Graves' hyperthyroidism and the effect on fetal thyroid function.[100] MMI use in the first trimester has been associated with congenital malformation, specifically aplasia cutis congenital, omphalocele, omphalomesenteric duct anomaly, and esophageal/choanal atresia.[101,102] The rate of major congenital anomalies associated with MMI use was 4.1% and significantly higher than the rate of 2.1% in a control group composed of pregnant patients with GD not treated with ATDs during pregnancy.[101] A recent population-based analysis in Denmark showed a higher incidence of birth defects in women exposed to either PTU or MMI in early pregnancy, although a different pattern of birth defects was noted with PTU compared with MMI.[103] Because of a higher risk of embryopathy with MMI, the current recommendations are that PTU be used in the first trimester of pregnancy and then MMI resumed in the second trimester after organogenesis is complete.[98,104] However, given the recent findings of birth defects in women treated with either agent, definitive therapy before pregnancy is preferable to ATD therapy in early pregnancy.[105]

CPGS VERSUS CURRENT CLINICAL PRACTICE

In 2011, the ATA/AACE's hyperthyroidism CPGs were published simultaneously in the peer-reviewed journals of the 2 societies, *Thyroid* and *Endocrine Practice*, respectively.[8,11] Developed over the course of 5 years by a panel of 12 experts, including 9 adult endocrinologists, one pediatric endocrinologist, one nuclear medicine physician, and one endocrine surgeon, the guidelines addressed all aspects of the diagnosis and management of thyrotoxicosis of all causes. Among the 100 recommendations made by the committee, more than one-half dealt with the diagnosis and management of GD. The task of the guideline committee was made challenging by the dearth of high-quality published evidence in this area. Among the 100 recommendations made by the committee, 83 were classified as *strong*, defined as applying to most patients in most circumstances and having benefits that clearly outweighed the risk for positive recommendations and vice versa for negative recommendations. However, even among the strong recommendations, 68% were deemed to be based on weak data, defined as low-quality evidence consisting of observational studies, case series, or expert opinion; 31% were based on moderate-quality evidence; and only 1% were based on what was thought to be high-quality evidence.

Comparison of Guidelines with Current Practice Trends

Following the publication of the ATA/AACE's hyperthyroidism CPGs, a survey of endocrinologists who were members of the Endocrine Society, the AACE, and the ATA was conducted.[12] The survey explored current clinical practice in many of the clinical circumstances addressed by the guideline committee, including the diagnostic and management practices in uncomplicated GD, the approach to hyperthyroidism management in patients with concurrent GO, and the management of GD in pregnancy. The sections that follow compare and contrast the recommendations in the ATA/AACE's 2011 hyperthyroidism guidelines with the current clinical practice as assessed by responses to the GD management survey. For the purposes of illustration, the case scenarios used in the 2011 GD survey are the focus of the discussion that follows.

Index case (GD management survey)

A 42-year-old woman presents with moderate hyperthyroid symptoms of 2 months duration. She is otherwise healthy, takes no medications, and does not smoke cigarettes. She has 2 children, the youngest of whom is 10 years old, and does not plan on being pregnant again. This is her first episode of hyperthyroidism. She has a diffuse goiter of approximately 2 to 3 times the normal size, a pulse rate of 105 beats per minute, and a normal eye examination. Thyroid hormone levels are found to be twice the upper limit of normal (free T4 = 3.6 ng/dL; normal range = 1.01–1.79 ng/dL), with an undetectable thyrotropin level (TSH <0.01 mIU/L).

DIAGNOSIS

The ATA/AACE's hyperthyroid guidelines state that in the presence of obvious clinical features of GD, as in the index case discussed earlier, a thyroid scan and/or thyroid uptake is not specifically needed for diagnostic purposes. Likewise, in this circumstance, routine TRAb testing was deemed superfluous. Further, the routine use of thyroid ultrasound in the initial evaluation of patients with GD was not endorsed by the guideline committee in the absence of sufficient data to support a beneficial impact of this modality on patient care. However, respondents to the GD management survey noted frequent diagnostic use of scintigraphy in the index case, with 47% selecting either ^{123}I or ^{131}I radioactive iodine uptake, and 42% obtaining either a ^{123}I or Technetium-99m scan. Ultrasound was selected by 26% of survey respondents, 52% of whom would forgo nuclear thyroid imaging. Similarly, TSH-receptor antibody testing was selected by 58% of respondents, most of whom (72%) would use the thyroid-stimulating immunoglobulin assay.

PRIMARY TREATMENT MODALITY

The ATA/AACE's hyperthyroidism guidelines did not advocate in favor of any given modality for the primary treatment of hyperthyroidism caused by GD.[8,11] Rather, the committee recommended an individualized patient-centered approach, with consideration of specific patient features (such as a small goiter and mild hyperthyroidism favoring the use of ATDs) (**Box 1**) as well as patient values (such as reluctance to receive radioiodine or undergo surgery) that would favor a given modality over

---

Box 1
Clinical factors that favor a particular treatment modality

ATDs
- Patients with high likelihood of remission (women, mild disease, small goiter, negative or small titer thyrotropin receptor antibody)
- Elderly or those with comorbidities with increased surgical risk or low life expectancy
- Patients with moderate to severe active Graves' ophthalmopathy

Radioiodine
- Women planning pregnancy more than 4 to 6 months following RAI
- Patients with increased surgical risk (comorbidities, prior neck surgery, or radiation)
- Lack of access to high-volume thyroid surgeon
- Contraindication to ATD use

Surgery
- Patients with symptomatic compression or large goiters ($\geq$80 g)
- Patients with low RAIU
- When concurrent thyroid malignancy is suspected
- Patients with moderate to severe active Graves' ophthalmopathy
- Women planning pregnancy in less than 4 to 6 months

Adapted from Bahn RS, Burch HB, Cooper DS, et al. Hyperthyroidism and other causes of thyrotoxicosis: management guidelines of the American Thyroid Association and American Association of Clinical Endocrinologists. Thyroid 2011;21(6):600–1.

another (**Table 2**). The committee noted that any of the 3 treatment modalities, including ATDs, radioiodine, and thyroidectomy, were acceptable approaches to GD.

Survey respondents expressed a slightly more directed approach, with 58.6% of North American respondents selecting radioiodine, 40.5% ATDs, and only 0.9% thyroidectomy in the uncomplicated case of GD.[12] The use of RAI therapy for uncomplicated GD decreased from a survey performed 20 years earlier, at which time 69% of respondents selected this modality.[68] Further, the current survey found continued international differences in preferred primary modality, with only 13% of European respondents selecting radioiodine as the primary treatment modality, and 86% selecting prolonged therapy with antithyroid medications.

PREFERRED ATD

At the time the ATA/AACE's 2011 hyperthyroidism guidelines were being formulated, a heightened awareness of the association between the use of PTU and severe hepatotoxicity emerged.[106] A review of liver transplant registries in the United States revealed that PTU was the third most common drug linked to a need for liver transplantation and that between 1990 and 2007 there were 1 to 3 cases of liver failure per year linked to the use of this medication.[107] As noted earlier, these guidelines recommended that MMI be selected over PTU, with certain exceptions as previously noted. Survey respondents likewise favored MMI over PTU, with only 2.7% of respondents selecting PTU. This finding represented a striking change from the ATA's member survey 20 years earlier at which time 73% of respondents stated a preference for PTU. Finally, current survey respondents noted that, in response to a persistent cutaneous reaction to an ATD, 55.3% would switch to the alternate drug in this class.

MONITORING FOR ADVERSE EFFECTS OF ATD THERAPY

The ATA/AACE's hyperthyroidism guideline committee suggested that baseline liver function tests and complete cell count be obtained in all patients before the initiation

Table 2		
Patient values that favor a particular treatment modality		
Modality	**Higher Value**	**Lower Value**
ATDs	• Possibility of remission • Avoidance of lifelong thyroid hormone treatment • Avoidance of surgical risk • Avoidance of radioactivity exposure	• Avoidance of ATD adverse effects • Need for monitoring • Possibility of disease recurrence
Radioiodine	• Definitive therapy • Avoidance of surgical risk • Avoidance of ATD adverse effects	• Need for lifelong thyroid hormone replacement • Potential worsening/development of Graves' ophthalmopathy
Surgery	• Rapid and definitive resolution • Avoidance of radioactivity exposure • Avoidance of ATD adverse effects	• Surgical risk • Need for lifelong thyroid hormone replacement

Adapted from Bahn Chair RS, Burch HB, Cooper DS, et al. Hyperthyroidism and other causes of thyrotoxicosis: management guidelines of the American Thyroid Association and American Association of Clinical Endocrinologists. Thyroid 2011;21(6):601.

of ATD therapy in order to detect baseline abnormalities in these indices that are known to occur with increased frequency with GD and to ensure these abnormalities are not incorrectly attributed to the ATD.[8,11] However, the committee recommended no routine laboratory monitoring for either leukocyte abnormalities or hepatic dysfunction in patients taking ATDs. The rationale for this recommendation was that both agranulocytosis and severe hepatotoxicity may occur rapidly and unpredictably; therefore, in essence, routine monitoring does not provide reliable assurance against or warning of these adverse effects. Rather, an emphasis was placed by the committee on patient education regarding signs and symptoms relating to adverse drug effects, with immediate notification of their physician should these occur.

Survey respondents showed a distinctly different practice pattern in regard to monitoring for adverse effects from ATDs, with 54% of respondents routinely monitoring liver-associated enzymes and 48% routinely monitoring complete blood counts during a course of ATDs.[12]

MANAGEMENT OF HYPERTHYROIDISM IN PATIENTS WITH GRAVES' OPHTHALMOPATHY

Following the administration of RAI to patients with GD, there is a sustained increase in TRAb levels, lasting months to years before eventually declining.[108] This aggravation of the autoimmune response in GD is thought to be a contributor to the development of new or worsened GO following RAI, as has been demonstrated in 3 large randomized controlled trials.[94,109] The prophylactic use of corticosteroids to prevent worsening ophthalmopathy following radioiodine has been championed by Bartalena and colleagues, who have shown the utility of this approach to prevent new or worsened ophthalmopathy.[94,110,111] In addition to RAI, other risk factors for the development of Graves' ophthalmopathy are tobacco smoking, high TSH-R antibody titers, and high T3 levels (worse thyrotoxicosis).

The ATA/AACE's 2011 hyperthyroidism guidelines provide guidance on the approach to hyperthyroidism in patients with ophthalmopathy.[8,11] In patients with mild active ophthalmopathy, it was suggested that risk factors for the development of ophthalmopathy be considered and, if present, that prophylactic corticosteroid therapy accompany radioactive iodine therapy. These guidelines also advised that radioiodine be avoided in patients with moderate to severe active ophthalmopathy.

The GD management survey included a patient with non–vision threatening but moderate active ophthalmopathy.[12] Respondents showed a strong desire to avoid RAI in this setting, with only 2% selecting radioiodine alone, 17% selecting radioiodine plus prophylactic corticosteroids, 18.5% selecting thyroidectomy, and 63% selecting a prolonged course of ATDs as the primary treatment modality for the patients' hyperthyroidism (**Fig. 1**).

MANAGEMENT OF GD DURING PREGNANCY

Pregnancy presents unique challenges to the management of GD. The optimal control of hyperthyroidism with ATDs during pregnancy must be balanced against the effect of fetal exposure to these medications, which freely cross the placenta.[69] Although lower doses of ATDs can generally be used without affecting the fetus, there is a dose-related occurrence of both fetal goiter and fetal hypothyroidism with the use of ATDs in pregnancy.[69] Therefore, the guiding principle in the use of ATDs during pregnancy is to use the lowest effective doses needed to bring the mother from overt to subclinical hyperthyroidism while closely monitoring fetal well-being for evidence of overexposure to ATDs. Another important aspect related to the use of ATDs during

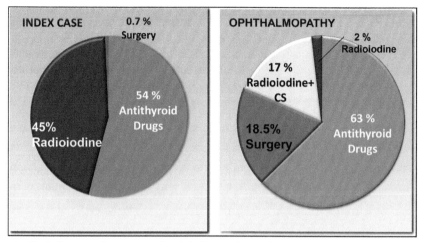

Fig. 1. The influence of presence of ophthalmopathy on the selection of therapy for hyperthyroidism in patients with GD. (*Adapted from* Burch HB, Burman KD, Cooper DS. A 2011 survey of clinical practice patterns in the management of Graves' disease. J Clin Endocrinol Metab 2012;97(12):4549–58; with permission.)

pregnancy is the association between MMI use during the first trimester and fetal embryopathy, as noted previously.[69,102]

The ATA/AACE's 2011 hyperthyroidism guidelines suggested that PTU, rather than MMI, should be used during the first trimester of pregnancy and then on entering the second trimester, MMI be substituted for the PTU.[8,11] Therefore, for a woman receiving MMI before becoming pregnant, this would necessitate a change to PTU for the first trimester and then back to MMI for the remainder of pregnancy. Because it is not clear to what extent ATD switching leads to loss of control of hyperthyroidism during pregnancy, these guidelines stated that an alternative is to continue PTU throughout the remainder of pregnancy while closely monitoring for hepatic dysfunction. The guidelines also noted that thyroid surgery was a reasonable option in women desiring pregnancy over the next 4 to 6 months, rather than radioiodine, because the latter is associated with an increase in TSH-receptor antibodies[108] that could potentially affect the fetal thyroid.

The GD management survey contained a section dealing with the management of hyperthyroidism during pregnancy.[12] Respondents were asked which primary mode of therapy they would recommend for GD in a women planning on becoming pregnant over the next 6 to 12 months. Half (50%) of the respondents would use ATDs in women planning pregnancy, 30% would use RAI, and 20% would send patients for thyroidectomy (**Fig. 2**). Respondents choosing ATDs before pregnancy were next asked which ATD they preferred in this setting. More than half (54%) of respondents would use PTU in women planning pregnancy (counter to the advice of the ATA/AACE's guidelines), and 46% would use MMI. Next respondents treating with MMI before pregnancy were asked whether they would switch to PTU when pregnancy is diagnosed. Seventy-six percent said they would switch to PTU, and 24% said they would continue MMI. Finally, respondents who switched to PTU during the first trimester were asked whether they would switch back to MMI during the second trimester, per the ATA/AACE's guidelines. Surprisingly, more than half (54%) of respondents said they would continue PTU for the remainder of pregnancy rather than switching back to MMI on entering the second trimester.

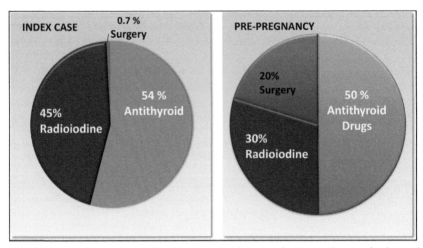

Fig. 2. The effect of pregnancy planning on the selection of primary therapy for hyperthyroidism caused by GD. (*Adapted from* Burch HB, Burman KD, Cooper DS. A 2011 survey of clinical practice patterns in the management of Graves' disease. J Clin Endocrinol Metab 2012;97(12):4549–58; with permission.)

SUMMARY

In summary, over the last century much has been learned about the pathogenesis, manifestations, and management of GD leading to the establishment of evidence-based CPGs. These joint CPGs from the ATA and AACE give recommendations on both the diagnosis and treatment of hyperthyroidism. A survey of clinicians performed that same year, however, revealed that current practices diverge from these recently published guidelines in multiple areas. These differences will need to be assessed serially to determine the impact of the guidelines on future clinical practice and perhaps vice versa.

REFERENCES

1. Cooper DS. Hyperthyroidism. Lancet 2003;362(9382):459–68.
2. Franklyn JA, Boelaert K. Thyrotoxicosis. Lancet 2012;379(9821):1155–66.
3. Laurberg P, Pedersen KM, Hreidarsson A, et al. Iodine intake and the pattern of thyroid disorders: a comparative epidemiological study of thyroid abnormalities in the elderly in Iceland and in Jutland, Denmark. J Clin Endocrinol Metab 1998; 83(3):765–9.
4. Biondi B, Kahaly GJ. Cardiovascular involvement in patients with different causes of hyperthyroidism. Nat Rev Endocrinol 2010;6(8):431–43.
5. Brandt F, Thvilum M, Almind D, et al. Graves' disease and toxic nodular goiter are both associated with increased mortality but differ with respect to the cause of death: a Danish population-based register study. Thyroid 2013;23(4):408–13.
6. Shu X, Ji J, Li X, et al. Cancer risk in patients hospitalised for Graves' disease: a population-based cohort study in Sweden. Br J Cancer 2010;102(9):1397–9.
7. Pellegriti G, Mannarino C, Russo M, et al. Increased mortality in patients with differentiated thyroid cancer associated with Graves' disease. J Clin Endocrinol Metab 2013;98(3):1014–21.
8. Bahn Chair RS, Burch HB, Cooper DS, et al. Hyperthyroidism and other causes of thyrotoxicosis: management guidelines of the American Thyroid Association

and American Association of Clinical Endocrinologists. Thyroid 2011;21(6): 593–646.

9. Garber JR, Cobin RH, Gharib H, et al. Clinical practice guidelines for hypothyroidism in adults: cosponsored by the American Association of Clinical Endocrinologists and the American Thyroid Association. Thyroid 2012;22(12):1200–35.

10. Cooper DS, Doherty GM, Haugen BR, et al. Revised American Thyroid Association management guidelines for patients with thyroid nodules and differentiated thyroid cancer. Thyroid 2009;19(11):1167–214.

11. Bahn RS, Burch HB, Cooper DS, et al. Hyperthyroidism and other causes of thyrotoxicosis: management guidelines of the American Thyroid Association and American Association of Clinical Endocrinologists. Endocr Pract 2011; 17(3):456–520.

12. Burch HB, Burman KD, Cooper DS. A 2011 survey of clinical practice patterns in the management of Graves' disease. J Clin Endocrinol Metab 2012;97(12):4549–58.

13. Tomer Y, Davies TF. The genetic susceptibility to Graves' disease. Baillieres Clin Endocrinol Metab 1997;11(3):431–50.

14. Brix TH, Kyvik KO, Hegedus L. What is the evidence of genetic factors in the etiology of Graves' disease? A brief review. Thyroid 1998;8(8):727–34.

15. Harvald B, Hauge M. A catamnestic investigation of Danish twins; a preliminary report. Dan Med Bull 1956;3(5):150–8.

16. Chopra IJ, Solomon DH, Chopra U, et al. Abnormalities in thyroid function in relatives of patients with Graves' disease and Hashimoto's thyroiditis: lack of correlation with inheritance of HLA-B8. J Clin Endocrinol Metab 1977;45(1):45–54.

17. Burek CL, Hoffman WH, Rose NR. The presence of thyroid autoantibodies in children and adolescents with autoimmune thyroid disease and in their siblings and parents. Clin Immunol Immunopathol 1982;25(3):395–404.

18. Hall R, Stanbury JB. Familial studies of autoimmune thyroiditis. Clin Exp Immunol 1967;2(Suppl):719–25.

19. Sunthornthepvarakul T, Hayashi Y, Refetoff S. Polymorphism of a variant human thyrotropin receptor (hTSHR) gene. Thyroid 1994;4(2):147–9.

20. Gu LQ, Zhu W, Zhao SX, et al. Clinical associations of the genetic variants of CTLA-4, Tg, TSHR, PTPN22, PTPN12 and FCRL3 in patients with Graves' disease. Clin Endocrinol (Oxf) 2010;72(2):248–55.

21. Tomer Y, Barbesino G, Keddache M, et al. Mapping of a major susceptibility locus for Graves' disease (GD-1) to chromosome 14q31. J Clin Endocrinol Metab 1997;82(5):1645–8.

22. Shi W, Liu W, Zhou X, et al. Associations of Helicobacter pylori infection and cytotoxin-associated gene A status with autoimmune thyroid diseases: a meta-analysis. Thyroid 2013;23(10):1294–300.

23. Pedersen IB, Knudsen N, Carle A, et al. Serum selenium is low in newly diagnosed Graves' disease: a population-based study. Clin Endocrinol (Oxf) 2013; 79(4):584–90.

24. Prummel MF, Strieder T, Wiersinga WM. The environment and autoimmune thyroid diseases. Eur J Endocrinol 2004;150(5):605–18.

25. Klein I, Ojamaa K. Thyroid hormone and the cardiovascular system. N Engl J Med 2001;344(7):501–9.

26. Klein I, Danzi S. Thyroid disease and the heart. Circulation 2007;116(15):1725–35.

27. Danzi S, Klein I. Thyroid hormone-regulated cardiac gene expression and cardiovascular disease. Thyroid 2002;12(6):467–72.

28. Hegazi MO, Ahmed S. Atypical clinical manifestations of Graves' disease: an analysis in depth. J Thyroid Res 2012;2012:768019.

29. Bogaard HJ, Al Husseini A, Farkas L, et al. Severe pulmonary hypertension: the role of metabolic and endocrine disorders. Pulm Circ 2012;2(2):148–54.
30. Roffi M, Cattaneo F, Topol EJ. Thyrotoxicosis and the cardiovascular system: subtle but serious effects. Cleve Clin J Med 2003;70(1):57–63.
31. Volzke H, Schwahn C, Wallaschofski H, et al. Review: the association of thyroid dysfunction with all-cause and circulatory mortality: is there a causal relationship? J Clin Endocrinol Metab 2007;92(7):2421–9.
32. Goswami R, Tandon RK, Dudha A, et al. Prevalence and significance of steatorrhea in patients with active Graves' disease. Am J Gastroenterol 1998;93(7):1122–5.
33. Milla CE, Zirbes J. Pulmonary complications of endocrine and metabolic disorders. Paediatr Respir Rev 2012;13(1):23–8.
34. Pino-Garcia JM, Garcia-Rio F, Diez JJ, et al. Regulation of breathing in hyperthyroidism: relationship to hormonal and metabolic changes. Eur Respir J 1998; 12(2):400–7.
35. Boelaert K, Torlinska B, Holder RL, et al. Older subjects with hyperthyroidism present with a paucity of symptoms and signs: a large cross-sectional study. J Clin Endocrinol Metab 2010;95(6):2715–26.
36. Ebert EC. The thyroid and the gut. J Clin Gastroenterol 2010;44(6):402–6.
37. Daher R, Yazbeck T, Jaoude JB, et al. Consequences of dysthyroidism on the digestive tract and viscera. World J Gastroenterol 2009;15(23):2834–8.
38. Malik R, Hodgson H. The relationship between the thyroid gland and the liver. QJM 2002;95(9):559–69.
39. Kubota S, Amino N, Matsumoto Y, et al. Serial changes in liver function tests in patients with thyrotoxicosis induced by Graves' disease and painless thyroiditis. Thyroid 2008;18(3):283–7.
40. Gurlek A, Cobankara V, Bayraktar M. Liver tests in hyperthyroidism: effect of antithyroid therapy. J Clin Gastroenterol 1997;24(3):180–3.
41. Thompson P Jr, Strum D, Boehm T, et al. Abnormalities of liver function tests in tyrotoxicosis. Mil Med 1978;143(8):548–51.
42. Ch'ng CL, Biswas M, Benton A, et al. Prospective screening for coeliac disease in patients with Graves' hyperthyroidism using anti-gliadin and tissue transglutaminase antibodies. Clin Endocrinol (Oxf) 2005;62(3):303–6.
43. Bunevicius R, Prange AJ Jr. Psychiatric manifestations of Graves' hyperthyroidism: pathophysiology and treatment options. CNS Drugs 2006;20(11):897–909.
44. Bunevicius R, Velickiene D, Prange AJ Jr. Mood and anxiety disorders in women with treated hyperthyroidism and ophthalmopathy caused by Graves' disease. Gen Hosp Psychiatry 2005;27(2):133–9.
45. Chattopadhyay C, Chakrabarti N, Ghosh S. An assessment of psychiatric disturbances in Graves disease in a medical college in eastern India. Niger J Clin Pract 2012;15(3):276–9.
46. Brownlie BE, Rae AM, Walshe JW, et al. Psychoses associated with thyrotoxicosis - 'thyrotoxic psychosis.' A report of 18 cases, with statistical analysis of incidence. Eur J Endocrinol 2000;142(5):438–44.
47. Krassas GE, Poppe K, Glinoer D. Thyroid function and human reproductive health. Endocr Rev 2010;31(5):702–55.
48. Carani C, Isidori AM, Granata A, et al. Multicenter study on the prevalence of sexual symptoms in male hypo- and hyperthyroid patients. J Clin Endocrinol Metab 2005;90(12):6472–9.
49. Krassas GE, Pontikides N, Deligianni V, et al. A prospective controlled study of the impact of hyperthyroidism on reproductive function in males. J Clin Endocrinol Metab 2002;87(8):3667–71.

50. Benson RC, Dailey ME. The menstrual pattern in hyperthyroidism and subsequent posttherapy hypothyroidism. Surg Gynecol Obstet 1955;100(1):19–26.
51. Krassas GE, Pontikides N, Kaltsas T, et al. Menstrual disturbances in thyrotoxicosis. Clin Endocrinol (Oxf) 1994;40(5):641–4.
52. Nicholls JJ, Brassill MJ, Williams GR, et al. The skeletal consequences of thyrotoxicosis. J Endocrinol 2012;213(3):209–21.
53. Vestergaard P, Mosekilde L. Hyperthyroidism, bone mineral, and fracture risk–a meta-analysis. Thyroid 2003;13(6):585–93.
54. Prabhakar BS, Bahn RS, Smith TJ. Current perspective on the pathogenesis of Graves' disease and ophthalmopathy. Endocr Rev 2003;24(6):802–35.
55. Burch HB, Wartofsky L. Graves' ophthalmopathy: current concepts regarding pathogenesis and management. Endocr Rev 1993;14(6):747–93.
56. Ponto KA, Merkesdal S, Hommel G, et al. Public health relevance of Graves' orbitopathy. J Clin Endocrinol Metab 2013;98(1):145–52.
57. Cooper DS, Ladenson PW. The thyroid gland. In: Gardner DG, Shoback D, editors. Greenspan's basic & clinical endocrinology. 9th edition. China: McGraw-Hill Companies; 2007. p. 285–328.
58. Werner SC. Classification of the eye changes of Graves' disease. Am J Ophthalmol 1969;68(4):646–8.
59. Mourits MP, Koornneef L, Wiersinga WM, et al. Clinical criteria for the assessment of disease activity in Graves' ophthalmopathy: a novel approach. Br J Ophthalmol 1989;73(8):639–44.
60. Mourits MP, Prummel MF, Wiersinga WM, et al. Clinical activity score as a guide in the management of patients with Graves' ophthalmopathy. Clin Endocrinol (Oxf) 1997;47(1):9–14.
61. Bartalena L, Baldeschi L, Dickinson AJ, et al. Consensus statement of the European group on Graves' orbitopathy (EUGOGO) on management of Graves' orbitopathy. Thyroid 2008;18(3):333–46.
62. Fatourechi V, Bartley GB, Eghbali-Fatourechi GZ, et al. Graves' dermopathy and acropachy are markers of severe Graves' ophthalmopathy. Thyroid 2003;13(12):1141–4.
63. Schwartz KM, Fatourechi V, Ahmed DD, et al. Dermopathy of Graves' disease (pretibial myxedema): long-term outcome. J Clin Endocrinol Metab 2002;87(2):438–46.
64. Fatourechi V. Thyroid dermopathy and acropachy. Best Pract Res Clin Endocrinol Metab 2012;26(4):553–65.
65. Trivalle C, Doucet J, Chassagne P, et al. Differences in the signs and symptoms of hyperthyroidism in older and younger patients. J Am Geriatr Soc 1996;44(1):50–3.
66. Teelucksingh S, Pendek R, Padfield PL. Apathetic thyrotoxicosis in adolescence. J Intern Med 1991;229(6):543–4.
67. Grewal RP. Apathetic hyperthyroidism in an adolescent. J Psychiatry Neurosci 1993;18(5):276.
68. Solomon B, Glinoer D, Lagasse R, et al. Current trends in the management of Graves' disease. J Clin Endocrinol Metab 1990;70(6):1518–24.
69. Cooper DS. Antithyroid drugs. N Engl J Med 2005;352(9):905–17.
70. Nakamura H, Miyauchi A, Miyawaki N, et al. Analysis of 754 cases of antithyroid drug-induced agranulocytosis over 30 years in Japan. J Clin Endocrinol Metab 2013;98(12):4776–83.
71. Sundaresh V, Brito JP, Wang Z, et al. Comparative effectiveness of therapies for Graves' hyperthyroidism: a systematic review and network meta-analysis. J Clin Endocrinol Metab 2013;98(9):3671–7.

72. Williams KV, Nayak S, Becker D, et al. Fifty years of experience with propylthiouracil-associated hepatotoxicity: what have we learned? J Clin Endocrinol Metab 1997;82(6):1727–33.

73. Emiliano AB, Governale L, Parks M, et al. Shifts in propylthiouracil and methimazole prescribing practices: antithyroid drug use in the United States from 1991 to 2008. J Clin Endocrinol Metab 2010;95(5):2227–33.

74. Abraham P, Avenell A, Park CM, et al. A systematic review of drug therapy for Graves' hyperthyroidism. Eur J Endocrinol 2005;153(4):489–98.

75. Cappelli C, Gandossi E, Castellano M, et al. Prognostic value of thyrotropin receptor antibodies (TRAb) in Graves' disease: a 120 months prospective study. Endocr J 2007;54(5):713–20.

76. Anagnostis P, Adamidou F, Polyzos SA, et al. Predictors of long-term remission in patients with Graves' disease: a single center experience. Endocrine 2013; 44(2):448–53.

77. Laurberg P, Berman DC, Andersen S, et al. Sustained control of Graves' hyperthyroidism during long-term low-dose antithyroid drug therapy of patients with severe Graves' orbitopathy. Thyroid 2011;21(9):951–6.

78. de Rooij A, Vandenbroucke JP, Smit JW, et al. Clinical outcomes after estimated versus calculated activity of radioiodine for the treatment of hyperthyroidism: systematic review and meta-analysis. Eur J Endocrinol 2009;161(5):771–7.

79. Akamizu T, Satoh T, Isozaki O, et al. Diagnostic criteria, clinical features, and incidence of thyroid storm based on nationwide surveys. Thyroid 2012;22(7): 661–79.

80. Lee SL. Radioactive iodine therapy. Curr Opin Endocrinol Diabetes Obes 2012; 19(5):420–8.

81. Acharya SH, Avenell A, Philip S, et al. Radioiodine therapy (RAI) for Graves' disease (GD) and the effect on ophthalmopathy: a systematic review. Clin Endocrinol (Oxf) 2008;69(6):943–50.

82. Yip J, Lang BH, Lo CY. Changing trend in surgical indication and management for Graves' disease. Am J Surg 2012;203(2):162–7.

83. Palit TK, Miller CC 3rd, Miltenburg DM. The efficacy of thyroidectomy for Graves' disease: a meta-analysis. J Surg Res 2000;90(2):161–5.

84. Wilhelm SM, McHenry CR. Total thyroidectomy is superior to subtotal thyroidectomy for management of Graves' disease in the United States. World J Surg 2010;34(6):1261–4.

85. Werga-Kjellman P, Zedenius J, Tallstedt L, et al. Surgical treatment of hyperthyroidism: a ten-year experience. Thyroid 2001;11(2):187–92.

86. Erbil Y, Ozluk Y, Giris M, et al. Effect of lugol solution on thyroid gland blood flow and microvessel density in the patients with Graves' disease. J Clin Endocrinol Metab 2007;92(6):2182–9.

87. Erbil Y, Giris M, Salmaslioglu A, et al. The effect of anti-thyroid drug treatment duration on thyroid gland microvessel density and intraoperative blood loss in patients with Graves' disease. Surgery 2008;143(2):216–25.

88. Shinall MC Jr, Broome JT, Baker A, et al. Is potassium iodide solution necessary before total thyroidectomy for graves disease? Ann Surg Oncol 2013;20(9): 2964–7.

89. Geffner DL, Hershman JM. Beta-adrenergic blockade for the treatment of hyperthyroidism. Am J Med 1992;93(1):61–8.

90. Wiersinga WM, Touber JL. The influence of beta-adrenoceptor blocking agents on plasma thyroxine and triiodothyronine. J Clin Endocrinol Metab 1977;45(2): 293–8.

91. Perrild H, Hansen JM, Skovsted L, et al. Different effects of propranolol, alprenolol, sotalol, atenolol and metoprolol on serum T3 and serum rT3 in hyperthyroidism. Clin Endocrinol (Oxf) 1983;18(2):139–42.

92. Zang S, Ponto KA, Kahaly GJ. Clinical review: intravenous glucocorticoids for Graves' orbitopathy: efficacy and morbidity. J Clin Endocrinol Metab 2011; 96(2):320–32.

93. Marcocci C, Bartalena L, Tanda ML, et al. Comparison of the effectiveness and tolerability of intravenous or oral glucocorticoids associated with orbital radiotherapy in the management of severe Graves' ophthalmopathy: results of a prospective, single-blind, randomized study. J Clin Endocrinol Metab 2001;86(8): 3562–7.

94. Bartalena L, Marcocci C, Bogazzi F, et al. Relation between therapy for hyperthyroidism and the course of Graves' ophthalmopathy. N Engl J Med 1998; 338(2):73–8.

95. Naik V, Khadavi N, Naik MN, et al. Biologic therapeutics in thyroid-associated ophthalmopathy: translating disease mechanism into therapy. Thyroid 2008; 18(9):967–71.

96. Salvi M, Vannucchi G, Campi I, et al. Treatment of Graves' disease and associated ophthalmopathy with the anti-CD20 monoclonal antibody rituximab: an open study. Eur J Endocrinol 2007;156(1):33–40.

97. Savino G, Balia L, Colucci D, et al. Intraorbital injection of rituximab: a new approach for active thyroid-associated orbitopathy, a prospective case series. Minerva Endocrinol 2013;38(2):173–9.

98. Stagnaro-Green A, Abalovich M, Alexander E, et al. Guidelines of the American Thyroid Association for the diagnosis and management of thyroid disease during pregnancy and postpartum. Thyroid 2011;21(10):1081–125.

99. Azizi F, Amouzegar A. Management of hyperthyroidism during pregnancy and lactation. Eur J Endocrinol 2011;164(6):871–6.

100. Momotani N, Noh JY, Ishikawa N, et al. Effects of propylthiouracil and methimazole on fetal thyroid status in mothers with Graves' hyperthyroidism. J Clin Endocrinol Metab 1997;82(11):3633–6.

101. Yoshihara A, Noh J, Yamaguchi T, et al. Treatment of Graves' disease with antithyroid drugs in the first trimester of pregnancy and the prevalence of congenital malformation. J Clin Endocrinol Metab 2012;97(7):2396–403.

102. Clementi M, Di Gianantonio E, Cassina M, et al. Treatment of hyperthyroidism in pregnancy and birth defects. J Clin Endocrinol Metab 2010;95(11): E337–41.

103. Andersen SL, Olsen J, Wu CS, et al. Birth defects after early pregnancy use of antithyroid drugs: a Danish nationwide study. J Clin Endocrinol Metab 2013; 98(11):4373–81.

104. Karras S, Tzotzas T, Kaltsas T, et al. Pharmacological treatment of hyperthyroidism during lactation: review of the literature and novel data. Pediatr Endocrinol Rev 2010;8(1):25–33.

105. Rivkees SA. Propylthiouracil versus methimazole during pregnancy: an evolving tale of difficult choices. J Clin Endocrinol Metab 2013;98(11):4332–5.

106. Bahn RS, Burch HS, Cooper DS, et al. The role of propylthiouracil in the management of Graves' disease in adults: report of a meeting jointly sponsored by the American Thyroid Association and the Food and Drug Administration. Thyroid 2009;19(7):673–4.

107. Cooper DS, Rivkees SA. Putting propylthiouracil in perspective. J Clin Endocrinol Metab 2009;94(6):1881–2.

108. Laurberg P, Wallin G, Tallstedt L, et al. TSH-receptor autoimmunity in Graves' disease after therapy with anti-thyroid drugs, surgery, or radioiodine: a 5-year prospective randomized study. Eur J Endocrinol 2008;158(1):69–75.

109. Tallstedt L, Lundell G, Torring O, et al. Occurrence of ophthalmopathy after treatment for Graves' hyperthyroidism. The Thyroid Study Group. N Engl J Med 1992;326(26):1733–8.

110. Lai A, Marcocci C, Bogazzi F, et al. Lower dose prednisone prevents radioiodine-associated exacerbation of initially mild or absent graves' orbitopathy: a retrospective cohort study. J Clin Endocrinol Metab 2010;95(3):1333–7.

111. Bartalena L, Sassi L, Compri E, et al. Use of corticosteroids to prevent progression of Graves' ophthalmopathy after radioiodine therapy for hyperthyroidism. N Engl J Med 1989;321(20):1349–52.

Thyroid Disease and the Cardiovascular System

Sara Danzi, PhD[a],*, Irwin Klein, MD[b,c]

KEYWORDS

- Hypothyroidism • Hyperthyroidism • Subclinical • Thyroid hormone
- Triiodothyronine • Heart • Cardiac myocyte

KEY POINTS

- Thyroid dysfunction may significantly impair cardiac and cardiovascular health.
- Chronic diseases, such as heart disease, may lead to the low T_3 syndrome.
- More severe heart disease (NYS Heart Association classification stages 3 and 4) is associated with an increased prevalence of low T_3 syndrome.
- Regardless of the cause, in this context decreased serum T_3 levels are associated with poor prognosis, especially in heart disease.

INTRODUCTION

There is an intimate relationship between the thyroid gland and the heart. Thyroid dysfunction, including subclinical thyroid disease, has significant effects on cardiovascular function and health. Likewise, chronic disease states, such as heart disease, may lead to reduced serum thyroid hormone levels, specifically T_3 (low T_3 syndrome) causing a synergistic negative effect on cardiac and cardiovascular function. Therefore, diagnosis and treatment of the patient with heart disease may benefit from analysis of thyroid status, including levels of serum total T_3.

THYROID HORMONE REGULATION AND METABOLISM

The thyroid gland produces 2 biologically active hormones, thyroxine (T_4) and triiodothyronine (T_3). Although T_4 has some documented nongenomic effects, it is largely considered a prohormone. Most of T_4 is converted to T_3 by 5′-monodeiodination in the liver, kidneys, and skeletal muscle.[1,2] T_3 is then delivered to the circulation so that it is available for tissues and organs that rely solely or predominantly on serum T_3, such as the heart.

---

[a] Department of Biological Sciences and Geology, Queensborough Community College, 222-05 56th Avenue, Bayside, NY 11364, USA; [b] Department of Medicine and Cell Biology, NYU School of Medicine, New York, NY 10016, USA; [c] Private Office, 935 Northern Boulevard, Great Neck, NY 11021, USA
* Corresponding author.
E-mail address: saradanzi@gmail.com

Endocrinol Metab Clin N Am 43 (2014) 517–528
http://dx.doi.org/10.1016/j.ecl.2014.02.005
0889-8529/14/$ – see front matter © 2014 Elsevier Inc. All rights reserved.

Expression and activity of relevant monodeiodinases are also regulated in part by T_3.[3] Serious chronic illness, such as heart disease, is often associated with decreased serum T_3 levels. This is known as low T_3 syndrome or nonthyroidal illness and is frequently caused by impaired deiodinase activity, primarily from congestion in the liver.[1] The hepatic type 1 iodothyronine deiodinase (D1) is induced at the transcriptional level by T_3, but in illness, a cytokine-mediated effect blocks the induction, resulting in decreased serum T_3 levels.[4]

The regulation of thyroid hormone synthesis and secretion is primarily dependent on thyrotropin (thyroid stimulating hormone or TSH), synthesized and released by the anterior pituitary in a negative feedback loop. This feedback is largely driven by serum T_4 levels and thus, serum T_3 levels decline without promoting a compensatory response from the pituitary. In the low T_3 syndrome, however, increased T_4 production would not be beneficial because it is the conversion to T_3 that is impaired. The consequences of this and potentially significant implications for the heart and cardiovascular system are discussed.

THYROID HORMONE ACTION AT THE CELLULAR LEVEL

The actions of T_3 include genomic transcriptional activation and repression and nongenomic actions targeted to specific membrane proteins, organelles, and cytoskeletal components. Membrane proteins include solute transporters for ions (Ca^{2+}, Na^+) and glucose among many others.[5] Together, the nongenomic and genomic actions of T_3 on cardiac myocytes and vascular smooth muscle are responsible for significant effects on the heart and cardiovascular system function.

The transcriptional actions of T_3 are mediated by nuclear receptor proteins that bind to specific thyroid hormone response elements in the upstream region of T_3 responsive genes.[6] These nuclear receptors, which include TRα and TRβ, activate expression of positively regulated genes in the presence of T_3 and in the absence of T_3, repress transcription of negatively regulated genes. A survey of the list of T_3-responsive genes in the cardiac myocyte can explain why the heart is so sensitive to serum levels of T_3 (**Table 1**).[1,7] Our studies demonstrate that it is T_3 and not T_4 that enters the cardiac myocyte (Sara Danzi, PhD, and Irwin Klein, MD, personal communication). Measures of α-MHC heteronuclear RNA (hnRNA), the first product of transcription (prespliced), serve as a rapid, sensitive measure of T_3-mediated transcription in the rodent myocyte.[8] Cardiac α-MHC hnRNA is detectable within 30 minutes after T_3 administration. However, after T_4 administration, detectable α-MHC hnRNA expression is delayed by almost 12 hours coinciding with rising serum T_3 levels. These data support the premise that T_4 is not transported into the cardiac myocyte, and adequate serum T_3 is required for maximum α-MHC expression.

Table 1
Effect of T_3 on cardiac-specific genes

Positively Regulated	Negatively Regulated
Alpha-myosin heavy chain	Beta-myosin heavy chain
Sarcoplasmic reticulum Ca^{2+}-ATPase	Phospholamban
Na^+/K^+-ATPase	Adenylyl cyclase catalytic subunits
Beta1-adrenergic receptor	Thyroid hormone receptor alpha-1
Atrial natriuretic hormone	Na^+/Ca^{2+} exchanger
Voltage-gated potassium channels	Thyroid hormone transporters (MCT8,10) Adenine nucleotide translocase-1 (ANT1)

Despite the fact that the regulation of α-MHC has been carefully studied in rodent cardiac myocytes, it is the calcium cycling proteins in the human heart that appear to be the most important target of thyroid hormone action. The sarcoplasmic reticulum calcium ATPase (SERCA2) functions to sequester calcium in the sarcoplasmic reticulum during the relaxation phase of myocyte contraction. The SERCA2 ion transporter is regulated by the presence and phosphorylation state of membrane protein phospholamban (PLB). Phosphorylation of PLB alters the conformational state of the protein, which in turn affects SERCA2 function.[9,10] Expression of both these proteins is regulated by T_3. SERCA2 expression is positively regulated and PLB expression is negatively regulated. In addition, the degree of PLB phosphorylation is regulated by T_3. The net effect is that, in the presence of T_3, myocyte calcium cycling is enhanced leading to improved cardiac myocyte relaxation and improved overall cardiac diastolic function. This is the mechanism by which T_3 acts as a unique lusitropic agent. With insufficient serum T_3 levels, impaired diastolic function may result. The low T_3 syndrome may be a significant factor in heart disease, specifically diastolic dysfunction.

Thyroid hormone analogues are of clinical interest for potential therapeutic value in lipid lowering and weight loss. The development for clinical use has heretofore been hampered by the untoward cardiac effects despite being designed for thyroid hormone receptor selectivity.[11] However, a recent study of the TRβ specific ligand, eprotirome, has shown the novel ability to lower serum cholesterol levels without affecting heart rate or cardiac function.[12] This class of drugs will require further study as a novel addition to the therapeutic armamentarium for reducing cardiovascular risk through lowered low density lipoprotein (LDL) cholesterol and Lp(a).[13] To date, the development of eprotirome has been halted as a result of untoward histologic findings in cartilage from animals treated with the drug for 12 months.

THYROID HORMONE ACTION ON THE HEART AND CARDIOVASCULAR SYSTEM

Thyroid function can be assessed in various ways including measurement of thyroid hormones, free and total T_4 and T_3 and of TSH. Most often, the measurement of serum TSH levels is the only test ordered, as TSH is considered the gold standard for thyroid function. However, despite the narrowing of the reference range for TSH (from 0.3–3.5 mU/L), variations in thyroid hormone levels within the normal range are associated with predictable affects on cardiac function.[14,15] Measurement of other thyroid hormones, specifically total T_3, demonstrates associations with impaired cardiac function and serum brain natriuretic peptide in patients with cardiac disease and heart failure (especially diastolic dysfunction).[16]

Cellular T_3 uptake from serum depends on members of the monocarboxylate transporter (MCT) and organic anion transporter family of plasma membrane transporters.[16,17] These proteins transport a variety of ligands but only MCT8 and MCT10 (also known as TAT1) are highly specific for iodothyronines and are expressed in heart (Sara Danzi, PhD, and Irwin Klein, MD, personal communication).[18] Most data indicate that the cardiac myocyte cannot metabolize T_4 to T_3. The observed cardiac myocyte nuclear actions and changes in gene expression result from changes in blood levels of T_3.[8] The cardiac myocyte is very sensitive to changes in serum T_3, and this is evidenced by rapid changes in the expression of T_3 mediated genes.[8]

Through effects on cardiac myocytes and vascular smooth muscle cells, increased serum T_3 levels are associated with enhanced contractility and diastolic function and lower systemic vascular resistance (SVR).[1,19] Data from the Framingham Heart Study confirm that TSH is inversely related to left ventricular contractility.[20] Clearly heart rate is positively associated with serum T_3 levels and heart rate remains one of the most sensitive physiologic measures of thyroid hormone action.

The effects of thyroid hormone on the heart and cardiovascular system are the most informative and sensitive signs of thyroid dysfunction. Thyroid disease states have predictable cardiac and hemodynamic consequences. These are discussed later.

HYPERTHYROIDISM

Many of the classic signs and symptoms of hyperthyroidism are the cardiac and hemodynamic manifestations and include palpitations, tachycardia, exercise intolerance, dyspnea on exertion, widened pulse pressure, and sometimes atrial fibrillation (**Table 2**).[21,22] In patients with hyperthyroidism, whether endogenous or exogenous in origin, cardiac output may be increased by 50% to 300% over that of normal subjects due to the combined effect of increased resting heart rate, contractility, ejection fraction, and blood volume with decreased SVR.[1] Vascular tissue in the pulmonary system does not appear to respond similarly, and pulmonary hypertension has been noted with hyperthyroidism.[23] Pulmonary artery hypertension in hyperthyroidism may be associated with signs of right-sided heart failure, including neck vein distension and peripheral edema.[24,25]

Cardiac contractility is enhanced, including both systolic and diastolic function, and cardiac output and resting heart rate are increased in hyperthyroidism.[26] A decrease in SVR decreases afterload and improves myocardial efficiency. An increase in blood volume and an increase in venous return cause the preload of the heart to increase, further augmenting cardiac output. The increase in cardiovascular hemodynamics allows for increased blood flow leading to enhanced perfusion to provide for the substrate and oxygen demands of peripheral tissues (**Fig. 1**).

The cardiovascular manifestations of hyperthyroidism are independent of the cause of the increased levels of thyroid hormone.[27] Tachycardia is the most common finding. Heart rate is increased both at rest and with exercise and palpitations are common. Atrial arrhythmias, including atrial fibrillation can occur but this is more common in older patients. Other findings include widened pulse pressure, increased systolic and lowered diastolic pressure, and dyspnea on exertion. Exercise intolerance with limitations such as climbing one flight of stairs results from both skeletal muscle and respiratory weakness as well as a decrement in cardiac reserve capacity.

Table 2 Cardiovascular signs and symptoms associated with hyperthyroidism and hypothyroidism	
Hyperthyroidism	**Hypothyroidism**
Palpitations	Fatigue
Anginal chest pain	Decreased endurance
Exercise intolerance	Increased serum cholesterol
Atrial fibrillation	Impaired cardiac contractility
Exertional dyspnea	Impaired diastolic function
Cardiac hypertrophy	Increased SVR
Systolic hypertension	Bradycardia
Peripheral edema	Decreased endothelial-derived relaxation factor
Hyperdynamic precordium	Increased homocysteine
Pulmonary hypertension	Increased C-reactive protein
Heart failure	

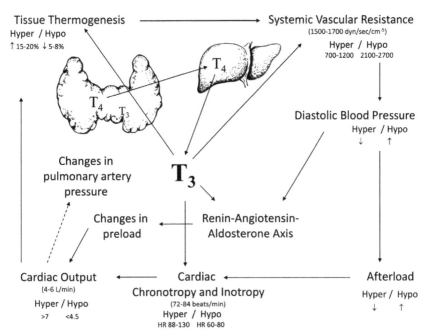

Fig. 1. Effects of thyroid hormone on cardiovascular hemodynamics. T_3 affects tissue thermogenesis, systemic vascular resistance, blood volume, cardiac contractility, heart rate, and cardiac output as indicated by the arrows.

Signs and symptoms of heart failure may rarely occur in patients with thyrotoxicosis, usually in the setting of prolonged and severe hyperthyroidism or after the onset of atrial fibrillation. Because cardiac output at rest is increased in hyperthyroidism, the increased output that normally accompanies exercise is blunted. Pulmonary and peripheral edema can occur as atrial filling pressure increases, causing a congested circulation.[13] True heart failure in hyperthyroidism, characterized by decreased cardiac contractility, abnormal diastolic compliance, and pulmonary congestion, is most likely the result of rate-related heart failure because sustained tachycardia impairs left ventricular contractility. This finding should be confirmed by noninvasive cardiac measures such as echocardiography followed by the usual course of diuretics. Beta-adrenergic blocking drugs are indicated to control the heart rate and should be used as part of the initial therapy within an intensive care unit setting if the degree of heart failure is significant enough to impair cardiovascular hemodynamics. Although propranolol is the most commonly used agent, intravenous use should be avoided and the short-acting agent esmolol can be used if concern about negative inotropy outweighs the goal of rate reduction. Attention to other potential medical comorbidities, such as infection, should also be addressed. Although β-adrenergic blockade can provide improvement in many, if not all of the cardiovascular findings, definitive treatment is necessary to normalize serum T_4, T_3, and TSH. Treatment of the hyperthyroidism in these circumstances is best accomplished with [131]Iodine or alternatively methimazole, and in almost all cases, this returns cardiac function to normal.[28] In the setting of multinodular goiter, pretreatment with methimazole may be beneficial, but this does not appear to be the case in patients with classical Grave disease.

Sinus tachycardia is the most common rhythm disturbance in young, otherwise healthy patients with hyperthyroidism. Atrial fibrillation caused by hyperthyroidism (especially subclinical hyperthyroidism) is observed more frequently with advancing age.[29] Although the prevalence of abnormal thyroid function testing, including a subnormal serum TSH level, is low in patients with new onset atrial fibrillation, the benefit associated with the ability to restore thyrotoxic patients to a euthyroid state and sinus rhythm justifies routine TSH testing in this setting.

Symptomatic treatment of thyrotoxic atrial fibrillation includes β-adrenergic blockade[13]; this can be accomplished rapidly whereas treatments including radioiodine and methimazole leading to restoration of the euthyroid state require a longer time. Digitalis has been used to control the ventricular response in hyperthyroidism-associated atrial fibrillation but usually requires higher doses of this medication. Anticoagulation in patients with hyperthyroidism and atrial fibrillation is controversial because the potential for systemic or cerebral embolization must be weighed against the risk of bleeding and complications. The major risk factor for systemic embolization in thyrotoxicosis seems to be age and not the presence of atrial fibrillation. Therefore, unless there is a separate cardiac indication for warfarin or other forms of anticoagulation, either no treatment or aspirin can be used especially in younger individuals, as needed.

Successful treatment of hyperthyroidism to restore normal serum levels of T_4 and T_3 leads to reversion to sinus rhythm in most younger patients within a few months. In the setting of atrial fibrillation of longer duration and in older patients, the rate of reversion to sinus rhythm is lower and electrical or pharmacologic cardioversion should therefore be attempted after the patient has been rendered euthyroid.

HYPOTHYROIDISM

In contrast to the dramatic clinical signs and symptoms of hyperthyroidism, the cardiovascular manifestations of hypothyroidism are more subtle.[22] Thus, although bradycardia, diastolic hypertension, a narrow pulse pressure, and a relatively quiet precordium are characteristic findings, the correct diagnosis is often established when a serum TSH level is obtained for one of a variety of clinical indications. These may include fatigue, myalgias, elevated cholesterol, or the feeling of puffiness (see **Table 2**). Hemodynamic changes of hypothyroidism are diametrically opposite to those of hyperthyroidism.[30] Treatment of hypothyroid patients with restoration of a euthyroid state resolves these changes in parallel with a resolution of clinical symptoms.

Hypothyroidism also produces increases in total and LDL cholesterol as well as apolipoprotein B through multiple mechanisms, but in general, in magnitude proportional to the severity of the hypothyroidism. Thus, the finding of a direct relationship between the level of TSH as a measure of hypothyroidism and serum total cholesterol and LDL cholesterol is not surprising.[31]

Serum creatine kinase is elevated by 50% to 10-fold in as many as 30% of patients with hypothyroidism. Isoform specificity indicates that more than 96% is the muscle form, consistent with a skeletal muscle origin of increased enzyme release.[32] Pericardial effusions can occur, consistent with the observation that patients with hypothyroidism have an increase in volume of distribution of albumin and a decrease in lymphatic clearance function. Occasionally, the pericardial effusions are quite large, and echocardiography demonstrates small to moderate effusions in as many as 30% of overtly hypothyroid patients. The presence of pericardial fluid in hypothyroid patients does not usually compromise cardiac output. Cardiac tamponade is exceedingly rare, and after initiation of T_4 therapy, the effusion resolves over a period of weeks to months.

The electrocardiogram in hypothyroidism is characterized by sinus bradycardia, low voltage, and prolongation of the action potential duration and the QT interval. The latter, in turn, predisposes patients to ventricular arrhythmias. There are case reports of patients with acquired torsades de pointes that completely resolved with thyroid hormone therapy.[1]

As a result of an increase in risk factors, including hypercholesterolemia, hypertension, and elevated levels of homocysteine, patients with hypothyroidism may have increased risk for atherosclerosis.[32,33] Studies have shown increases in abdominal aortic atherosclerosis in patients with even mild hypothyroidism.[34] Whether patients with hypothyroidism have an increase in coronary artery disease is an important clinical issue.

In otherwise healthy patients younger than 50 years, it is possible to initiate full replacement doses of L-thyroxine (100–150 μg/d or 1.5 μg/kg). In patients older than 50 years with known or suspected coronary artery disease, the issue is more complicated and treatment should be started with low dose (25–50 μg) T_4 and increased slowly, no more than every 6 to 12 weeks.

In all patients, thyroid hormone replacement should continue until serum TSH is normal and the patients are clinically euthyroid. The concept that these patients benefit from maintenance of "mild hypothyroidism" is not supported by the known effects of thyroid hormone on the heart and cardiovascular system. Thyroid hormone replacement should be accomplished with purified preparations of levothyroxine sodium. Preparations containing T_4 with T_3 (eg, thyroid extract) or the existing purified preparations of T_3 do not appear to offer benefit in the majority of patients. The short half-life of T_3 and the inability to maintain serum levels within normal range in patients so treated can add to cardiac risk.[35,36]

The leading causes of hypothyroidism include Hashimoto disease, previous radioiodine therapy for Graves' disease, and iodine deficiency (in parts of the world where that remains a public health problem). Thyroid gland failure in turn produces diagnostic elevations in serum TSH.[14] Thus, the finding of elevated TSH is sufficient to establish the diagnosis and form the basis for treatment. Thus, TSH screening can be advised for all adults and particularly patients demonstrating hypertension, hypercholesterolemia, hypertriglyceridemia, coronary or peripheral vascular disease, unexplained pericardial or pleural effusions, and a variety of musculoskeletal syndromes.[1,32]

SUBCLINICAL THYROID DISEASE

In contrast to overt symptomatic thyroid disease, subclinical thyroid disease implies the absence of classical hyper- or hypothyroidism-related symptoms in patients with thyroid dysfunction. The definition has been further refined to include the demonstration of an abnormal TSH level in the presence of normal serum levels of total T_4 and free T_4.[37,38] A recent study confirmed that heart failure risks are increased in subclinical thyroid disease, with both higher and lower TSH levels.[39] With the advent of widespread TSH screening, the prevalence of subclinical thyroid disease may exceed that of overt disease by three- to four-fold.

SUBCLINICAL HYPOTHYROIDISM

Subclinical hypothyroidism, defined by a TSH level above the upper range of the reference population (usually >5 mU/L), is seen in as many as 9% of unselected populations, and prevalence clearly increases with advancing age.[40] In contrast to younger patients, in whom there is a strong female predilection, this difference is lost in older populations. Studies of lipid metabolism, atherosclerosis, cardiac contractility, and SVR are altered in subclinical hypothyroidism. Cholesterol levels rise in parallel with increments in TSH elevations starting at 5 mU/L. In a large study of women in Rotterdam, it was noted that atherosclerosis and myocardial infarction were increased with odds ratios of 1.7 and 2.3, respectively, in women with subclinical hypothyroidism. Interestingly, the presence of antithyroid antibodies indicated heightened risk.[34] Restoration of serum TSH to normal after thyroid hormone replacement improved lipid levels, lowered SVR, and improved cardiac contractility.[38] In patients with subclinical hypothyroidism, isovolumic relaxation times are prolonged, whereas systolic contractile function is unchanged. Replacement with L-thyroxine sodium at a mean dose of 68 ug/d (range 50–100 ug/d) restored isovolumic relaxation times to normal, and compared with those in the same patients before therapy, SVR declined and systolic function was significantly improved.[38] A variety of studies have indicated that the changes in SVR may result from alterations in endothelium-dependent vasodilation.[41,42] Taking these findings together, it seems appropriate to recommend thyroid hormone replacement for all patients with subclinical hypothyroidism from a cardiovascular perspective.[13,43,44] The lack of untoward cardiac effects observed when serum TSH levels have been restored to normal indicates that the potential benefits far outweigh the risks of treatment.[1,33,37,44]

Because hypothyroidism is known to produce a variety of modifiable cardiovascular risk factors, it seemed quite attractive to suggest that thyroid hormone treatment of all degrees of hypothyroidism would result in a cardiovascular benefit.[1] However, a prospective randomized, controlled trial to test this hypothesis would be potentially unethical to undertake in overtly hypothyroid patients and require an inordinate number of subjects to study subclinical hypothyroidism. With the increasing magnitude of health care costs related to the diagnosis and treatment of heart failure, especially in the aging population, this has important clinical implications. Similarly, the increasing prevalence of subclinical hypothyroidism in the aging population makes the question of when and for whom thyroid hormone therapy should be recommended, an ongoing clinical challenge.

As a test of this hypothesis, the report from Razvi and colleagues[44] using The United Kingdom General Practitioner research database to identify individuals with subclinical hypothyroidism and serum TSH levels in a range of 5 to 10 mU/L was of special interest. In that "real-world" study, 53% of the subclinical hypothyroid patients were treated with levothyroxine and treatment led to a significant reduction in both ischemic heart disease events and cardiovascular mortality. In contrast, the older patients (older than 70 years) did not demonstrate the same therapeutic benefit.

DIAGNOSIS AND TREATMENT

Several studies have attempted to address the possibility of combination T_4, T_3 therapy for hypothyroidism with mixed results. The potential application in a small percentage of hypothyroid patients with impaired deiodinase (D2) function has been acknowledged. A properly conducted study with these selected patients may indicate a benefit of combination therapy where deiodinase activity has been compromised.[45,46] (This seems in contrast to your statement above that combination T_4 and T_3 should not be used; also contrary to ATA guidelines, but I think correctly reflects the discussions of last year's Spring ATA meeting.)

ALTERATIONS IN THYROID HORMONE METABOLISM THAT ACCOMPANY HEART DISEASE

The intimate relationship between thyroid hormones and the heart are evident in thyroid dysfunction with the observed effects on the heart and cardiovascular system. In addition, altered thyroid hormone metabolism occurs in the setting of heart disease, after cardiac surgery, or after acute myocardial infarction, resulting in low serum T_3 levels despite normal TSH and T_4 levels, which appears to result from a cytokine-induced blockade of iodothyronine deiodinase synthesis and activity, characteristic of chronic illness.[4,47,48] Interleukin 6 and tumor necrosis factor α levels are increased in the low T_3 syndrome.

In patients with heart failure, the decrease in serum T_3 concentration is proportional to the severity of the heart disease as assessed by the New York Heart Association (NYHA) functional classification.[49] T_3 is an important regulator of cardiac gene expression and, in fact, the list of T_3-mediated genes that are altered in overt hypothyroidism is almost identical to the changes in gene expression in heart failure.[50,51] These include the genes that encode the contractile proteins, α-MHC and β-MHC, the sodium calcium exchanger (NCX1), SERCA2, PLB, and the β-adrenergic receptor (β-AR). The net effect of these alterations in gene expression is to alter cardiac contractility, calcium cycling, and diastolic relaxation of the myocardium.

The low T_3 syndrome is a strong prognostic, independent predictor of death in patients with acute and chronic heart disease.[49,52,53] In human and animal studies, T_3 replacement in heart failure improved left ventricular function and restored myocyte gene expression to euthyroid levels, similar to that seen in the treatment of hypothyroidism (**Fig. 2**).[49,54–56]

In addition to heart disease, the presence of coronary artery disease, per se, in a population of chemically euthyroid subjects was associated with low levels of freeT$_3$. This low T_3 state was also associated with a poor prognosis.[57]

AMIODARONE-INDUCED THYROID DYSFUNCTION

Amiodarone is an iodine-rich antiarrhythmic agent effective for the treatment of ventricular and atrial tachyarrhythmias. Because of its iodine content and structural similarity to thyroid hormones, amiodarone can cause abnormalities in thyroid function tests. However, the risk is increased in patients with underlying autoimmune thyroid disease. Amiodarone may inhibit the 5′-monodeiodination of T_4 in the liver and pituitary thereby decreasing serum T_3 and increasing serum T_4 levels. Although serum TSH levels initially remain normal, there may be a progression to overt hypothyroidism. Overt hypothyroidism should be treated with levothyroxine.[58]

Less commonly, but more challenging to treat, amiodarone may cause hyperthyroidism (amiodarone-induced thyrotoxicosis; AIT). The new onset or recurrence of ventricular irritability, the return or worsening of heart failure symptoms, and changes in Coumadin dose requirements may be the first indication. Type 1 AIT is more

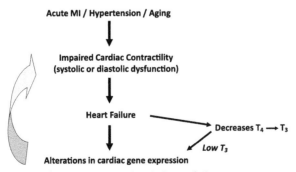

Fig. 2. Alterations in cardiac gene expression in heart failure.

common in iodine-deficient areas and is associated with preexisting thyroid abnormalities. Type II is a destructive thyroiditis. Treatment of AIT may include corticosteroids or antithyroid drugs, but the discontinuation of amiodarone will not remedy the thyroid dysfunction because the half-life of amiodarone is quite long.[59,60]

REFERENCES

1. Klein I, Danzi S. Thyroid disease and the heart. Circulation 2007;116:1725–35.
2. Koenig RJ. Regulation of type 1 iodothyronine deiodinase in health and disease. Thyroid 2005;15:835–40.
3. Bianco AC, Kim BW. Deiodinases: implications of the local control of thyroid hormone action. J Clin Invest 2006;116:2571–9.
4. Yu J, Koenig RJ. Induction of type 1 iodothyronine deiodinase to prevent the nonthyroidal illness syndrome in mice. Endocrinology 2006;147:3580–5.
5. Davis PJ, Davis FB. Nongenomic actions of thyroid hormone on the heart. Thyroid 2002;12:459–66.
6. Dillmann WH. Cellular action of thyroid hormone on the heart. Thyroid 2002;12: 447–52.
7. Danzi S, Klein I, Portman MA. Effect of triiodothyronine on gene transcription during cardiopulmonary bypass in infants with ventricular septal defect. Am J Cardiol 2005;95:787–9.
8. Danzi S, Ojamaa K, Klein I. Triiodothyronine mediated myosin heavy chain gene transcription in the heart. Am J Physiol Heart Circ Physiol 2003;284:H2255–63.
9. Gustavsson M, Verardi R, Mullen DG, et al. Allosteric regulation of SERCA by phosphorylation-mediated conformational shift of phospholamban. Proc Natl Acad Sci U S A 2013;110:17338–43.
10. Ojamaa K, Kenessey A, Klein I. Thyroid hormone regulation of phospholamban phosphorylation in the rat heart. Endocrinology 2000;141:2139–44.
11. Danzi S, Klein I. Cardiac specific effects of thyroid hormone analogues. Horm Metab Res 2011;43:1–6.
12. Ladenson PW, Kristensen JD, Ridgway EC, et al. Use of the thyroid hormone analogue eprotirome in statin-treated dyslipidemia. N Engl J Med 2010;362:906–16.
13. Klein I, Ojamaa K. Thyroid hormone and the cardiovascular system. N Engl J Med 2001;344:501–9.
14. Demers LM, Spencer CA. Laboratory medicine practice guidelines: laboratory support for the diagnosis and monitoring of thyroid disease. Thyroid 2003;13:3–126.
15. Roef GL, Taes YE, Kaufman JM, et al. Thyroid hormone levels within the reference range are associated with heart rate, cardiac structure, and function in middle-aged men and women. Thyroid 2013;23:947–54.
16. Selvaraj S, Klein I, Danzi S, et al. Association of Serum Triiodothyronine with B-type natriuretic peptide and severe left ventricular diastolic dysfunction in heart failure with preserved ejection fraction. Am J Cardiol 2012;110:234–9.
17. Visser WE, Friesema EC, Visser TJ. Minireview: thyroid hormone transporters: the knowns and the unknowns. Mol Endocrinol 2011;25:1–14.
18. Friesema EC, Jansen J, Jachtenberg JW, et al. Effective cellular uptake and efflux of thyroid hormone by human monocarboxylate transporter 10. Mol Endocrinol 2008;22:1357–69.
19. Danzi S, Klein I. Thyroid hormone and the cardiovascular system. Med Clin North Am 2012;96:257–68.
20. Pearce EN, Yang Q, Benjamin EJ, et al. Thyroid function and left ventricular structure and function in the Framingham Heart Study. Thyroid 2010;20:367–73.

21. Dahl P, Danzi S, Klein I. Thyrotoxic cardiac disease. Curr Heart Fail Rep 2008;5: 170–6.

22. Klein I. Endocrine disorders and cardiovascular disease. In: Bonow RO, Mann DL, Zipes DP, et al, editors. Braunwald's heart disease, chapter 86. 9th edition. St. Louis (MO): WB Saunders and Company; 2011. p. 1829–43.

23. Marvisi M, Brianti M, Marani G, et al. Hyperthyroidism and pulmonary hypertension. Respir Med 2002;96:215–20.

24. Ismail HM. Reversible pulmonary hypertension and isolated right-sided heart failure associated with hyperthyroidism. J Gen Intern Med 2007;22:148–50.

25. Danzi S, Klein I. Thyroid hormone and blood pressure regulation. Curr Hypertens Rep 2003;5:513–20.

26. Mintz G, Pizzarello R, Klein I. Enhanced left ventricular diastolic function in hyperthyroidism: noninvasive assessment and response to treatment. J Clin Endocrinol Metab 1991;73:146–50.

27. Klein I, Danzi S. The cardiovascular system in thyrotoxicosis. In: Braverman L, Utiger R, editors. Werner & Ingbar's the thyroid: a fundamental and clinical text, chapter 31. 10th edition. Philadelphia: Lippincott Williams & Wilkins; 2012. p. 559–68.

28. Bahn RS, Burch HB, Cooper DS, et al. Hyperthyroidism and other causes of thyrotoxicosis: management guidelines of the American Thyroid Association and American Association of Clinical Endocrinologists. Endocr Pract 2011;17:456–520.

29. Sawin CT, Geller A, Wolf PA, et al. Low serum thyrotropin levels as a risk factor for atrial fibrillation in older persons. N Engl J Med 1994;33:1249–52.

30. Klein I, Danzi S. The cardiovascular system in hypothyroidism. In: Braverman L, Utiger R, editors. Werner & Ingbar's the thyroid: a fundamental and clinical text. 10th edition. Philadelphia: Lippincott Williams & Wilkins; 2012. p. 774–80 Chapter 53.

31. Parle JV, Maisonneuve P, Sheppard MC, et al. Prediction of all-cause and cardiovascular mortality in elderly people from one low serum thyrotropin result: a 10-year cohort study. Lancet 2001;358:861.

32. Rush J, Danzi S, Klein I. Role of thyroid disease in the development of statin-induced myopathy. Endocrinologist 2006;16:279.

33. Cappola AR, Ladenson PW. Hypothyroidism and atherosclerosis. J Clin Endocrinol Metab 2003;88:2438.

34. Hak AE, Pols HA, Visser TJ, et al. Subclinical hypothyroidism is an independent risk factor for atherosclerosis and myocardial infarction in elderly women: the Rotterdam Study. Ann Intern Med 2000;132:270.

35. Kim SD, Kim SH, Park KS, et al. Regression of the increased common carotid artery-intima media thickness in subclinical hypothyroidism after thyroid hormone replacement. Endocr J 2009;56:753.

36. Garber JR, Cobin RH, Gharib H, et al. Clinical practice guidelines for hypothyroidism in adults; cosponsored by the American Association of Clinical Endocrinologists and the American Thyroid Association. Thyroid 2012;22:1200–35.

37. Rodondi N, den Elzen WP, Bauer DC, et al. Subclinical hypothyroidism and the risk of coronary heart disease and mortality. JAMA 2010;304:1365.

38. Biondi B, Cooper DS. The clinical significance of subclinical thyroid dysfunction. Endocr Rev 2008;29:76.

39. Gencer B, Collet TH, Virgini V, et al. Subclinical thyroid dysfunction and the risk of heart failure events: an individual participant data analysis from 6 prospective cohorts. Circulation 2012;126:1040–9.

40. Cappola AR, Fried LP, Arnold AM, et al. Thyroid status, cardiovascular risk, and mortality in older adults. JAMA 2006;295:1033.

41. Biondi B, Klein I. Hypothyroidism as a risk factor for hypothyroidism. Endocrine 2004;24:1–13.
42. Taddei S, Caraccio N, Virdis A, et al. Impaired endothelium-dependent vasodilatation in subclinical hypothyroidism: beneficial effect of levothyroxine therapy. J Clin Endocrinol Metab 2003;88:3731.
43. Iervasi G, Molinaro S, Landi P, et al. Association between increased mortality and mild thyroid dysfunction in cardiac patients. Arch Intern Med 2007;167:1526–32.
44. Razvi S, Weaver JU, Butler TJ, et al. Levothyroxine treatment of subclinical hypothyroidism, fatal and nonfatal cardiovascular events, and mortality. Arch Intern Med 2012;172:811–7.
45. Wartofsky L. Combination L-T3 and L-T4 therapy for hypothyroidism. Curr Opin Endocrinol Diabetes Obes 2013;20:460–6.
46. Klein I, Danzi S. Thyroid hormone treatment to mend a broken heart. J Clin Endocrinol Metab 2008;93:1172–4.
47. Boelen A, Maas MA, Lowik CW, et al. Induced illness in interleukin-6 (IL-6) knock-out mice: a causal role of IL-6 in the development of the low 3,5,3'-triiodothyronine syndrome. Endocrinology 1996;137:5250–4.
48. Lubrano V, Pingitore A, Carpi A, et al. Relationship between triiodothyronine and proinflammatory cytokines in chronic heart failure. Biomed Pharmacother 2010;64:165–9.
49. Iervasi G, Pingitore A, Landi P, et al. Low-T3 syndrome: a strong prognostic predictor of death in patients with heart disease. Circulation 2003;107:708–13.
50. Danzi S, Klein I. Changes in thyroid hormone metabolism and gene expression in the failing heart: therapeutic implications. In: Iervasi G, Pingitore A, editors. Thyroid and heart failure, from pathophysiology to clinics. Italy: Springer-Verlag; 2009. p. 97–107 Chapter 10.
51. Danzi S, Klein I. Alterations in thyroid hormones which accompany cardiovascular disease. Clinical Thyroidology 2009;21:3–5.
52. Zhang B, Peng W, Wang C, et al. A low fT3 level as a prognostic marker in patients with acute myocardial infarctions. Intern Med 2012;51:3009–15.
53. Nicolini G, Pitto L, Kusmic C, et al. New insights into mechanisms of cardioprotection mediated by thyroid hormones. J Thyroid Res 2013;2013:264387.
54. Henderson K, Danzi S, Paul JT, et al. Physiological replacement of T_3 improves left ventricular function in an animal model of myocardial infarction-induced congestive heart failure. Circ Heart Fail 2009;2:243–52.
55. Pingitore A, Galli E, Barison A, et al. Acute effects of triiodothyronine (T3) replacement therapy in patients with chronic heart failure and low-T3 syndrome: a randomized, placebo-controlled study. J Clin Endocrinol Metab 2008;93:1351–8.
56. DeGroot LJ. Non-thyroidal illness syndrome is a manifestation of hypothalamic-pituitary dysfunction, and in view of current evidence, should be treated with appropriate replacement therapies. Crit Care Clin 2006;22:57–86.
57. Coceani M, Iervasi G, Pingitore A, et al. Thyroid hormone and coronary artery disease: from clinical correlations to prognostic implications. Clin Cardiol 2009;32:380–5.
58. Cohen-Lehman J, Dahl P, Danzi S, et al. Effects of amiodarone on thyroid function. Nat Rev Endocrinol 2010;6:34–41.
59. Bogazzi F, Bartalena L, Cosci C, et al. Treatment of type II amiodarone-induced thyrotoxicosis by either iopanoic acid or glucocorticoids: a prospective, randomized study. J Clin Endocrinol Metab 1999;88:2003.
60. Danzi S, Klein I. Amiodarone-induced thyroid dysfunction. J Intensive Care Med 2013. [Epub ahead of print].

Thyroid Disease and Cognition

Mary H. Samuels, MD

KEYWORDS

- Hypothyroidism • Thyrotoxicosis • Subclinical hypothyroidism
- Subclinical thyrotoxicosis • Mood • Cognition

KEY POINTS

- Alterations in mood and cognitive function are common in overt hypothyroidism and usually improve with therapy. These alterations can include anxiety, depression, and widespread cognitive decrements, particularly in memory functions.
- Alterations in mood and cognitive function are common in overt thyrotoxicosis and usually improve with therapy. These alterations can include anxiety and depression, and cognitive decrements in attention, concentration, and executive function.
- Subtle alterations in mood and cognitive function may exist in subclinical hypothyroidism and subclinical thyrotoxicosis, but major decrements are not seen. Cognitive deficits are primarily in working memory and executive function.

INTRODUCTION

The occurrence of psychological and cognitive changes in adults with altered thyroid function has been known for many years. In the late nineteenth century, reports first described hypothyroid and thyrotoxic patients with a range of mental disturbances.[1,2] In modern times, earlier diagnosis of thyroid disorders has reduced the incidence of severe clinical disease, but patients still occasionally present with profound mental and behavioral changes.

Advances in neuroscience have led to validated neurocognitive tests that measure specific cognitive domains, mapped to critical brain regions. These advances allow for sensitive and targeted investigations of cognitive function, which reveal the presence of subtle affective and cognitive disturbances in hypothyroidism and thyrotoxicosis. The purpose of this review is to synthesize current data on central nervous system dysfunction in altered thyroid states and to provide clinical recommendations based on these data. Only adult-onset disease will be considered, as effects of congenital and childhood onset thyroid dysfunction are beyond the scope of this review.

There are 4 categories of thyroid dysfunction considered here, based on laboratory testing of free thyroxine (fT4), triiodothyronine (T3), and thyroid stimulating hormone

The author has nothing to disclose.
Division of Endocrinology, Diabetes, and Clinical Nutrition, Oregon Health & Science University, 3181 Southwest Sam Jackson Park Road, Portland, OR 97239, USA
E-mail address: samuelsm@ohsu.edu

(TSH) levels. Overt hypothyroidism is defined as a low-serum fT4 and elevated TSH level, whereas overt thyrotoxicosis is defined as a high-serum fT4 and/or T3 and suppressed TSH level. More subtle degrees of altered thyroid status include subclinical hypothyroidism (elevated TSH, normal fT4) and subclinical thyrotoxicosis (suppressed TSH, normal fT4 and T3). Although these entities are discussed separately, in reality they represent a continuum of thyroid function and dysfunction.

It is important to include affective disorders in a discussion of cognitive effects of altered thyroid status because thyroid dysfunction can directly alter mood, and mood decrements, in turn, can impair cognition. Therefore, effects of thyroid dysfunction on mood will also be considered in each section.

Before discussing specific types of thyroid dysfunction, it is helpful to emphasize issues that pertain to the entire field. The literature can be divided into larger cross-sectional or longitudinal studies and smaller interventional studies. Many older studies of either type were limited by small sample sizes, heterogeneous subject groups, or cognitive tests of limited sensitivity. For these reasons, much of the literature is inconclusive or inconsistent. More recent influential studies have been larger and/or have used more modern cognitive tests. This review briefly summarizes the older literature and emphasizes in more detail recent studies that have advanced the field. **Table 1** provides a broad summary of mood and cognitive alterations in the 4 types of thyroid dysfunction considered herein.

Table 1
Summary of effects of altered thyroid status on mood and cognitive function

Thyroid Condition	Effects on Mood	Effects on Cognitive Function
Overt hypothyroidism	Likely increased rates of anxiety, depression Largely reversible with L-T4 treatment Rarely, "myxedema madness"	Widespread mild to moderate decrements, especially in memory Largely reversible with L-T4 treatment
Subclinical hypothyroidism	Mild symptoms of depression or anxiety may be present, not reliably improved with L-T4 treatment Some symptoms may be related to self-knowledge of thyroid disease Moderate to severe mood alterations not typical	Mild defects in memory, executive function Reverse with L-T4 treatment Major cognitive deficits not seen
Overt thyrotoxicosis	Symptoms of irritability, agitation are common May have increased rates of depression or anxiety Affective symptoms usually improve with β-blockers or definitive therapy Rarely, "thyroid storm"	May have decrements in attention/concentration and executive function Largely reversible with therapy
Subclinical thyrotoxicosis	No consistent increased rates of anxiety or depression Some symptoms may be related to self-knowledge of thyroid disease	Inconsistent associations with mild cognitive decrements Major cognitive decrements not seen May be associated with increased risk for development of dementia

Finally, there are several related topics that have clinical relevance. They include effects of variation in thyroid hormone levels within the normal range on central nervous system function, the use of combined L-T4/L-T3 therapy to improve mood and cognition in hypothyroid patients, associations between altered thyroid function and the development of dementia, and the entity of Hashimoto encephalopathy. These topics are covered separately at the end of this review.

MECHANISMS OF PSYCHIATRIC AND COGNITIVE EFFECTS OF HYPOTHYROIDISM

A large body of evidence from animal studies supports clinical observations of thyroid hormones' importance to central nervous system function. Thyroid hormone is critical for structural and functional development of the brain, including areas that control affective and cognitive processes.[3,4] Thyroid hormone continues to be critical for normal function in the mature brain. To this end, the transport of thyroid hormone into the brain, region-specific regulation of T4 to T3 conversion, and regional T3 receptor levels are tightly regulated.[5–7]

Animal models show that abnormal thyroid function alters brain morphology and function in areas that subserve cognition. Adult-onset hypothyroidism in rats reduces the numbers of granule cells of the dentate gyrus and pyramidal cells of the hippocampal CA1 region, decreases the apical dendritic spine density of hippocampal CA1 pyramidal neurons, reduces hippocampal synaptic plasticity, and impairs learning.[8] Thyroid dysfunction also alters the expression of neurotransmitter, neuromodulator, and growth factor systems in the adult rat brain, indirectly affecting brain function, including areas that subserve affective and cognitive functions.[4,9] For example, thyroid hormone deficiency alters the expression of hippocampal enzymes that regulate catecholamine, serotonin, and GABA systems.[4,10,11] These findings provide a mechanistic framework for the clinical studies reviewed in the following sections.

PSYCHIATRIC AND COGNITIVE EFFECTS OF OVERT HYPOTHYROIDISM
Mood Effects

Subjective psychological complaints in adults with overt hypothyroidism are common. Slowing of thought and speech, decreased attentiveness, apathy, and poor concentration often occur, and the diagnosis may be confused with depression. Other patients may report symptoms consistent with anxiety. Rarely, severely hypothyroid patients present with agitation, leading to frank psychosis ("myxedema madness").[12]

Hypothyroid patients without such overt psychiatric symptoms may have more subtle alterations in mood. In some studies, objective testing reveals increased scores on anxiety or depression scales, which reverse with levothyroxine (L-T4) therapy.[13–16] In contrast, one large, population-based study failed to find an association between hypothyroidism and anxiety or depression.[17] However, the scales used in this study were relatively insensitive to subtle effects, and individuals likely vary in their susceptibility to central nervous system effects of hypothyroidism.

Cognitive Effects

Adult-onset overt hypothyroidism can affect a wide range of cognitive domains.[13,14,16,18] Cross-sectional studies report decrements in general intelligence, as well as attention/concentration, memory, perceptual function, language, psychomotor function, and executive function. Memory is the most consistently affected domain.[16,19–23] Recent studies using sensitive, specific tests documented a specific deficit in verbal memory.[16,19] L-T4 treatment is usually effective in treating these cognitive decrements, although there may not be complete reversal.[14,22–25]

Functional imaging studies provide objective evidence that brain function is altered in hypothyroid patients, with decreased cerebral blood flow and function globally and in regions that mediate attention, visuospatial processing, working memory, and motor speed.[26–29] In a recent report using functional magnetic resonance imaging (fMRI), deficits in working memory in hypothyroid patients were no longer present after 6 months of therapy with L-T4.[29]

Because overt hypothyroidism may present with mood or cognitive decrements, serum TSH measurement should be performed in patients with syndromes of affective illness or impaired cognitive function. It may be difficult to distinguish thyroid-related neurocognitive decrements from other disease processes in hypothyroid patients. Observation during L-T4 therapy may clarify these issues, because deficits due to hypothyroidism are largely reversible.

PSYCHIATRIC AND COGNITIVE EFFECTS OF SUBCLINICAL HYPOTHYROIDISM
Mood Effects

Symptoms of depression or anxiety are reported to be more common in subclinical hypothyroid patients, compared with the general population (reviewed in Refs.[13,30,31]). However, many of these studies have limitations, and this is not a universal finding.[17,30–36] In fact, the largest cross-sectional studies of mood in subclinical hypothyroidism found no differences in depression or anxiety between euthyroid and subclinical hypothyroid subjects.[17,32–34,37] There are several strengths to these latter studies, including large sample sizes, broad age ranges that included large numbers of older subjects, and absence of bias (population-based).

There are 3 randomized, placebo-controlled, blinded studies of L-T4 therapy in subjects with subclinical hypothyroidism, which showed no improvement in depression or psychological distress scores.[38–40] In one study, therapy actually worsened anxiety.[39]

These studies suggest that mood alterations in subclinical hypothyroidism may be more apparent when subjects are aware of their thyroid status, suggesting that at least some symptoms are not related to thyroid hormone levels, but rather the self-knowledge of a thyroid disease process. Mild affective symptoms may be more prevalent in subclinical hypothyroidism, but if so, they are not reliably improved with L-T4 treatment. Moderate to severe affective symptoms are unlikely to be due to subclinical hypothyroidism and need to be evaluated and treated as separate disorders.

Cognitive Effects

Unlike overt hypothyroidism, subclinical hypothyroidism is not associated with widespread or severe cognitive dysfunction (reviewed in Refs.[30,31]) and has been shown in large and rigorous cross-sectional and longitudinal population-based (ie, unbiased) studies.[32,33,41] A widely quoted example is the cross-sectional study of mood and cognition in almost 6000 older subjects referenced above.[32] All subjects underwent an extensive battery of screening tests for cognitive function, including attention and orientation, learning, memory, perception, and language skills. No differences were found in any of these tests between the subjects with subclinical hypothyroidism and euthyroid subjects.

These large studies indicate that subjects with subclinical hypothyroidism do not have major cognitive impairments. However, the administered tests were often designed to screen large numbers of subjects and might not detect subtle deficits. Indeed, smaller-scale studies using labor-intensive, sensitive measures report that specific cognitive domains may be mildly impaired in subclinical hypothyroidism, although not all studies are consistent.[16,23,24,30,35,36,42–45] The most commonly affected cognitive domains are memory and executive function.

Functional neuroimaging has provided a neuroanatomical basis for this defect in working memory and executive function. In a recent study,[46] subjects with subclinical hypothyroidism (mean TSH = 14.7 mU/L) were found to have impaired working memory and abnormal fMRI results in frontal brain areas responsible for executive function. A subset of the subjects were treated with L-T4 for 6 months (mean TSH = 1.35 mU/L), at which point working memory and fMRI results normalized. Further objective evidence is a recent report using positron emission tomography.[26,47,48] Untreated subclinical hypothyroid subjects had lower regional glucose metabolism than controls in specific brain areas important for cognition (mean TSH = 16.9 mU/L). Metabolic activity was restored after 3 months of L-T4 treatment (mean TSH = 2.8 mU/L). Likely explanations for the positive results in these experimental studies include higher mean TSH levels and more sensitive measures of working memory.

Given the subtlety of cognitive impairments documented in these studies, it is not surprising that L-T4 treatment often does not lead to marked clinical improvement. Several studies have reported that treatment leads to minor improvements, usually in memory, as in the fMRI study described above.[16,35,44–46] Lending some clarity to this topic, there are 2 rigorous, double-blind, placebo-controlled interventional studies reported in the past 7 years.[38,40] In both studies, subjects with subclinical hypothyroidism underwent an extensive battery of cognitive testing and then were randomized to placebo or L-T4 for 12 months. Repeat cognitive testing showed no effect of L-T4 compared with placebo. There were a few limitations to these studies, including relatively mild degrees of subclinical hypothyroidism in both studies (up to 8.5 or 10 mU/L), and a high rate of normalization of TSH levels in the placebo group in one study.[40] However, these 2 studies strongly argue against major effects of subclinical hypothyroidism on cognitive function.

In conclusion, global cognitive dysfunction does not occur in subclinical hypothyroidism, and major decrements in specific cognitive domains are unlikely. However, subtle deficits exist in memory and executive function. Sensitive and specific tests are required to delineate these abnormalities, and their clinical significance is likely to be minor or additive to other cognitive issues. Therefore, patients with subclinical hypothyroidism and significant cognitive dysfunction have independent diagnoses that should be evaluated and treated separately.

PSYCHIATRIC AND COGNITIVE EFFECTS OF OVERT THYROTOXICOSIS
Mood Effects

Clinical observations indicate that thyrotoxic patients often appear irritable, jittery, or agitated. Thoughts and words can be disjointed. Although this may mimic manic behavior, fully developed mania is rare. When true mania or hypomania occurs,[49] the patients typically have a previous diagnosis or strong family history of bipolar disorder. With the onset of thyrotoxic storm (a rare manifestation of severe thyrotoxicosis), delirium, restlessness, and agitation can appear.[50]

In contrast with the typical presentation of a thyrotoxic patient with irritability and anxiety, some patients present with "apathetic thyrotoxicosis."[51] This presentation is more common in elderly patients, although it has been described in young adults. Apathetic thyrotoxicosis mimics a depressive disorder,[49,51] characterized by apathy, lethargy, weight loss, depressed mood, and pseudodementia. The diagnosis can be overlooked, because many of the common physical manifestations of thyrotoxicosis are lacking.

Most studies indicate that thyrotoxic subjects have high rates of depression and anxiety,[18,49,52–54] with rates of either condition greater than 60%[53,54] and often with emotional lability. In contrast, a Norwegian study in an unselected population of more than 30,000 individuals reported no association between thyrotoxicosis and self-reported levels of depression and anxiety,[17] although the psychiatric measure used was relatively insensitive for subtle symptoms.

In terms of treatment, administration of a β-blocker can provide rapid relief from symptoms of anxiety and irritability associated with thyrotoxicosis. Definitive treatment usually leads to significant improvement in affective symptoms,[52] although they may not completely resolve.

Cognitive Effects

Some cross-sectional studies of overt thyrotoxicosis have shown specific decrements in attention/concentration and executive function compared with euthyroid subjects, although other studies have failed to find cognitive deficits.[52,54–56] Most treatment studies report improvement in cognitive function,[52,54,57] although some studies have shown residual attention deficits after euthyroidism was achieved.[58,59] Functional imaging studies have provided objective measures of cerebral dysfunction in thyrotoxicosis. Several studies have shown that Graves' disease subjects have abnormal cerebral metabolism by magnetic resonance spectroscopy in the parieto-occipital, midoccipital, and midfrontal regions, which map to executive function and working memory domains.[60,61] Schreckenberger and colleagues[62] reported that positive emission tomography scanning in patients with Graves' disease revealed abnormal glucose metabolism in the right hemispheric limbic system, a primary site for long-term memory. In contrast, the study by Zhu and colleagues[46] described earlier found no difference in a sensitive and specific test of working memory or changes in fMRI in subjects with thyrotoxicosis.

In aggregate, these studies suggest that impaired mood (increased depressive and anxiety symptoms) may occur in thyrotoxic subjects. There are also intriguing suggestions that cerebral metabolism in specific brain regions is abnormal, in regions corresponding to memory and executive functions. However, the clinical data on functional correlates of these observations on cognition are less clear, and major cognitive deficits are not expected in overt thyrotoxicosis outside of attention and concentration, unless there is coexistent psychiatric or cognitive morbidity.

PSYCHIATRIC AND COGNITIVE EFFECTS OF SUBCLINICAL THYROTOXICOSIS
Mood Effects

Some studies suggest that subjects with subclinical thyrotoxicosis have increased rates of depression, anxiety, and irritability.[15,63,64] These findings are qualitatively similar but quantitatively less severe than those in overt thyrotoxicosis. However, recent large cross-sectional studies have not confirmed these findings in unselected populations.[17,32] Interestingly, the large Netherlands study did show decrements in subclinical thyrotoxic subjects who knew they had thyroid disease.[65] As in subclinical hypothyroidism, this suggests that subjects' self-awareness of a thyroid diagnosis may contribute to higher reporting rates of affective symptoms.

Cognitive Effects

Several observational studies have examined the association between subclinical thyrotoxicosis and cognitive measures. The studies were heterogeneous in terms of sample sizes, exclusion criteria, age range, degree of TSH suppression, and cognitive measurements. Results were also heterogeneous, with some reporting lower cognitive function in subclinical thyrotoxicosis or when T3 or T4 levels were higher.[64,66–68] On the other hand, other studies did not show an association between subclinical thyrotoxicosis and cognitive measures,[32,37,69] including the 2 largest rigorously conducted studies.[32,37] Longitudinal studies have more consistently reported associations between subclinical thyrotoxicosis and the development of dementia in older subjects, although this is not a universal finding (see later discussion) (reviewed in Ref.[66]).

In terms of interventional studies, 2 studies recruited subjects with L-T4-treated hypothyroidism and increased L-T4 doses in a randomized, blinded fashion, to induce subclinical thyrotoxicosis. Walsh and colleagues[70] found no deficits in a battery of cognitive tests that included attention, motor function, working memory, cognitive efficiency, and executive function. Samuels[71] also found no effects on mood or working or long-term memory, but did report improvements in motor learning.

From a clinical standpoint, based on these studies, major abnormalities in mood or cognitive function in patients with subclinical thyrotoxicosis are not expected and should be evaluated and treated as separate disorders.

EFFECT OF THYROID FUNCTION VARIATIONS WITHIN THE NORMAL RANGE ON MOOD AND COGNITION

In euthyroid subjects without thyroid disease, depression or anxiety has been linked to variations in TSH or fT4 levels within the normal range.[65,69,72,73] However, the correlations were in different directions depending on the report, and recent large and well-conducted studies found no correlations between TSH levels and depression or anxiety.[17,32,33] Similarly, performance on tests of cognitive function has been inconsistently associated with variations in TSH, fT4, or fT3 levels within the normal range.[32,33,41,66–69,74–78] When such effects are reported, the magnitude is generally small. In one pertinent treatment study, symptomatic euthyroid subjects with no history of thyroid disease were given L-T4 in a blinded, placebo-controlled fashion, with no improvement in psychological symptoms.[79]

Many hypothyroid patients receiving L-T4 therapy continue to complain of impaired mood and cognitive function, despite normal TSH levels. This finding has been inconsistently supported with validated testing in the literature.[65,80–84] In the largest study of more than 30,000 subjects, there was no overall correlation between thyroid function and self-reported depression or anxiety, but the subgroup with known thyroid disease had an increased risk of both affective disorders.[65] There is only one study whereby L-T4 doses were varied within the normal range in hypothyroid subjects receiving L-T4, with no changes in cognitive measures.[70] These subjects were blinded to their L-T4 doses, highlighting biases that may exist when subjects are aware that they have a diagnosis of thyroid disease, which may lead to overreporting symptoms in cross-sectional studies.

Another possible explanation for variations in patients' symptoms may be polymorphisms in the deiodinase 2 or thyroid hormone transporter genes.[85,86] L-T4-treated hypothyroid patients with one specific polymorphism in the deiodinase 2 gene had decrements in mood and cognition compared with similar patients without these polymorphisms, possibly related to expected lower tissue T3 levels (although these have not been directly measured).[85] These findings require further exploration in controlled studies. In the meantime, persistent affective or cognitive deficits in adequately treated hypothyroid patients likely represent independent diagnoses that require separate evaluation and therapy.

Finally, the presence or titer of antithyroid antibodies in euthyroid subjects has been linked to alterations in mood or cognition, although the postulated mechanism is unclear.[87–90] On the other hand, in the largest study to date of more than 30,000 subjects, no association between antithyroid antibodies and depression or anxiety was found,[91] although the results of this study are limited by the fact that relatively insensitive measures of mood were used.

IMPACT OF T4/T3 COMBINATION THERAPY ON MOOD AND COGNITION IN HYPOTHYROIDISM

Although T4 is the main product of the thyroid gland, T3 is the active thyroid hormone at the cellular level. Most T3 is produced via deiodination of circulating T4 in peripheral tissues, but about 20% of T3 is produced directly by the thyroid gland. As mentioned above, many L-T4-treated hypothyroid subjects continue to have mood and cognitive complaints despite normalization of TSH levels. Therefore, the question has been raised as to whether these patients might benefit from combined L-T3 and L-T4 therapy, rather than L-T4 monotherapy. This question has been addressed in several placebo-controlled, blinded interventional studies (reviewed in Ref.[92]). Most failed to find significant improvements in mood or cognitive function with combined therapy. However, trials have been limited by the fact that there is no available sustained release L-T3 preparation that mimics endogenous serum levels.

In addition to these trials of L-T4/L-T3 combination therapy, one recent study compared desiccated thyroid extract (which contains a relatively high L-T3/L-T4 ratio) to L-T4 monotherapy in hypothyroid patients.[93] Subjects were treated with either desiccated thyroid extract or L-T4 for 6 weeks in a randomized, blinded, crossover fashion. There were no differences in validated measures of symptoms, quality of life, depression, or memory. These results suggest that desiccated thyroid extract is not superior to L-T4 for central nervous system function.

Finally, L-T4 patients with the same polymorphism in the deiodinase 2 gene mentioned above have a better response to combined L-T4/L-T3 therapy compared with L-T4 alone (reviewed in Ref.[92]). These findings raise the possibility that patients with this (or other) polymorphisms could have relatively lower tissue T3 levels and perhaps derive clinical benefit from T3 therapy. Such a conjecture is theoretical, however, and requires confirmation before clinical application.

POSSIBLE ASSOCIATIONS BETWEEN ALTERED THYROID FUNCTION AND THE DEVELOPMENT OF DEMENTIA

Given the known effects of thyroid hormone on brain function, it is reasonable to ask whether altered thyroid status is a risk factor for the development of dementia (reviewed in Ref.[66]). Results from cross-sectional studies have been divergent, with some reports that high or low TSH levels, or variations in TSH levels within the normal range, were correlated with the presence of dementia.[66] These studies were limited by confounding factors present in cross-sectional analyses of ill patients, and therefore, cannot be considered conclusive.

Prospective community-based studies of older subjects have provided more useful data regarding this issue. Most report increased risks of dementia in subjects with subclinical thyrotoxicosis or higher fT4 levels within the normal range.[66,94] Additional studies report associations between higher fT4 levels and increased rates of hippocampal and amygdala atrophy on MRI and more extensive neocortical neuritic plaques and neurofibrillary tangles at autopsy.[66,95] Finally, long-term follow-up of a subset of the Framingham cohort reported that women with the lowest and highest tertiles of TSH had an increased risk of developing dementia (reviewed in Ref.[66]). No relationship was found in men. At this time, it is not yet determined whether or how altered thyroid function predisposes to the development of dementia, although these studies provide intriguing evidence that higher thyroid function may be a risk factor.

HASHIMOTO ENCEPHALOPATHY

Patients with autoimmune thyroiditis can rarely manifest a subacute onset of confusion leading to delirium or dementia. Patients are euthyroid, but have measurable antithyroid antibodies. This clinical entity has been called "Hashimoto encephalitis" or "steroid-responsive encephalopathy with autoimmune thyroiditis (SREAT)" (reviewed in Ref.[96]). The clinical presentation is variable, but often includes memory loss, seizures, tremor, myoclonus, and ataxia. The MRI is normal or nonspecific, whereas the electroencephalogram shows nonspecific slowing and epileptiform discharges. Most patients have elevated cerebrospinal fluid protein levels, but there are no diagnostic laboratory tests. SREAT is a diagnosis of exclusion once vasculitic, paraneoplastic, infectious, and psychiatric causes have been ruled out. High-dose glucocorticoids are the mainstay of therapy, with most patients showing response within weeks, some within a few doses.

Although by definition SREAT includes positive antithyroid antibodies, there is no relationship between antibody titer and severity of the disease. There is also no evidence that the antibodies react with brain tissue or affect nerve function. These patients may have specific central nervous system tissue autoantigens not present in Hashimoto patients without encephalopathy or in patients with other thyroid diseases.[97] At present, the entity is best considered a nonspecific autoimmune encephalopathy, and the presence of antithyroid antibodies is best considered an epiphenomenon.

SUMMARY

Given the variety of findings in the literature summarized above, what conclusions can be drawn regarding mood and cognition in thyroid dysfunction (see **Table 1**)? First, overt hypothyroidism is often associated with clinically significant decrements in mood and cognitive function (especially memory). Second, mood alterations are also common in overt thyrotoxicosis, particularly depression and anxiety, and mild decrements in attention, concentration, and executive function may be seen. Third, major affective and cognitive dysfunction, affecting numerous domains, is not typical of subclinical thyroid disease, either subclinical hypothyroidism or subclinical thyrotoxicosis. However, subtle deficits in specific cognitive domains (primarily working memory and executive function) likely exist in subclinical thyroid disease. The degree of mood or cognitive dysfunction is probably related to the degree of thyroid dysfunction, and subclinical thyroid disease is unlikely to cause major clinical problems in most patients.

Therapy for overt hypothyroidism and thyrotoxicosis is indicated, regardless of the presence of mood or cognitive complaints, and these symptoms will improve with therapy. Therapy for subclinical thyroid dysfunction is a more complicated decision. Consideration should be given to treat patients with subclinical thyroid disease and complaints of mood or cognitive alterations. However, because deficits are usually mild, patients with mild thyroid disease and significant distress related to mood or cognition most likely have independent diagnoses that should be evaluated and treated separately.

REFERENCES

1. Gull WW. On a cretinoid state supervening in adult life in women. Trans Clin Soc Lond 1873;7:180.
2. Graves RJ. Newly observed affection of the thyroid gland in females. Lond Med Surg J 1835;7:516.
3. Williams GR. Neurodevelopmental and neurophysiological actions of thyroid hormone. J Neuroendocrinol 2008;20:784–94.
4. Koromilas C, Liapi C, Schulpis K, et al. Structural and functional alterations in the hippocampus due to hypothyroidism. Metab Brain Dis 2010;25:339–54.
5. Ceballos A, Belinchon MM, Sanchez-Mendoza E, et al. Importance of monocarboxylate transporter 8 for the blood-brain barrier-dependent availability of 3,5,3'-triiodo-L-thyronine. Endocrinology 2009;150:2491–6.
6. Courtin F, Zrouri H, Lamirand A, et al. Thyroid hormone deiodinases in the central and peripheral nervous system. Thyroid 2005;15:931–42.
7. Puymirat J, Miehe M, Marchand R, et al. Immunocytochemical localization of thyroid hormone receptors in the adult rat brain. Thyroid 1991;1:173–84.
8. Fernández-Lamo I, Montero-Pedrazuela A, Delgado-García JM, et al. Effects of thyroid hormone replacement on associative learning and hippocampal synaptic plasticity in adult hypothyroid rats. Eur J Neurosci 2009;30:679–92.
9. Smith JW, Evans AT, Costall B, et al. Thyroid hormones, brain function and cognition: a brief review. Neurosci Biobehav Rev 2002;26:45–60.
10. Carageorgiou H, Pantos C, Zarros A, et al. Changes in acetylcholinesterase, Na+,K+-ATPase, and Mg2+-ATPase activities in the frontal cortex and the hippocampus of hyper- and hypothyroid adult rats. Metabolism 2007;56:1104–10.
11. Tousson E, Ibrahim W, Arafa N, et al. Monoamine concentrations changes in the PTU induced hypothyroid rat brain and the ameliorating role of folic acid. Hum Exp Toxicol 2012;31:282–9.
12. Easson WM. Myxedema with psychosis. Arch Gen Psychiatry 1966;14:277.
13. Davis JD, Tremont G. Neuropsychiatric aspects of hypothyroidism and treatment reversibility. Minerva Endocrinol 2007;32:49–65.
14. Constant EL, Adam S, Seron X, et al. Anxiety and depression, attention, and executive functions in hypothyroidism. J Int Neuropsychol Soc 2005;11:535–44.
15. Gulseren S, Gulseren L, Hekimsoy Z, et al. Depression, anxiety, health-related quality of life, and disability in patients with overt and subclinical thyroid dysfunction. Arch Med Res 2006;37:133–9.
16. Correia N, Mullally S, Cooke G, et al. Evidence for a specific defect in hippocampal memory in overt and subclinical hypothyroidism. J Clin Endocrinol Metab 2009;94:3789–97.
17. Engum A, Bjaro T, Mykletun A, et al. An association between depression, anxiety and thyroid function–a clinical fact or an artefact? Acta Psychiatr Scand 2002;106:27–34.
18. Samuels MH. Cognitive function in untreated hypothyroidism and hyperthyroidism. Curr Opin Endocrinol Diabetes Obes 2008;15:429–33.
19. Miller KJ, Parsons TD, Whybrow PC, et al. Verbal memory retrieval deficits associated with untreated hypothyroidism. J Neuropsychiatry Clin Neurosci 2007;19:132–6.
20. Burmeister LA, Ganguli M, Dodge HH, et al. Hypothyroidism and cognition: preliminary evidence for a specific defect in memory. Thyroid 2001;11:1177–85.

21. Botella-Carretero JI, Galán JM, Caballero C, et al. Quality of life and psychometric functionality in patients with differentiated thyroid carcinoma. Endocr Relat Cancer 2003;10:601–10.

22. Mennemeier M, Garner RD, Heilman KM. Memory, mood and measurement in hypothyroidism. J Clin Exp Neuropsychol 1993;15:822–31.

23. Osterweil D, Syndulko K, Cohen SN, et al. Cognitive function in non-demented older adults with hypothyroidism. J Am Geriatr Soc 1992;40:325–35.

24. Nystrom E, Hamburger A, Lindstedt G, et al. Cerebrospinal fluid proteins in subclinical and overt hypothyroidism. Acta Neurol Scand 1997;95:311–4.

25. Miller KJ, Parsons TD, Whybrow PC, et al. Memory improvement with treatment of hypothyroidism. Int J Neurosci 2006;116:895–906.

26. Bauer M, Silverman DH, Schlagenhauf F, et al. Brain glucose metabolism in hypothyroidism: a positron emission tomography study before and after thyroid hormone replacement therapy. J Clin Endocrinol Metab 2009;94:2922–9.

27. Lass P, Slawek J, Derejko M, et al. Neurological and psychiatric disorders in thyroid dysfunctions. The role of nuclear medicine: SPECT and PET imaging. Minerva Endocrinol 2008;33:75–84.

28. Constant EL, de Volder AG, Ivanoiu A, et al. Cerebral blood flow and glucose metabolism in hypothyroidism: a positron emission tomography study. J Clin Endocrinol Metab 2001;86:3864–70.

29. He XS, Ma N, Pan ZL, et al. Functional magnetic resource imaging assessment of altered brain function in hypothyroidism during working memory processing. Eur J Endocrinol 2011;164:951–9.

30. Samuels MH. Cognitive function in subclinical hypothyroidism. J Clin Endocrinol Metab 2010;95:3611–3.

31. Joffe RT, Pearce EN, Hennessey JV, et al. Subclinical hypothyroidism, mood, and cognition in older adults: a review. Int J Geriatr Psychiatry 2012;28:111–8.

32. Roberts LM, Pattison H, Roalfe A, et al. Is subclinical thyroid dysfunction in the elderly associated with depression or cognitive dysfunction? Ann Intern Med 2006;145:573–81.

33. Gussekloo J, van Exel E, de Craen AJ, et al. Thyroid status, disability and cognitive function, and survival in old age. JAMA 2004;292:2591–9.

34. Bell RJ, Rivera-Woll L, Davison SL, et al. Well-being, health-related quality of life and cardiovascular disease risk profile in women with subclinical thyroid disease—a community-based study. Clin Endocrinol (Oxf) 2007;66:548–56.

35. Baldini IM, Vita A, Mauri MC, et al. Psychopathological and cognitive features in subclinical hypothyroidism. Prog Neuropsychopharmacol Biol Psychiatry 1997; 21:925–35.

36. Park YJ, Lee EJ, Lee YJ, et al. Subclinical hypothyroidism (SCH) is not associated with metabolic derangement, cognitive impairment, depression or poor quality of life (QoL) in elderly subjects. Arch Gerontol Geriatr 2010;50: 68–73.

37. de Jongh RT, Lips P, van Schoor NM, et al. Endogenous subclinical thyroid disorders, physical and cognitive function, depression, and mortality in older individuals. Eur J Endocrinol 2011;165:545–54.

38. Jorde R, Waterloo K, Storhaug H, et al. Neuropsychological function and symptoms in subjects with subclinical hypothyroidism and the effect of thyroxine treatment. J Clin Endocrinol Metab 2006;91:145–53.

39. Kong WM, Sheikh MH, Lumb PJ, et al. A 6-month randomized trial of thyroxine treatment in women with mild subclinical hypothyroidism. Am J Med 2002;112: 348–54.

40. Parle J, Roberts L, Wilson S, et al. A randomized controlled trial of the effect of thyroxine replacement on cognitive function in community-living elderly subjects with subclinical hypothyroidism: the Birmingham Elderly Thyroid Study. J Clin Endocrinol Metab 2010;95:3623–32.

41. St John JA, Henderson VW, Gatto NM, et al. Mildly elevated TSH and cognition in middle-aged and older adults. Thyroid 2009;19:111–7.

42. Manciet G, Dartigues F, Decamps A, et al. The PAUID survey and correlates of subclinical hypothyroidism in elderly community residents in the southwest of France. Age Ageing 1995;24:235–41.

43. Luboschitzky R, Obregon MJ, Kaufman N, et al. Prevalence of cognitive dysfunction and hypothyroidism in an elderly community population. Isr J Med Sci 1996;2:60–5.

44. Jaeschke R, Guyatt G, Herstein H, et al. Does treatment with L-thyroxine influence health status in middle-aged and older adults with subclinical hypothyroidism? J Gen Intern Med 1996;11:744–9.

45. Bono G, Fancellu R, Blandini F, et al. Cognitive and affective status in mild hypothyroidism and interactions with L-thyroxine treatment. Acta Neurol Scand 2004;110:59–66.

46. Zhu DF, Wang ZX, Zhang DR, et al. fMRI revealed neural substrate for reversible working memory dysfunction in subclinical hypothyroidism. Brain 2006;129:2923–30.

47. Samuels MH, Schuff KG, Carlson NE, et al. Health status, mood, and cognition in experimentally induced subclinical hypothyroidism. J Clin Endocrinol Metab 2007;92:2545–51.

48. Jensovsky J, Ruzicka E, Spackova N, et al. Changes of event related potential and cognitive processes in patients with subclinical hypothyroidism after thyroxine treatment. Endocr Regul 2002;36:115–22.

49. Brownlie BE, Rae AM, Walshe JW, et al. Psychoses associated with thyrotoxicosis—'thyrotoxic psychosis.' A report of 18 cases, with statistical analysis of incidence. Eur J Endocrinol 2000;142:438–44.

50. Klubo-Gwiezdzinska J, Wartofsky L. Thyroid emergencies. Med Clin North Am 2012;96:385–403.

51. Wagle AC, Wagle SA, Patel AG. Apathetic form of thyrotoxicosis. Can J Psychiatry 1998;43:747–8.

52. Vogel A, Elberling TV, Hørding M, et al. Affective symptoms and cognitive functions in the acute phase of Graves' thyrotoxicosis. Psychoneuroendocrinology 2007;32(1):36–43.

53. Kathol RG, Delahunt JW. The relationship of anxiety and depression to symptoms of hyperthyroidism using operational criteria. Gen Hosp Psychiatry 1986;8:23–8.

54. Trzepacz PT, McCue M, Klein I, et al. A psychiatric and neuropsychological study of patients with untreated Graves' disease. Gen Hosp Psychiatry 1988;10:49–55.

55. Yudiarto FL, Muliadi L, Moeljanto D, et al. Neuropsychological findings in hyperthyroid patients. Acta Med Indones 2006;38:6–10.

56. Wallace JE, MacCrimmon DJ. Acute hyperthyroidism: cognitive and emotional correlates. J Abnorm Psychol 1980;4:519–27.

57. Whybrow PC, Prange AJ, Treadway CR. Mental changes accompanying thyroid gland dysfunction. Arch Gen Psychiatry 1969;20:48–63.

58. Trzepacz PT, McCue M, Klein I, et al. Psychiatric and neuropsychological response to propranolol in Graves' Disease. Biol Psychiatry 1988;23:678–88.

59. Fahrenfort JJ, Wilterdink AM, van der Veen EA. Long-term residual complaints and psychosocial sequelae after remission of hyperthyroidism. Psychoneuroendocrinology 2000;25:201–11.
60. Elberling TV, Danielsen ER, Rasmussen AK, et al. Reduced myo-inositol and total choline measured with cerebral MRS in acute thyrotoxic Graves' disease. Neurology 2003;60:142–5.
61. Danielsen ER, Elberling TV, Rasmussen AK, et al. Reduced parietooccipital white matter glutamine measured by proton magnetic resonance spectroscopy in treated Graves' disease patients. J Clin Endocrinol Metab 2008;93:3192–8.
62. Schreckenberger MF, Egle UT, Drecker S, et al. Positron emission tomography reveals correlations between brain metabolism and mood changes in hyperthyroidism. J Clin Endocrinol Metab 2006;91:4786–91.
63. Rockel M, Teuber J, Schmidt R, et al. Preclinical hyperthyroidism and its correlation with clinical and psychological symptoms. Klin Wochenschr 1987;65:264–73 [in German, abstract in English].
64. Ceresini G, Laurentani F, Maggio M, et al. Thyroid function abnormalities and cognitive impairment in elderly people: results of the Invecchiare in Chianti Study. J Am Geriatr Soc 2009;57:89–93.
65. Panicker V, Evans J, Bjoro T, et al. A paradoxical difference in relationship between anxiety, depression and thyroid function in subjects on and not on T4: findings from the HUNT study. Clin Endocrinol 2009;71:574–80.
66. Gan EH, Pearce HS. The thyroid in mind: cognitive function and low thyrotropin in older people. J Clin Endocrinol Metab 2012;97:3438–49.
67. Prinz PN, Scanlan JM, Vitaliano PP, et al. Thyroid hormones: positive relationships with cognition in healthy, euthyroid older men. J Gerontol A Biol Sci Med Sci 1999;54:M111–6.
68. Beydoun MA, Beydoun HA, Kitner-Triolo MH, et al. Thyroid hormones are associated with cognitive function: moderation by sex, race, and depressive symptoms. J Clin Endocrinol Metab 2013;98:3470–81.
69. Van Boxtel MP, Menheere PP, Bekers O, et al. Thyroid function, depressed mood, and cognitive performance in older individuals: the Maastricht Aging Study. Psychoneuroendocrinology 2004;29:891–8.
70. Walsh JP, Ward LC, Burke V, et al. Small changes in thyroxine dosage do not produce measurable changes in hypothyroid symptoms, well-being, or quality of life: results of a double-blind, randomized clinical trial. J Clin Endocrinol Metab 2006;91:2624–30.
71. Samuels MH, Schuff KG, Carlson NE, et al. Health status, mood, and cognition in experimentally induced subclinical thyrotoxicosis. J Clin Endocrinol Metab 2008;93:1730–6.
72. Joffe RT, Levitt AJ. Basal thyrotropin and major depression: relation to clinical variables and treatment outcome. Can J Psychiatry 2008;53:833–8.
73. Williams MD, Harris R, Dayan CM, et al. Thyroid function and the natural history of depression: findings from the Caerphilly Prospective Study (CaPS) and a meta-analysis. Clin Endocrinol (Oxf) 2009;70:484–92.
74. Livner A, Wahlin A, Backman L. Thyroid stimulating hormone and prospective memory functioning in old age. Psychoneuroendocrinology 2009;34:1554–9.
75. Hogervorst E, Huppert R, Matthews FE, et al. Thyroid function and cognitive decline in the MRC Cognitive Function and Ageing Study. Psychoneuroendocrinology 2008;33:1013–22.
76. Grigorova M, Sherwin BB. Thyroid hormones and cognitive functioning in healthy, euthyroid women: a correlational study. Horm Behav 2012;61:617–22.

77. Wahlin A, Bunce D, Wahlin TB. Longitudinal evidence of the impact of normal thyroid stimulating hormone variations on cognitive functioning in very old age. Psychoneuroendocrinology 2005;30:625–37.

78. Booth T, Deary IJ, Starr JM. Thyroid stimulating hormone, free thyroxine and cognitive ability in old age: the Lothian Birth Cohort Study 1936. Psychoneuroendocrinology 2013;38:597–601.

79. Pollock MA, Sturrock A, Marshall K, et al. Thyroxine treatment in patients with symptoms of hypothyroidism but thyroid function tests within the reference range: randomised double blind placebo controlled crossover trial. BMJ 2001;323:891–5.

80. Saravanan P, Chau WF, Roberts N, et al. Psychological well-being in patients on 'adequate' doses of l-thyroxine: results of a large, controlled community-based questionnaire study. Clin Endocrinol (Oxf) 2002;57:577–85.

81. Saravanan P, Visser TJ, Dayan CM. Psychological well-being correlates with free thyroxine but not free 3,5,3'-triiodothyronine levels in patients on thyroid hormone replacement. J Clin Endocrinol Metab 2006;91:3389–93.

82. Wekking EM, Appelhof BC, Fliers E, et al. Cognitive functioning and well-being in euthyroid patients on thyroxine replacement therapy for primary hypothyroidism. Eur J Endocrinol 2005;153:747–53.

83. Samuels MH, Schuff KG, Carlson NE, et al. Health status, psychological symptoms, mood and cognition in L-thyroxine treated hypothyroid subjects. Thyroid 2007;17:249–58.

84. Kramer CK, von Muhlen D, Kritz-Silverstein D, et al. Treated hypothyroidism, cognitive function, and depressed mood in old age: the Rancho Bernardo Study. Eur J Endocrinol 2009;161:917–21.

85. Panicker V, Saravanan P, Vaidya B, et al. Common variation in the DIO2 gene predicts baseline psychological well-being and response to combination thyroxine plus triiodothyronine therapy in hypothyroid patients. J Clin Endocrinol Metab 2009;94:1623–9.

86. van der Deure WM, Appelhof BC, Peeters RP, et al. Polymorphisms in the brain-specific thyroid hormone transporter OATP1C1 are associated with fatigue and depression in hypothyroid patients. Clin Endocrinol (Oxf) 2008;69:804–11.

87. Carta MG, Hardoy MC, Carpiniello B, et al. A case control study on psychiatric disorders in Hashimoto disease and euthyroid goiter: not only depressive but also anxiety disorders are associated with thyroid autoimmunity. Clin Pract Epidemiol Ment Health 2005;1:23–7.

88. Grabe HJ, Volzke H, Ludemann J, et al. Mental and physical complaints in thyroid disorders in the general population. Acta Psychiatr Scand 2005;112:286–93.

89. Ott J, Promberger R, Kober F, et al. Hashimoto's thyroiditis affects symptom load and quality of life unrelated to hypothyroidism: a prospective case-control study in women undergoing thyroidectomy for benign goiter. Thyroid 2011;21:161–7.

90. Leyhe T, Müssig K, Weinert C, et al. Increased occurrence of weaknesses in attention testing in patients with Hashimoto's thyroiditis compared to patients with other thyroid illnesses. Psychoneuroendocrinology 2008;33:1432–6.

91. Engum A, Bjøro T, Mykletun A, et al. Thyroid autoimmunity, depression and anxiety; are there any connections? An epidemiological study of a large population. J Psychosom Res 2005;59:263–8.

92. Biondi B, Wartofsky L. Combination treatment with T4 and T3: toward personalized replacement therapy in hypothyroidism? J Clin Endocrinol Metab 2012;97:2256–71.

93. Hoang TD, Olsen CH, Mai VQ, et al. Desiccated thyroid extract compared with levothyroxine in the treatment of hypothyroidism: a randomized, double-blind, crossover study. J Clin Endocrinol Metab 2013;98:1982–90.
94. Yeap BB, Alfonso H, Chubb SA, et al. Higher free thyroxine levels predict increased incidence of dementia in older men: the Health in Men Study. J Clin Endocrinol Metab 2012;97:E2230–7.
95. de Jong FJ, Masaki K, Chen H, et al. Thyroid function, the risk of dementia and neuropathologic changes: the Honolulu Asia Aging Study. Neurobiol Aging 2009;30:600–6.
96. Castillo P, Woodruff B, Caselli R, et al. Steroid-responsive encephalopathy associated with autoimmune thyroiditis. Arch Neurol 2006;63:197–202.
97. Gini B, Lovato L, Cianti R, et al. Novel autoantigens recognized by CSF IgG from Hashimoto's encephalitis revealed by a proteomic approach. J Neuroimmunol 2008;196:153–8.

Ethical Issues in the Management of Thyroid Disease

M. Sara Rosenthal, PhD

KEYWORDS

- Clinical ethics • Informed consent • Autoimmune thyroid disease • Thyroid cancer
- Radioablation • Adjuvant radioactive iodine therapy

KEY POINTS

- The focus of this article is on clinical ethics issues in the thyroid disease context.
- In the context of thyroid disease management, clinical ethics dilemmas affect a wide range of health care providers: endocrinologists, primary care physicians, surgeons, oncologists, nuclear medicine specialists and technologists, genetic counselors, nurses, and physician assistants.
- In autoimmune thyroid disease, there are unique challenges to informed consent, and potential duties to warn in severe hypothyroidism.
- In thyroid cancer, the most common ethical issues revolve around truth-telling and advance care planning, and genetic screening for medullary thyroid cancer.
- Novel ethical issues in thyroid disease include end of life discussions in poorly differentiated thyroid cancers; priority-setting for drug shortages; and resolving clinical disagreement over standards of care.

INTRODUCTION

Clinical ethics is a subspecialty of bioethics that deals with ethical dilemmas that specifically involve the provider-patient relationship. Clinical ethics issues comprise weighing therapeutic benefits against risks and side effects, innovative therapies, end-of-life care, unintended versus intentional harms to patients or patient populations, medical error, health care access, cultural competency, and professional virtues and integrity. Clinical ethics issues may also involve moral distress and there are distinct clinical ethics issues that arise in different thyroid disease management contexts and patient populations.

Program for Bioethics, Department of Internal Medicine, University of Kentucky, 740 S. Limestone Street, Suite K-522, Lexington, KY 40506, USA
E-mail address: m.sararosenthal@uky.edu

Endocrinol Metab Clin N Am 43 (2014) 545–564
http://dx.doi.org/10.1016/j.ecl.2014.02.013
0889-8529/14/$ – see front matter © 2014 Elsevier Inc. All rights reserved.

Moral distress refers to a situation in which the health care provider knows the ethical course of action, but is constrained from acting on it; constraints may stem from patient/surrogate decisions; institutional power relations, regulations, or policies; or legal issues. Unresolved moral distress can lead to moral residue; this is a particular problem for health care providers with less moral agency, such as nurses, residents, or other health care trainees but also affects physicians in all specialties (see, in particular: Epstein EG, Hamric AB. Moral distress, moral residue, and the crescendo effect. J Clin Ethics 2009;20(4):330–42. Available at: http://www.ncbi.nlm.nih.gov/pmc/articles/PMC3612701/).

This article reviews core ethical principles for practice, as well as the moral and legal requirements of informed consent. It then discusses the range of ethical issues and considerations that present in the management of autoimmune thyroid disease and thyroid cancer. In addition, ethical issues concerning vulnerable populations and resource allocation are explored.

CORE ETHICAL PRINCIPLES

Thyroid practitioners need to understand core principles in medical ethics[1] that are often competing. The Principle of Respect for Persons, first articulated in The Belmont Report[2] (http://www.hhs.gov/ohrp/humansubjects/guidance/belmont.html) is a dual obligation of health care providers to respect autonomous patients, but protect nonautonomous patients. Although sometimes used synonymously with the Principle of Respect for Autonomy[1] (aka Principle of Autonomy), what distinguishes respect for persons from respect for autonomy is the explicit obligation to protect those who do not have decision-making capacity (**Box 1**). Both principles stipulate that care should be guided according to patients' wishes, values, beliefs, and preferences, which is determined through the process of informed consent. Both principles stipulate that autonomous patients (those with decision-making capacity) guide their own care. However, the Principle of Respect for Persons is inclusive of nonautonomous patients, and deals with patients without decision-making capacity. In these cases, this principle obligates health care providers to ensure there is a surrogate decision maker available to make decisions based on patient preferences, if known (substitute judgment), or, if not known, based on the patient's best interests. Informed consent (discussed later) supports both the principles of respect for persons and autonomy, and establishes whether patients are autonomous agents or whether patients require surrogate decision makers.

The Principle of Beneficence obligates practitioners to weigh therapeutic benefits over therapeutic risks, or to maximize clinical goods and minimize clinical harms. Beneficent care necessarily recognizes that there may be limits to autonomy when patients request (or demand) therapies or interventions that are medically inappropriate. However, respecting autonomy also necessarily recognizes that there may be limits to beneficence. Patients may request therapies that are potentially harmful, risky, or nonexistent. Practitioners need to use their clinical judgment to balance autonomy and beneficence so that attempts to satisfy one do not violate the other. Informed consent thus also supports the Principle of Beneficence by requiring truth telling: a full disclosure of therapeutic options to be discussed, and all associated risks and benefits. This process also entails a discussion of what is not an option or medically appropriate. Informed consent helps to educate autonomous patients or surrogates about what constitutes a beneficent care plan. The antiquated concept of truth-telling as a harm or beneficent deception[3] derives from a paternalistic model in which the practitioner used therapeutic privilege to withhold information from the patient in the belief

---

Box 1
Criteria for decision-making capacity

Distinct from competency (which is a legal determination, made by a judge for decision-making authority), decision-making capacity is a medical determination that can be made by the attending or responsible physician; all competent persons have presumption of capacity. Decision-making capacity can change over short periods of time and be affected by physiologic changes.

The criteria to assess capacity are U-ARE:

- Understanding: do patients understand their medical status, treatment options, and risks associated with the various options? Is there a basic understanding of the facts involved in that decision? Are there language or literacy barriers?

- Appreciation: does the patient have some appreciation of the nature and significance of the decision?

- Rationality (or ability to reason): is the patient able to reason with the information in order to make a decision? Can the patient engage in reasoning and manipulate information rationally? Does the patient make rational decisions, or offer a rationale for a seemingly irrational decision, based on preferences, beliefs, culture, and so forth? In patients with dementia or mental health status changes, look for decisional stability over time, in contrast with vacillation, which indicates an absence of capacity.

- Expression of choice: can patients communicate a decision or express themselves in some way (orally, in written form, in gestures, or blinking)? This is important for patients with aphasia or who cannot speak.

Some patients require a more formal capacity assessment, which may need to involve a psychiatric consultation or an ethics consultation.

Standards for capacity

Decision-making capacity relates to a particular decision at a particular time, may exist for simple but not complex decisions, and may exist for medical but not other decisions. Decision-making capacity operates on a sliding scale that permits lesser standards of capacity for less consequential medical decisions (such as getting a flu shot), and requires higher standards of capacity for greater consequential decisions such as consenting to radioactive iodine or total thyroidectomy. The more serious the expected harm to the patient from acting on a choice, the higher should be the standard of decision-making capacity. However, no single standard for capacity is adequate for all decisions. The standard of capacity necessary depends on the risk involved, and varies from low to high.

Data from Refs.[12,97–100]

---

that it was a clinical good. However, this is no longer considered ethically defensible unless there are exceptional circumstances, and, in such cases, an ethics consultation is advised.

The Principle of Nonmaleficence obligates practitioners not to intentionally harm patients through acts of commission or omission. Satisfying this principle thus entails a duty to warn at-risk third parties if the patient is an agent of harm, as well as disclosing unintentional harms or errors. The distinction between the principles of beneficence and nonmaleficence is that the former involves an intention to offer a benefit (active beneficence) and avoid a harm (passive nonmaleficence),[1] which may not prevent some harm from occurring; this is the case in radioiodine ablation in a patient with Graves' disease who develops postablative hypothyroidism. The benefit is in the outcome of lessening patient suffering by resolving hyperthyroidism and providing thyroid hormone replacement to achieve euthyroidism for the patient's benefit.

Thus, the goal of improving the patient's well-being has been achieved. Beneficence therefore involves a balancing of benefits and harms with a minimizing of harms as a means to a benefit. The latter is a direct obligation not to cause harm that has no known beneficial outcome, or does not lead to an improved patient status. In the same Graves' disease example, performing radioablation without any follow-up or replacement of thyroid hormone would be a clear violation of the Principle of Nonmaleficence.

In addition, the Principle of Justice in the context of clinical ethics concerns distributive justice issues, which comprise equality of treatment (eg, cultural competence issues), access to health care, and resource allocation. Numerous socioeconomic and psychosocial factors such as income, literacy, numeracy, education and culture, and psychological health may present barriers to both informed consent and health care access.

Origins of the 4 Principles

The current framework for medical ethics guidelines began as a response to the Nuremberg Trials; in 1947 American authors drafted the Nuremberg Code (http://www.hhs.gov/ohrp/archive/nurcode.html), which originally stipulated guidelines for biomedical research. It was published by the Government Printing Office as part of a 15-volume series in 1949.[4] The Nuremberg Code set out specific guidelines for informed consent and also established that children were never appropriate human research subjects. This American-authored document did not sufficiently protect even American patients from unethical clinical trials, and several egregious violations of the Nuremberg Code continued throughout the postwar period until the 1970s in US patient populations. Infamous clinical trials included the Tuskegee Syphilis Study,[2,3,5] the Guatemalan Syphilis trial,[5] Willowbrook, and the Brooklyn Jewish Chronic Disease Hospital.[3,6] Thyroid disease investigators are included among Nuremberg Code violators. In 1996, a report was released about nontherapeutic doses of I-131 given to Alaskan natives from 1955 to 1957 without their informed consent. This report documented a covert thyroid disease study conducted by the United States Air Force, known as The Arctic Aeromedical Laboratory's Thyroid Function Study. In this study, one or more doses of 50 µCi of I-131 were given to 101 native Alaskans and 19 military personnel who had no evidence of thyroid disease, placing them at potential risk for thyroid cancers.[7]

The continued Nuremberg violations paved the way for the formation of the National Commission for Human Subjects Protections, and the Belmont Report (1978), which published agreed-on principles for medical research involving human subjects.[2] The Belmont Report schema was to identify a principle with a corresponding guideline.[8] The Principle of Respect for Persons was the underlying principle for informed consent practices; the Principle of Beneficence was the underlying principle for trial design and the risk/benefit analysis; and the Principle of Justice dealt with patient/subject selection, ensuring that the "burdens and benefits of research were evenly distributed."[2,8] The author of the Belmont principles was simultaneously working on a deeper treatise on core ethical principles for medicine, which eventually was published as *The Principles of Biomedical Ethics* (first edition, 1979, now in its sixth edition).[1] This work took hold as the dominant framework for everyday practitioners looking for an applied set of ethical principles for practice (known as principlism). Although there are continuing critiques by other philosophers about whether the principlism approach sufficiently accounts for all ethical behaviors and issues in medicine,[9] the 4 principles outlined by Beauchamp and Childress[1] are well defended and practical foundations for clinical ethics guidelines and frameworks.

Informed Consent

Informed consent can be understood as both a moral and legal requirement that supports (if not, upholds) the Principle of Respect for Persons. As a moral requirement, the history of informed consent was first articulated in the Nuremberg Code: "The voluntary consent of the human subject is absolutely essential."[4] It was further expanded in the Belmont Report,[2] which established a moral framework for medical research and practice, boundaries between accepted medical practice and research, and the moral necessity of protecting vulnerable populations who cannot provide valid consent. Informed consent comprises 3 components[10]: (1) full disclosure[11] of all treatment options, and their associated risks and benefits; (2) capacity and competency,[12] meaning that patients must be considered to meet the legal standard of competence (autonomous adults or autonomous emancipated minors) as well as have decision-making capacity (see **Box 1**); and (3) consent must be voluntary,[13] meaning that patients should be free of coercion in making their decisions.

The legal doctrine of informed consent has its roots in common law, tort law, and constitutional law. Precedent-setting cases include[3] *Schloendorff v Society of New York Hospital* (1914),[14] which introduced self determination; *Salgo v Leland Stanford Jr University Board of Trustees* (1957),[15] which introduced the term informed consent and criteria for disclosure; and *Natanson v Kline* (1960),[16] which first proposed that failure to disclose risks constituted negligence.[3] Three landmark 1972 cases (*Canterbury v Spence*,[17] *Cobbs v Grant*,[18] and *Wilkinson v Vesey*[19]) most firmly established informed consent as a legal requirement. All 3 cases involved patients who were not sufficiently informed about the risks of procedures. In *Canterbury v Spence* the court stated that, "informed consent is a basic social policy..."[17] In *Cobbs v Grant*, the court emphasized "a duty of reasonable disclosure of the available choices ...[and] the dangers inherently and potentially involved in each."[18] In *Wilkinson v Vesey*, the court stated: "a physician is bound to disclose all the known material risks peculiar to the proposed procedure."[19]

Informed consent is not absolute; exceptions to informed consent include public health emergencies, medical emergencies, therapeutic privilege, and patient waivers to consent.

Privacy and Confidentiality

Privacy and confidentiality support the principles of respect for persons, nonmaleficence (when privacy violation is a social harm), and justice, whereby medical information could be used in a discriminatory manner to affect social access, as in genetic information. The Health Insurance Portability and Accountability Act (HIPAA) Privacy Rules (Public Law 104–191, see: http://www.hhs.gov/ocr/privacy/hipaa/understanding/summary/index.html) govern how medical information may be used, but there are exceptions to confidentiality and HIPAA when public health is at risk and there is an ethical or legal duty to warn a third party of risk. The duty to warn is discussed further under the contexts of impaired hypothyroid patients and disclosure of RET mutations. Practitioners involved in genetic counseling should become familiar with the Genetic Information Nondiscrimination Act (GINA) (Public Law 110–233), which is intended to protect individuals against the misuse of genetic information for health insurance and employment.[20]

Professional Virtues and Integrity

Professional virtues and integrity in medicine (aka professionalism and humanism) refer to codes of behavior for clinical practice. They are not moral frameworks for the practice of medicine, but codes of professional conduct to maintain integrity and standards developed for persons claiming to possess special knowledge or skills. Professional codes exist in many professions, and medicine is no exception. In American medicine, the most significant professional code introduced was by Thomas Percival, in *Medical Ethics* (1803)[21]; it was initially drafted for hospitals and medical charities and focused on medical etiquette and gentlemanly conduct.[3] It was the model for the first AMA code of ethics.[3,21] Another work, produced by Worthington Hooker, *Physician and Patient* (1849), dealt with lying and deception, quackery, and charlatans.[3]

Professional virtues and integrity underpin all professional codes of ethics, and such virtues are best captured in the works of Edmund Pellegrino. (See, for example, Pellegrino E, Thomasma D. *Virtues in Medical Practice.* Oxford University Press, 1993) For thyroidology, the first dedicated professional code for practice was published in 2013,[22] which outlines conflicts of interest, and provides guidelines for a range of professionalism issues.

ETHICAL ISSUES IN AUTOIMMUNE THYROID DISEASES

When managing autoimmune thyroid disease, continuous ethical tensions between the principles of respect for persons and beneficence persist because there are unique challenges to informed consent. This challenge is particularly apparent in the management of Graves' disease.[23] With respect to severe hypothyroidism, ethical and legal duties to warn emerge as well.[24]

Unique Ethical Issues in Graves' Disease

The history of the use of radioactive iodine (RAI) to treat Graves' disease[25,26] is documented by Sawin and Becker.[27] Although radioablation for Graves' disease is a standard of care in some countries, it is not in others,[28,29] which has created ethical dilemmas in what constitutes beneficent care as well as obtaining valid consent to treatment.[23] The ethical use of RAI is only relative to whether it constitutes a beneficent treatment to which the autonomous patient fully consents.

The standard of care for Graves' disease is guided by patient preferences, under the principles of respect for persons, as well as patient candidacy under the principles of beneficence and nonmaleficence. Antithyroid medication, radioablation, or surgery have been shown to be equally effective in appropriate candidates.[28,30,31] For patients who are fearful of radioablation,[23] or who have conditions that may be contraindications for its use (such as compliance issues with posttreatment precautions, or severe Graves' ophthalmopathy with an intolerance to steroids), other options should be presented. In some patients, options may be limited. For patients who are at high risk for aplastic anemia (a risk of methimazole), or who do not meet criteria for liver transplantation, the risk of fulminant hepatic failure with propylthiouracil may not make it a more beneficent option.[30,31] For patients who are not surgical candidates because of the numerous contraindications that could be present (eg, severe obesity, cardiovascular risks, Jehovah's Witnesses who do not consent to blood transfusion), surgery cannot be presented as an option. Thus, patient preferences may have limits in situations in which there are other contraindications for therapy. For example, patients with severe obstructive goiters may require surgery, even if they do not prefer it. In addition, in patients with limited access to health care coverage or insurance who are equally good candidates for any option, RAI may be the most cost-effective therapy.[28] In addition, patients with Graves' disease treated with either surgery or ablation who later become pregnant after their hypothyroidism is treated are frequently not informed about the risk of autoantibodies persisting, transplacental stimulation of the fetal thyroid, and fetal thyrotoxicosis.[31,32] Patients who are fertile and planning a family after treatment need to be informed about these risks.

Complicating the informed consent process may be problems with decision-making capacity (see **Box 1**). Severe hyperthyroidism and thyrotoxicosis can cause distorted thinking and anxiety, and can result in psychiatric diagnoses such as psychosis and mania.[33,34]

Part of an adequate consent process in Graves' disease includes correcting patient misconceptions about treatment options, which proliferate on the Internet. These misconceptions may include unsubstantiated fears about RAI and cancer risks, and false information about hypothyroidism and thyroid hormone replacement (discussed later).

Informed consent for radioablation

Patients with Graves' disease who consent to radioablation frequently do not understand and appreciate the intent of the therapy and the expected clinical consequence of hypothyroidism, or that thyroid hormone replacement is necessary for euthyroidism.[23] Practitioners who attempt to obtain consent on the patient's first visit, or who promise that partial ablation will lead to euthyroidism without hypothyroidism or the need for thyroid hormone replacement are not engaging in an adequate informed consent process, or truth telling. Patients may perceive their eventual hypothyroidism as medical error, or a risk that was not adequately explained in the consent process, placing the practitioner at risk for an accusation of negligence.

Understanding and appreciation of radiation safety precautions after RAI ablation for Graves' disease is another factor in the informed consent process that affects RAI candidacy. Patients who would have difficulty complying with these precautions might not be suitable candidates, because they could be agents of harm to their families or third parties, although less than in radioiodine treatment of thyroid cancer.

Nuclear medicine technologists frequently report that they encounter patients who do not seem to understand or appreciate why they are being given radioisotopes.[35] In these circumstances, there is frequently institutional confusion about whose role it is to obtain informed consent and to explain procedures. Nuclear medicine technologists who do not have sufficient knowledge about autoimmune thyroid disease may find themselves in the position of obtaining consent for radioablation when they are not sufficiently trained or qualified to do so. In some of these cases, it may be ethically obligatory to delay the procedure until the appropriate attending physician can be available to reconsent the patient.[35]

Ethical Challenges with Hypothyroidism

The ethical issues that emerge in patients presenting with hypothyroidism (autoimmune or iatrogenic) concern impairment, which can be a barrier to informed consent and decision-making capacity. Even in patients with mild to moderate hypothyroidism, some impairment may be present.[24] In patients with severe hypothyroidism (defined here as a thyroid-stimulating hormone [TSH] of 30 Iμ/mL or higher[24]), practitioners may have a duty to warn the patient against driving or performing tasks that require alertness.[24] If the patient is an agent of harm, the Principle of Nonmaleficence obligates practitioners to warn third parties at risk, by contacting a legal surrogate decision maker, or even the appropriate authorities (eg, the Department of Motor Vehicles) until the patient is euthyroid. Imagine severely hypothyroid patients driving carpools with small children, buses, or commercial trucks, or working as airline pilots.[24]

In the typical clinical context, hypothyroid patients do not need to consent to a high-risk procedure or to a procedure involving radioisotopes, and thus a lesser standard of capacity (see **Box 1**) is ethically permissible, but the patient needs to understand and appreciate that the medication is lifesaving and mandatory. Patients do need to consent to take thyroid hormone replacement, and thus compliance is a factor, as well as access to medication. The standard of care that best meets the beneficence standard for thyroid hormone replacement is monotherapy with levothyroxine (LT4)[36] with a prescription for a generic or brand the patient can afford. However, because of a vast, confused alternative medicine literature[37] that has framed LT4 as synthetic or not optimal, and desiccated porcine thyroid hormone as better and supposedly natural, many patients insist on this lesser standard of care.[36] Moreover, combination therapy with T3, potentially a harmful therapy for many patients, is promoted by some practitioners as either equal or superior (based on a research literature replete with short-term studies of heterogeneous design that are not easily subject to meta-analysis and cannot be generalized to all patient populations[38]), and is also requested by patients. The ethical dilemma that presents is whether thyroid practitioners have an ethical or legal obligation to provide a lower standard of care because it is a patient's preference. Practitioners do not have to violate beneficence if they think that a patient is making a demand for inappropriate care; in such cases, practitioners may transfer care to a physician who is willing to prescribe what the patients wants. However, in a situation in which a patient is severely hypothyroid, and agrees only to an inferior formulation of thyroid hormone, it is ethically permissible to provide a lower standard of care if it is thought to be better than nothing.

When hypothyroid patients refuse thyroid hormone replacement therapy
Thyroid hormone replacement can be framed as a lifesaving therapy for severely hypothyroid patients using a presumed-consent framework reserved for emergency settings. This framework permits consent to be waived for a lifesaving procedure until the patient is stabilized and regains decision-making capacity. In all other cases of refusal, if the patient does not have capacity, a surrogate decision maker needs to be contacted. If the patient does have capacity and expresses a desire to live, but still refuses to take thyroid hormone, this indicates problems with meeting the criteria for capacity (see **Box 1**), and a psychiatric consult may be warranted.

Unique issues with diagnostic challenges
Ethical problems may be inherent in diagnostic challenges, in which patients show signs of either thyroiditis or Graves' disease that are ignored, misdiagnosed as something else (particularly when they have hashitoxicosis), or diagnosed in such a mild form that it may difficult to gauge when it is best to initiate therapy. Graves' ophthalmopathy can create diagnostic challenges when the eye problems precede any signs of hyperthyroidism, or when radioablation without steroids is recommended to patients with subclinical eye disease that worsens after radioablation.[31]

Diagnostic problems become ethical problems when they lead to negligently delayed diagnoses, improper follow-up, and prolonged patient suffering, which can create situations in which patients are highly distrustful, and may be unfairly labeled as "difficult" when they eventually encounter the appropriate practitioner.

There is also a controversial diagnosis of Hashimoto encephalopathy[39] (made by neurologists) that can further aggravate the misdiagnosis cycle.

More challenging still are euthyroid patients claiming to be hypothyroid despite no objective evidence, after ruling out TSH-inhibiting conditions, or other conditions that can create many of the same symptoms. In these cases, beneficent-based obligations require that practitioners engage in truth telling and trust building, and refrain from pre-scribing unnecessary medications, despite the patient's insistence.[40–42]

ETHICAL ISSUES IN THYROID CANCER

Managing thyroid cancer requires the involvement of multiple subspecialties that may include endocrinology, surgery, nuclear medicine, radiology, medical oncology, and genetic counseling (in hereditary medullary thyroid cancer). The most common ethical issues that emerge in thyroid cancer generally concern truth-telling and truthful prog-nostication,[43] which can interfere with both patient autonomy and beneficent care plans; it can also lead to practitioner moral distress. In cases of iodine-avid thyroid cancer, there is clinical disagreement among the community of experts over what con-stitutes beneficent care with no available data to settle the dispute (a circumstance known as clinical equipoise[44]). Thus, thyroid oncologists have an ethical duty to disclose all known treatment options, their expected benefits and risks, and conse-quences, which includes treatment approaches they may not entirely support or agree with, or even offer at their institutions, such as radioiodine dosimetry. There are distinct ethical issues in iodine-avid and iodine non-avid thyroid cancers. In iodine-avid thyroid cancer, clinical equipoise has become ethically problematic for patient care. Another common ethical issue in iodine-avid thyroid cancer is candidacy for either hypothyroid withdrawal or recombinant human TSH (rhTSH), and barriers to rhTSH, which may range from socioeconomic barriers to drug scarcity.

In iodine non-avid, poorly differentiated thyroid cancers (eg, anaplastic thyroid can-cer or medullary thyroid cancer), there are unique ethical issues that arise, even though there is general consensus regarding a range of treatment approaches.[45,46]

Because surgical ethics issues related to thyroidectomy are similar to any other sur-gical ethics context, involving surgical competency, candidacy, innovative proce-dures,[47] and informed consent, the discussion here is limited to ethical issues arising from the unique therapies and dilemmas in thyroid cancer. (For a thorough re-view of surgical ethics issues, see McCullough L, Jones J, Brody B. *Surgical ethics.* Oxford University Press, 1998.)

Ethical issues with treating iatrogenic hypothyroidism resulting from total thyroidec-tomy are similar in scope to treating primary hypothyroidism in the autoimmune context, as discussed above.

Ethical Issues in Adjuvant RAI Therapy

The moral frameworks used in assessing patient candidacy for adjuvant RAI therapy are the principles of beneficence and nonmaleficence. The option of RAI must ensure that there is a greater balance of benefits than harms, or that clinical goods are maxi-mized and clinical harms minimized. Systemic RAI has a small increased relative risk of secondary cancers, and a clinically insignificant absolute risk,[48] but this does not mean it cannot be a beneficent therapy if there is also a risk of morbidity from either recurrent or persistent disease without adjuvant systemic RAI therapy. (This has been the morally defensible framework for giving adjuvant chemotherapy for many years.) Because the thyroid oncology literature reports that long-term survival is maxi-mized and recurrence is minimized when adjuvant RAI therapy is used in metastatic iodine-avid thyroid cancers,[49] this therapy rises to the standard of beneficence; not offering it would beg the question of whether beneficence is being violated. The path-ologic nature of persistent iodine-avid thyroid cancer is to become iodine non-avid over time,[50] so, in the absence of any known, effective, systemic, tumoricidal thera-pies for metastatic differentiated thyroid cancer, the value of even a theoretical benefit of preventing recurrence is enhanced if there is also a theoretical risk of losing iodine avidity over time. Patients with thyroid cancer who are not advised of this when given the option of a watch–and-wait protocol (see, for example, Roshenstok and colleagues[51]) may not have informed consent, because potential loss of iodine avidity is a material risk. Watch–and-wait protocols, in which the prevailing standard of care is being withheld, demand greater ethical justification.[52]

There seems to be consensus that patients with unifocal papillary tumors less than 1 cm in diameter (micropapillary tumors) are not candidates for adjuvant RAI therapy.[53] However, there is wide variation in what patients are offered when they have multifocal papillary tumors of less than 1 cm, or when the tumors have one or more of the following features: (1) they have breached the thyroid capsule, (2) they have associated lymph node involvement; and/or (3) they are of a high-risk variant (eg, tall cell).[53,54] Data for the risks of secondary cancers following adjuvant RAI therapy for these groups do not even exceed the risk of daily life,[48] a common measure of minimal or low risk used in the research ethics context. Moreover, the long-term survival data on patients who did not receive RAI therapy do not account for morbidity from recurrence.[49,54–56] Qualitative data on young women with highly treatable differentiated thyroid cancers concluded that there were covert psychosocial consequences to not thriving versus surviving in repeated cycles of recurrent therapies.[57] Informed consent ultimately must disclose the theoretical risks associated with having[48] or not having[56] adjuvant RAI.

Medical candidacy for RAI therapy must also be balanced with both patient preferences and contraindications to RAI such as compliance with RAI preparation protocols (low-iodine diet; access to rhTSH; or, if no access, physical and psychosocial fitness for a hypothyroid withdrawal scan, including not driving) and compliance with posttreatment precautions and social distancing. Here, too, there may be additional duties to warn involved with impaired hypothyroid patients.[24]

Radioidine dosimetry

Radioidone dosimetry involves individualized dose calculation of RAI to gauge the safety limit for dosing RAI[58]; it is reserved for aggressive iodine-avid disease for which standard doses of RAI are medically inappropriate, either because they are too high or because they are too low. Dosimetry, as a means to therapy, is active beneficence; it is a treatment approach that is well documented, and rises to the standard of beneficence. The ethical obligation for practitioners with dosimetry candidates is 2-fold. First, there must be full disclosure that dosimetry is an option, with a referral site provided (because it is not offered at most institutions). Second, full disclosure of all risks and benefits, including the risks associated with not having dosimetry, must be part of the consent discussion. Patients with informed consent guide whether dosimetry continues to be offered; as with other RAI therapies, some patients may not be candidates because of compliance with posttreatment precautions.

Unique Ethical Issues in Iodine Non-avid Thyroid Cancer

Iodine non-avid thyroid cancers, such as medullary thyroid cancer (MTC), anaplastic thyroid cancer (ATC), or other poorly differentiated thyroid cancers unresponsive to therapy, raise distinct ethical issues. In these contexts, aggressive, overwhelming disease for which there is no curative treatment, or effective tumoristatic therapies, means that end-of-life discussions must take place.

The first ATC clinical practice guidelines published by Smallridge and colleagues[45] provide clear guidelines for advanced care planning discussions with patients using a team-based approach, in which the patient is provided, from the outset, with truthful prognostication and all available options, including the option of innovative therapies, clinical trials (even if the trial is at a different site), or palliative measures only (now legally required to be provided as an option in some states for patients with terminal prognoses; see the Palliative Care Information Act at: http://www.health.ny.gov/professionals/patients/patient_rights/palliative_care/information_act.htm). However, discussions about advance directives do not replace an advance care planning discussion.[22]

Thyroidologists can also help to craft an individualized palliative treatment plan, known as physician/medical orders for life-sustaining treatment (POLST/MOLST),[59] which can incorporate patient preferences and recognize the nuances of medical care that advance directives typically cannot. POLST orders follow the patient to various institutions, and forms may be obtained through www.polst.org.

The extensive body of literature regarding end of life confirms that truth-telling leads to better dying experiences for patients, who do not want to be lied to or "die deaths they deplore in locations they despise"[43(ppxiv)]. Truthful prognostication also reduces moral distress for practitioners,[60] who may be tempted to provide unrealistic, overly heroic therapies because they are unable to accept the patient's grim status.

The ethical use of tyrosine kinase inhibitors

Tyrosine kinase inhibitors (TKIs), which are tumoristatic therapies, are a promising new modality of care for aggressive metastatic cancers, and have been approved for use by the US Food and Drug Administration for MTC. However, they are expensive, and are generally only available to the wealthy unless there is a third-party payor willing to accept the costs (thousands of dollars per week). Thus, although they can be effective drugs, price restricts access for most uninsured patients (although compassionate use can be available). TKIs are not offered in many countries with universal health care because of their costs. Can clinicians ethically defend what they charge patients for TKIs, particularly in situations in which benefit is not absolute?[61] Some investigators have compared the price of TKIs with so-called price gouging.[62] TKIs can work well in a variety of patients with aggressive cancers, and can achieve greater longevity. When costs are unsustainable for any long-term use, this needs to be part of the informed consent process. Many patients elect to self-ration and opt not to spend their entire financial estates, intended for their children, to buy themselves a few more months.[63] The use of TKIs is difficult to defend as a beneficent therapy when patients have no access to them. Thus, unless it is available as a clinical trial, recommendation of TKIs must be balanced with access and the socioeconomic status of patients. Post-trial access is also a consideration.

Confidentiality, Genomics, and MTC

When genetic screening is done in cases of suspected hereditary MTC, a genetic counselor should be involved if possible, because thyroid practitioners are not typically trained in proper genetic counseling.[64] Ethical problems may involve socioeconomic or psychosocial barriers to screening; psychosocial harms consequent to positive results, which could include emotional distress and genetic discrimination.[65] Ethical dilemmas arise when the presenting patient either refuses genetic screening from the outset, or a patient who tests positive for the mutations refuses to disclose results to at-risk relatives. There are different considerations in the adult and pediatric contexts.[65] In adult populations the legal and ethical duty to warn identifiable third parties of foreseeable, serious harm was established in *Tarasoff. v Regents of the University of California*,[66,67] in which the court held that: "privacy ends where the public peril begins."[66] The duty to warn is an accepted ethical and legal standard used not just for public safety in the mental health context but in the infectious disease and highly penetrant genetic disease context. The legal doctrine of duty to warn is built on several pre-HIPAA cases, but HIPAA provides exceptions for warning in the same situations that existed before HIPAA, as does the American Society of Human Genetics. In 2013, the American College of Medical Genetics stated that warning of RET mutations should be mandatory in cases of whole-genome sequencing.[68] *Pate v Threlkel*,[67,69] a case about inherited MTC, established that physicians have a duty to warn a patient's children or other intended beneficiaries of genetic risk, but the duty could be satisfied by warning the patient.[67] *Safer v the Estate of Pack*,[70] another genetic risk case, helps to establish that physicians cannot satisfy the duty to warn by merely warning the patient, and that they must take "reasonable steps to guarantee that immediate family members are warned."[71] However, more recently, the legal and ethical concept of duty to rescue has been promoted in the genomics context as a more appropriate framework. The duty to rescue is based on the premise that a clinician or investigator must take action to try to prevent serious harm when she/he "discovers genetic information that clearly indicates a high probability of a serious condition for which there is an effective intervention." Other considerations in the genetic context can include the privilege to disclose,[72] the duty to share,[73] and the duty to disclose.[74]

In cases in which there are pediatric patients at high risk of developing MTC in childhood, practitioners should refer to the specific 2011 pediatric ethics guidelines for hereditary MTC published in the *International Journal of Pediatric Endocrinology*.[65]

ETHICAL FRAMEWORKS FOR VULNERABLE POPULATIONS

For thyroid practitioners dealing with prenatal, pediatric, or elderly populations, there are different ethical frameworks and considerations. Although there are other noted vulnerable patient populations that include the mentally ill, homeless, undocumented immigrants, and prisoners, this article does not deal with the complexity of ethical problems in such populations. Health disparities have not been adequately explored in the context of thyroid disease,[75] but, culled from other literature, any vulnerable population that does not have access to adequate health insurance[76] or primary care is not likely to have access to thyroid disease screening or adequate treatments.

An exhaustive and separate literature exists on health disparities in minority populations, which persist because of long-standing socioeconomic issues (education, income, insurance) and cultural distrust of institutionalized medicine in populations formerly abused. (See, for example, Washington HA. *Medical Apartheid, The Dark History of Medical Experimentation on Black Americans from Colonial Times to the Present*. Random House, 2008 or the works of Annette Dula.)

Prenatal Ethics Frameworks

In prenatal populations, prenatal ethics frameworks need to be adopted; such frameworks were established by the work of McCullough and Chervenak,[77,78] who outlined when the nonviable fetus is a patient, and even when the preimplanted embryo is a patient in the assisted conception context.[79] It is generally accepted that a previable fetus is considered to be a patient when the mother presents her fetus as a patient by declaring her interest in her fetus's well-being; here, the fetus needs to be morally considered in all treatment plans. The fetus does not have independent moral status, but rather dependent moral status, because fetal well-being cannot override maternal well-being. In this context, the practitioner must weigh the consequences of various therapies in pregnancy and during lactation. In contrast, viable fetuses are typically assumed to be patients unless there are extraordinary circumstances.

With the viable fetus, avoiding those harms not clearly outweighed by potential benefits is essential.

Preventative screening for maternal hypothyroidism

There is still debate over prophylactic screening for maternal hypothyroidism[80] despite the wide consensus that gestational hypothyroidism (particularly during the first 8 weeks of pregnancy) should be avoided, and that it leads to poor neonatal outcomes, impaired neuropsychological development in childhood, and fetal loss.[81,82] Cost-benefit analyses notwithstanding, when the fetus is a patient, health care providers have a clear ethical duty to prevent certain, probable, or imminent harms to a developing fetus. Although controversy remains over routinely screening pregnant women for thyroid dysfunction, most guidelines agree that screening should be done in pregnant women at high risk for thyroid dysfunction. However, clinical precedents exist for practitioners to adopt routine prenatal screenings in the absence of clear guidelines for conditions that occur less frequently than maternal hypothyroidism.[83–88] In this context, individual practitioners need to use medical judgment regarding prenatal screening.

Because hypothyroidism occurs in 2.5% of the fertile female population,[89] the moral obligation to avoid preventable and imminent harm is not ethically controversial.

Pediatric Ethics Frameworks

Pediatric ethicists support empowering pediatric patients, when possible, to make their own medical decisions. This framework is endorsed by the consensus statement "Informed Consent, Parental Permission, and Assent in Pediatric Practice" issued by the American Pediatric Association's Committee on Bioethics (see http://www.cirp.org/library/ethics/AAP/).[90] The document highlights the following: (1) children and adolescents should be included in all decisions, unless there is a good reason to exclude them. (2) Practitioners should empower children in decision making to the extent of the child's capacity (see **Box 1**); in the case of an adolescent, the capacity to make a decision is usually very high. (3) There is recognition that informed consent as a concept in adult care needs to be replaced with the dual concept of parental permission and pediatric assent.

Pediatric ethics uses a case-based system for empowering pediatric patients in making medical decisions, and there is no formal age of assent, although typically the criteria for decision-making capacity become pronounced in the adolescent years.

When to involve child protective services

Regardless of the capacity of the pediatric patient (see **Box 1**), there may be problems with parental refusal, and children cannot be treated without consent (understood as permission) from their legal guardians. The theoretical threshold to invoke state intervention is the harm principle.[91] The harm principle (from J. S. Mill, *On Liberty*, 1859) is an autonomy-limiting concept under the Principle of Nonmaleficence. The harm principle establishes that competent individuals have complete autonomy over their own beliefs and actions so long as those beliefs or actions do not create a significant likelihood of serious harm to another person. If one's actions or decisions place another in harm's way, state intervention is justified, and practitioners are obligated to prevent imminent harm under the Principle of Nonmaleficence. In the context of thyroid disease, the following examples merit invoking the harm principle: (1) parental refusal of thyroid hormone for hypothyroid children; (2) parental refusal of treatment of pediatric thyroid cancer, including prophylactic thyroidectomy in RET-positive children at risk for MTC before the age of 18 years; or (3) concerns that an adult patient's impairment or other actions places a child in harm's way, which could involve impaired hypothyroid parents who drive children or MTC adult patients who test positive for the RET mutation who refuse to have their at-risk children screened.

Practitioners need to understand that calling their respective state's child protective services (CPS) merely initiates an independent review by the state, but the determination of medical neglect is the sole responsibility of CPS and not the health care providers, the institutional ethics consultants, or institutional legal experts. Health care providers have a professional ethical duty to report all cases of suspected medical neglect to CPS, which is understood as an obligation under the Principle of Nonmaleficence.

Geriatric Ethics Frameworks

Geriatric ethics frameworks[92–94] emphasize decision-making capacity assessments during times of lucidity and physiologic comfort; signs of consistency in a patient's expressed values and preferences to help guide care during times when decision-making capacity is impaired or cannot be assessed. In this model, autonomy-based and beneficence-based obligations are to involve patients in decisions to the extent that they can, which includes truth telling and truthful prognostication[43]; shared decision-making models, in which the practitioner offers to help the patient reach a decision; and equality of therapeutic options so that the patient's age or limited capacity does not present a barrier to treatment. For example, thyroid screenings in elderly populations reveal a significant percentage of untreated thyroid disease contributing to age-related morbidity.[95] Thus, the diagnosis of dementia does not mean that TSH screening should be ignored, or that thyroid hormone should not be prescribed. Frail and elderly patients similarly should not automatically be relegated to comfort care only for thyroid cancer because of their age or capacity; however, aggressive treatments for micropapillary carcinomas, for example, need to be balanced using beneficence frameworks.

Special problems in geriatric populations involve behaviors known as counterdependence,[93] in which the patient mounts a defensive against dependence, denies needing help, and is hostile toward anyone who tries to help. There are also times in which the respective state's adult protective services (APS) need to be called. The theoretical threshold for involving APS is similar to that of CPS, and the harm principle,[91] which may be invoked in cases of guardianship. Guardians may be adult children of patients or may be state guardians. Signs of elder abuse, improper care at long-term care facilities, or guardian refusal of beneficent (not necessarily lifesaving) therapies are grounds for APS involvement. What constitutes beneficent care is any care that improves patient well-being, which must be balanced against quality of life or active life expectancy, meaning that a treatment would improve functionality and self-reliance, rather than further deteriorate it. Functional activities include independent bathing, dressing, mobility, and eating, whereas loss of these functional abilities represents loss of independence.[93]

RESOURCE ALLOCATION AND PRIORITY SETTING

Resource allocation in health care refers to the allocation of both abundant and scarce resources, which require different allocation frameworks. However, changes in pharmaceutical manufacturing processes and limited competition have led to scarcity in resources previously considered abundant. In the context of thyroid disease, drug shortages in rhTSH and even levothyroxine are seen, and shortages in medical radioisotopes caused by aging nuclear reactors are highly problematic,[96] prompting the passage by the US Congress of the American Medical Isotope Production Act, which is a 2013 bill that seeks to create facilities for domestic sources of medical radioisotopes.

The first proposed guideline for how to priority set for shortages in the thyroid context were published by the American Thyroid Association's Ethics Advisory Committee[22] in which a consequentialist framework is suggested. Consequentialist frameworks, in which both clinical and social criteria are used, consider both medical and psychosocial factors. These factors are critical when impairment is a consideration in patient selection for a scarce resource, particularly when impairment may affect intended beneficiaries of patients. In such frameworks the 23-year-old single mother with iodine-avid thyroid cancer, who cannot afford time off from work to support her special-needs child with cystic fibrosis, may take priority for rhTSH over the self-employed 50-year-old single man with no dependents, with the same diagnosis. Or consider two 55-year-old women with the same diagnosis; one takes care of her mother with advanced dementia; one is a retired widow with 2 grown, healthy adult children. The caregiver may be the best candidate for rhTSH. Using solely clinical criteria does not produce the same results. However, there may be exceptions when patients with thyroid cancer with pituitary defects do not have any other option except rhTSH.

In the context of nuclear disasters, panic buying of potassium iodide has occurred on the US west coast, without any rational or ethical distribution protocol. Potassium iodide distribution in areas in close proximity to nuclear power plants, or in the aftermath of a nuclear disaster, should be guided by a similar consequentialist framework.

Rationing protocols have developed over time, and are informed by poor protocols used in scarce resources, including protocols used in rationing insulin (1921), based on political persuasion; penicillin (1943), based on severity of infection without any selection transparency; hemodialysis (1961), based on subjective social worth criteria; and liver transplantation, before 1998, based on a first come, first served principle.[96]

SUMMARY

In the context of thyroid disease management, clinical ethics dilemmas affect a wide range of health care providers: endocrinologists, primary care physicians, surgeons, oncologists, nuclear medicine specialists and technologists, genetic counselors, nurses, and physician assistants.

Thyroid practitioners are more familiar with issues arising out of the treatment of autoimmune thyroid diseases, such as patient compliance with thyroid hormone replacement, or informed consent issues in the use of RAI. More recently, as the number of aggressive, iodine non-avid thyroid cancers increases, many thyroid practitioners are facing ethical dilemmas that are novel in the thyroid disease context but are classic in oncology and critical care contexts: end of life issues. For example, in the treatment of ATC, discussions need to be more concerned with palliative care, hospice, and code status than the relative merits of systemic RAI, which is a typical discussion in well-differentiated thyroid cancers.

New ethical dilemmas also present in hereditary MTC, in which questions concerning duties to pediatric populations have emerged, as well as other at-risk populations. In addition, with the increase in whole-genome sequencing, the recommendation of mandatory disclosure of the RET mutation in at-risk populations has presented new controversies.

Another novel ethical dilemma for thyroid practitioners concerns drug shortages, in which common drugs such as levothyroxine sodium, rhTSH, or medical isotopes go through periodic shortages prompting priority setting decisions typically seen in scarce resources contexts. Novel ethical issues are also arising with the passage of the US Affordable Care Act, which has increased access to thyroid screening through access to primary care services.

More difficult clinical ethics dilemmas also concern the standard of care in thyroid disease management, which has recently become more controversial because of the absence of well-designed clinical trials that can confirm what has been observed in clinical practice and in different patient populations. This absence has resulted in a situation in which there is frequent disagreement within the community of experts over whether treatment A is better than treatment B; this is known as clinical equipoise.

With a fuller understanding of core ethical principles, thyroid practitioners may have a deeper appreciation of how to frame ethical dilemmas and how to balance competing principles.

REFERENCES

1. Beauchamp TL, Childress JL. The principles of biomedical ethics. 6th edition. New York: Oxford University Press; 2008.
2. The National Commission for the Protection of Human Subjects of Biomedical and Behavioral Research. The Belmont report: ethical principles and guidelines for the protection of human subjects of research. Department of Health and Human Services; 1979.
3. Faden RR, Beauchamp TL. A history and theory of informed consent. New York: Oxford University Press; 1989.
4. Trials of war criminals before the Nuremberg Military Tribunals under control council law No. 10, vol. 2. Washington, DC: US Government Printing Office; 1949.
5. Reverby SM. Ethical failures and history lessons: The U.S. Public Health Service research studies in Tuskegee and Guatemala. Public Health Rev 2012;34.
6. Beecher HK. Ethics and clinical research. N Engl J Med 1966;274:1354.
7. Committee on Evaluation of the 1950s Air Force Human Health Testing in Alaska Using Radioactive Iodine 131, National Research Council. The Arctic Aeromedical Laboratory's thyroid function study: a radiological risk and ethical analysis. Washington, DC: National Academy Press; 1996.
8. Beauchamp TL. The origins and evolution of the Belmont report. In: Standing on Principles. New York: Oxford University Press; 2010. p. 4.
9. Gert B, Culver CM, Clouser KD. Bioethics, a systematic approach. 2nd edition. New York: Oxford University Press; 2006.
10. Etchells E, Sharpe G, Walsh P, et al. Bioethics for clinicians: 1. Consent. CMAJ 1996;155:177.
11. Etchells E, Sharpe G, Burgess MM, et al. Bioethics for clinicians: 2. Disclosure. CMAJ 1996;155:387.
12. Etchells E, Sharpe G, Elliott C, et al. Bioethics for clinicians: 3. Capacity. CMAJ 1996;155:657.
13. Etchells E, Sharpe G, Dykeman MJ, et al. Bioethics for clinicians: 4. Voluntariness. CMAJ 1996;155:1083.
14. *Schloendorff v Society of New York Hospital*, 211 NY. 125, 105 NE. 92 (1914).
15. *Salgo v Leland Stanford Jr. University Board of Trustees*, 317P 2d 170,181 (1957).
16. *Natanson v Klein*, 350 P 2d 1093 (1960).
17. *Canterbury v Spence*, 464 F 2d 772 (DC Cir 1972).

18. *Cobbs v Grant*, 8 Cal 3d 229, 502 P 2d 1, 104 Cal Rptr 505 (Cal 1972).
19. *Wilkinson v Vesey*, 110 RI 606, 624 (1972).
20. Clayton EW. Ethical, legal, and social implications of genomic medicine. N Engl J Med 2003;349:562.
21. Thomas Percival (1740-1804) Codifier of Medical Ethics. JAMA 1965;194:1319.
22. Rosenthal MS, Angelos P, Cooper DS, et al. Clinical and professional ethics guidelines for the practice of thyroidology. Thyroid 2013;23(10):1203-10.
23. Rosenthal MS. Patient misconceptions and ethical challenges in radioactive iodine scanning and therapy. J Nucl Med Technol 2006;34:143.
24. Rosenthal MS. The impaired hypothyroid patient: ethical considerations and obligations. Thyroid 2007;17:1261.
25. Chapman EM, Evans RD. The treatment of hyperthyroidism with radioactive iodine. J Am Med Assoc 1946;131:86.
26. Hertz S, Roberts A. Radioactive iodine in the study of thyroid physiology; the use of radioactive iodine therapy in hyperthyroidism. J Am Med Assoc 1946;131:81.
27. Sawin CT, Becker DV. Radioiodine and the treatment of hyperthyroidism: the early history. Thyroid 1997;7:163.
28. Wartofsky L, Glinoer D, Solomon B, et al. Differences and similarities in the diagnosis and treatment of Graves' disease in Europe, Japan, and the United States. Thyroid 1991;1:129.
29. Walsh JP. Management of Graves' disease in Australia. Aust N Z J Med 2000;30:559.
30. Singer PA, Cooper DS, Levy EG, et al. Treatment guidelines for patients with hyperthyroidism and hypothyroidism. Standards of Care Committee, American Thyroid Association. JAMA 1995;273:808.
31. Bahn RS, Burch HB, Cooper DS, et al. Hyperthyroidism and other causes of thyrotoxicosis: management guidelines of the American Thyroid Association and American Association of Clinical Endocrinologists. Endocr Pract 2011;17:456.
32. Zimmerman D. Fetal and neonatal hyperthyroidism. Thyroid 1999;9:727.
33. Brownlie BE, Rae AM, Walshe JW, et al. Psychoses associated with thyrotoxicosis – 'thyrotoxic psychosis.' A report of 18 cases, with statistical analysis of incidence. Eur J Endocrinol 2000;142:438.
34. Jadresic DP. Psychiatric aspects of hyperthyroidism. J Psychosom Res 1990;34:603.
35. Rosenthal MS. Informed consent in the nuclear medicine setting. J Nucl Med Technol 2011;39:1.
36. Garber JR, Cobin RH, Gharib H, et al. Clinical practice guidelines for hypothyroidism in adults: cosponsored by the American Association of Clinical Endocrinologists and the American Thyroid Association. Thyroid 2012;22:1200.
37. Ernst E, Cohen MH, Stone J. Ethical problems arising in evidence based complementary and alternative medicine. J Med Ethics 2004;30:156.
38. Escobar-Morreale HF, Botella-Carretero JI, Escobar del Rey F, et al. REVIEW: treatment of hypothyroidism with combinations of levothyroxine plus liothyronine. J Clin Endocrinol Metab 2005;90:4946.
39. Schiess N, Pardo CA. Hashimoto's encephalopathy. Ann N Y Acad Sci 2008;1142:254.
40. Veatch RM. Abandoning informed consent. Hastings Cent Rep 1995;25:5.
41. Tauber AI. Sick autonomy. Perspect Biol Med 2003;46:484.
42. Stirrat GM, Gill R. Autonomy in medical ethics after O'Neill. J Med Ethics 2005;31:127.

43. Christakis NA. Death foretold: prophecy and prognosis in medical care. Chicago: The University of Chicago Press; 1999.
44. Freedman B. Equipoise and the ethics of clinical research. N Engl J Med 1987; 317:141.
45. Smallridge RC, Ain KB, Asa SL, et al. American Thyroid Association guidelines for management of patients with anaplastic thyroid cancer. Thyroid 2012;22:1104.
46. Kloos RT, Eng C, Evans DB, et al. Medullary thyroid cancer: management guidelines of the American Thyroid Association. Thyroid 2009;19:565.
47. Biffl WL, Spain DA, Reitsma AM, et al. Responsible development and application of surgical innovations: a position statement of the Society of University Surgeons. J Am Coll Surg 2008;206:1204.
48. Sawka AM, Thabane L, Parlea L, et al. Second primary malignancy risk after radioactive iodine treatment for thyroid cancer: a systematic review and meta-analysis. Thyroid 2009;19:451.
49. Jonklaas J, Sarlis NJ, Litofsky D, et al. Outcomes of patients with differentiated thyroid carcinoma following initial therapy. Thyroid 2006;16:1229.
50. Ain KB. Management of undifferentiated thyroid cancer. Baillieres Best Pract Res Clin Endocrinol Metab 2000;14:615.
51. Robenshtok E, Fish S, Bach A, et al. Suspicious cervical lymph nodes detected after thyroidectomy for papillary thyroid cancer usually remain stable over years in properly selected patients. J Clin Endocrinol Metab 2012;97:2706.
52. Levine RJ. Ethics and regulation of clinical research. 2nd edition. New Haven (CT): Yale University Press; 1988.
53. Cooper DS, Doherty GM, Haugen BR, et al. Revised American Thyroid Association management guidelines for patients with thyroid nodules and differentiated thyroid cancer. Thyroid 2009;19:1167.
54. McLeod DS, Sawka AM, Cooper DS. Controversies in primary treatment of low-risk papillary thyroid cancer. Lancet 2013;381:1046.
55. Sawka AM, Goldstein DP, Brierley JD, et al. The impact of thyroid cancer and post-surgical radioactive iodine treatment on the lives of thyroid cancer survivors: a qualitative study. PLoS One 2009;4:e4191.
56. Mihailovic J, Stefanovic L, Stankovic R. Influence of initial treatment on the survival and recurrence in patients with differentiated thyroid microcarcinoma. Clin Nucl Med 2013;38:332.
57. Manuel SH. Surviving does not equal thriving: exploring the impact of thyroid cancer on young women's quality of life [thesis]. Ottawa (Canada): Library and Archives Canada; 2010.
58. Dorn R, Kopp J, Vogt H, et al. Dosimetry-guided radioactive iodine treatment in patients with metastatic differentiated thyroid cancer: largest safe dose using a risk-adapted approach. J Nucl Med 2003;44:451.
59. Hickman SE, Nelson CA, Moss AH, et al. Use of the physician orders for life-sustaining treatment (POLST) paradigm program in the hospice setting. J Palliat Med 2009;12:133.
60. Rushton CH. Defining and addressing moral distress: tools for critical care nursing leaders. AACN Adv Crit Care 2006;17:161.
61. Bible KC. Taking stock of therapeutic progress in metastatic radioactive iodine-refractory differentiated thyroid cancer: what's next? Thyroid 2013;23:383.
62. Experts in Chronic Myeloid Leukemia. The price of drugs for chronic myeloid leukemia (CML) is a reflection of the unsustainable prices of cancer drugs: from the perspective of a large group of CML experts. Blood 2013;121:4439.

63. Singer P. Why we must ration health care. New York Times 2009.
64. Demmer LA, O'Neill MJ, Roberts AE, et al. Knowledge of ethical standards in genetic testing among medical students, residents, and practicing physicians. JAMA 2000;284:2595.
65. Rosenthal MS, Diekema DS. Pediatric ethics guidelines for hereditary medullary thyroid cancer. Int J Pediatr Endocrinol 2011;847603:2011.
66. *Tarasoff v Regents of University of California*, in: 17 Cal 3d 425, 551 P 2d 334, 131 Cal Rptr 14 (1976).
67. Rosenthal MS, Pierce HH. Inherited medullary thyroid cancer and the duty to warn: revisiting Pate v. Threlkel in light of HIPAA. Thyroid 2005;15:140.
68. Green RC, Berg JS, Grody WW, et al. ACMG recommendations for reporting of incidental findings in clinical exome and genome sequencing. Genet Med 2013; 15:565.
69. *Pate v Threlkel*, in: 661 So 2d 278 (Fla 1995).
70. *Safer v Estate of T. Pack*, 677 A 2d 1188 (NJ Supp 1996).
71. Laberge AM, Burke W. Duty to warn at-risk family members of genetic disease. Virtual Mentor 2009;11:656.
72. Suter SM. Whose genes are these anyway?: familial conflicts over access to genetic information. Mich Law Rev 1854;91:1993.
73. Parker M, Lucassen AM. Genetic information: a joint account? BMJ 2004;329:165.
74. Callier S, Simpson R. Genetic diseases and the duty to disclose. Virtual Mentor 2012;14:640.
75. Golden SH, Brown A, Cauley JA, et al. Health disparities in endocrine disorders: biological, clinical, and nonclinical factors–an Endocrine Society scientific statement. J Clin Endocrinol Metab 2012;97:E1579.
76. Wilper AP, Woolhandler S, Lasser KE, et al. Health insurance and mortality in US adults. Am J Public Health 2009;99:2289.
77. Chervenak FA, McCullough LB. The fetus as a patient: an essential ethical concept for maternal-fetal medicine. J Matern Fetal Med 1996;5:115.
78. Chervenak FA, McCullough LB. The fetus as a patient: an essential concept for the ethics of perinatal medicine. Am J Perinatol 2003;20:399.
79. Chervenak FA, McCullough L. Ethical implications of the embryo as a patient. In: Kurjak A, Chervenak F, editors. The embryo as a patient. New York: Parthenon Publishing; 2001. p. 226.
80. Stagnaro-Green A, Abalovich M, Alexander E, et al. Guidelines of the American Thyroid Association for the diagnosis and management of thyroid disease during pregnancy and postpartum. Thyroid 2011;21:1081.
81. Krajewski DA, Burman KD. Thyroid disorders in pregnancy. Endocrinol Metab Clin North Am 2011;40:739.
82. American Thyroid Association. Consensus statement #2: American Thyroid Association statement on early maternal thyroidal insufficiency: recognition, clinical management and research directions. Thyroid 2005;15:77.
83. Delange F. Screening for congenital hypothyroidism used as an indicator of the degree of iodine deficiency and of its control. Thyroid 1998;8:1185.
84. Van Vliet G. Neonatal hypothyroidism: treatment and outcome. Thyroid 1999;9:79.
85. Kondo A, Kamihira O, Ozawa H. Neural tube defects: prevalence, etiology and prevention. Int J Urol 2009;16:49.
86. Collins JS, Kirby RS. Birth defects surveillance, epidemiology, and significance in public health. Birth Defects Res A Clin Mol Teratol 2009;85:873.
87. Wille MC, Weitz B, Kerper P, et al. Advances in preconception genetic counseling. J Perinat Neonatal Nurs 2004;18:28.

88. Solomon BD, Jack BW, Feero WG. The clinical content of preconception care: genetics and genomics. Am J Obstet Gynecol 2008;199:S340.
89. Wang C, Crapo LM. The epidemiology of thyroid disease and implications for screening. Endocrinol Metab Clin North Am 1997;26:189.
90. Bartholome WG. Informed consent, parental permission, and assent in pediatric practice. Pediatrics 1995;96:981.
91. Diekema DS. Parental refusals of medical treatment: the harm principle as threshold for state intervention. Theor Med Bioeth 2004;25:243.
92. Agich GJ. Autonomy and long-term care. New York: Oxford University Press; 1993.
93. Agich G. Dependence and autonomy in old age: an ethical framework for long-term care. Boston: Cambridge University Press; 2003.
94. Leuzy A, Gauthier S. Ethical issues in Alzheimer's disease: an overview. Expert Rev Neurother 2012;12:557.
95. Visser WE, Visser TJ, Peeters RP. Thyroid disorders in older adults. Endocrinol Metab Clin North Am 2013;42:287.
96. Rosenthal MS. Ethical issues in radioisotope shortages: rationing and priority setting. J Nucl Med Technol 2010;38:117.
97. Roth LH, Meisel A, Lidz CW. Tests of competency to consent to treatment. Am J Psychiatry 1977;134:279–84.
98. Buchanan AE, Brock DW. Deciding for others: the ethics of surrogate decision making. Cambridge (United Kingdom): Cambridge University Press; 1989.
99. Grisso T, Appelbaum PA. The assessment of decision-making capacity: a guide for physicians and other health professionals. Oxford (United Kingdom): Oxford University Press; 1998.
100. Culver CM, Gert B. The Inadequacy of Competence. Milbank Q 1990;68(4):619–43.

Management of Recurrent Cervical Papillary Thyroid Cancer

Rachna M. Goyal, MD[a,b,*], Jacqueline Jonklaas, MD, PhD[b],
Kenneth D. Burman, MD[a]

KEYWORDS

- Papillary thyroid cancer • Cervical lymph nodes • Ethanol injection
- Radioactive iodine • Cervical re-operation

KEY POINTS

- Thyroid cancer is the most common endocrine malignancy, and its incidence and prevalence are on the rise.
- Papillary thyroid cancer has been shown to metastasize and recur in the locoregional lymph nodes of the neck.
- Options for treatment of recurrent cervical papillary thyroid cancer include observation, surgery, radioactive iodine ablation, or percutaneous ethanol injection.

INTRODUCTION

Thyroid cancer is the most common endocrine malignancy, and its incidence and prevalence are on the rise. According to the American Cancer Society, the projected incidence of thyroid cancer for 2013 was 60,220 new cases (45,310 in women and 14,910 in men), with 1850 deaths from thyroid cancer (1040 women and 810 men).[1] Fortunately, most of these patients achieve good disease-specific outcomes if treated appropriately at the time of diagnosis. However, up to 30% of patients experience persistent disease or recurrences, often limited to cervical lymph nodes.[2] The management of these recurrent lymph nodes remains controversial, and the current guidelines do not clearly outline the best options. The existing literature consists of retrospective studies with small sample sizes; no prospective, large randomized trials are available that delineate the various treatment modalities. Currently, there are several approaches to patients with recurrent papillary thyroid cancer (PTC) in their cervical lymph nodes, including observation, radioactive iodine therapy, ethanol

[a] Division of Endocrinology, Washington Hospital Center, 110 Irving Street Northwest, Washington, DC 20010, USA; [b] Division of Endocrinology, Georgetown University Hospital, 4000 Reservoir Road Northwest, Building D Room 232, Washington, DC 20007, USA
* Corresponding author. Division of Endocrinology, Washington Hospital Center, 110 Irving Street Northwest, Washington, DC 20010.
E-mail address: RachnaMGoyal@gmail.com

Endocrinol Metab Clin N Am 43 (2014) 565–572
http://dx.doi.org/10.1016/j.ecl.2014.02.014
0889-8529/14/$ – see front matter © 2014 Elsevier Inc. All rights reserved.

injection, and surgery. The management approach should be a joint decision between the health care team and the patient.

BACKGROUND

The incidence of well-differentiated thyroid cancer continues to rise; in particular, the mortality rate of older men with differentiated thyroid cancer is increasing at an alarming rate. There are several risk factors associated with PTC. These include female gender (3 times more common in women), previous exposure to ionizing radiation, and rare hereditary conditions (eg, Cowden syndrome). Approximately 5% of patients with PTC will have familial PTC; the exact genetic cause has not yet been determined. Although mortality from thyroid cancer is low, the recurrence rate is 25% to 35%, making risk stratification a priority. Prognostic factors such as age less than 15 years or greater than or equal to 45 years, male gender, tumor size greater than 4 cm, follicular histology or tall and columnar cell variants, multifocality, initial local tumor invasion, and regional lymph node metastasis are associated with increased risk of recurrence.[3] Prediction of nodal metastases can also be determined based on several of the previously mentioned features, and additionally the genotype – BRAF-positive tumors are associated with higher rates of metastases, and therefore should not be solely observed but treated with more aggressive options.[4] Several risk factors for recurrence also include older age, follicular variant PTC, cervical lymph node involvement, T4 tumors, and stage greater than 4A.[5] Often, it may be difficult to distinguish between persistent and recurrent disease, and many of the patients thought to have recurrences may actually have had residual microscopic disease.

According to the American Thyroid Association (ATA) revised guidelines on the management and treatment of differentiated thyroid cancer from 2009, the initial surgical option for those with a tumor size of greater than 1 cm, is a near-total or total thyroidectomy. Thyroid lobectomy should be reserved for those with low-risk disease, micropapillary carcinoma, unifocality, absence of lymph nodes, and no personal history of head and neck irradiation. All patients with fine-needle aspiration proven differentiated thyroid cancer should be staged preoperatively and undergo a neck ultrasound with node mapping evaluating the contralateral lobe and lymph nodes for the presence of disease.[6] In the presence of metastatic disease in the central or lateral neck, regional lymph node dissection is often indicated.[7] However, performing prophylactic lymph node dissection at the time of thyroidectomy is controversial, and surgical expertise is warranted. However, it allows pathologic identification of metastases and leads to up-staging in patients over the age of 45. This can help guide further treatment options, including utility and dose of radioactive iodine.[8]

The thyroid gland has a rich lymphatic supply, allowing the possibility of thyroid cancer to spread to local lymph nodes in the central and lateral compartments of the neck. The lymph nodes of the neck are divided into 6 levels (**Fig. 1**). Level 1 is split into 2 sublevels: sublevel 1A (submental) and sublevel 2B (submandibular). Level 2 is upper jugular; level 3 is midjugular, and level 4 is lower jugular. Level 5 comprises the posterior triangle nodes including the supraclavicular nodes and spinal accessory nodes. The anterior compartment lymph nodes are located in level 6 and include the pretracheal and paratracheal lymph nodes, precricoid nodes, and perithyroidal lymph nodes.

Neck ultrasound is the imaging modality of choice to monitor well-differentiated thyroid cancer after total thyroidectomy. Certain sonographic features can help determine whether a lymph node is malignant or normal. Worrisome features for the presence of thyroid cancer include shape (taller than wide), irregular margins, lack of an echogenic hilus, the presence of calcifications, and enhanced perinodularvascularity.[9]

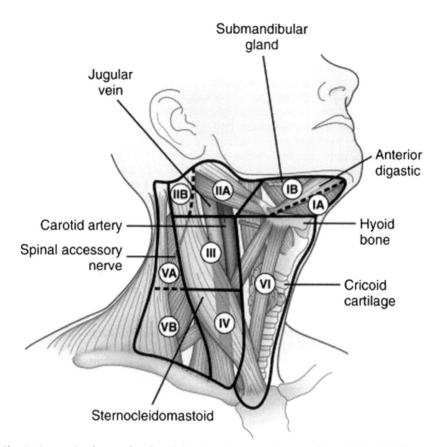

Fig. 1. Anatomic scheme of neck with lymph node compartments. (*From* Smith PW, Salomone LJ, Hanks JB. Thyroid. In: Sabiston DC, Townsend CM. Sabiston textbook of surgery: the biological basis of modern surgical practice. 19th edition. Philadelphia: Elsevier Saunders; 2012; with permission.)

Head and neck cancers tend to metastasize to specific lymph node clusters. Thyroid cancer in particular spreads to lymph nodes in the lower third of the neck in 67% of cases, the middle third in 20% of cases, and the superior third in13% of cases. This is in contrast to benign lymph nodes, which are more commonly seen the superior and middle thirds of the neck.[10] Flat, oval-shaped lymph nodes are considered benign, whereas round lymph nodes are often concerning for malignancy.[11] The type of border surrounding the lymph node and its correlation with cancer are somewhat controversial. In general, benign-appearing lymph nodes tend to have sharp borders, and cancerous nodes tend to have ill-defined borders on ultrasound.[12] The hilum of a normal lymph node appears as an eccentric, echogenic intranodal structure that is continuous with the adjacent perinodal fat. In malignant lymph nodes, this hilum frequently becomes obliterated. Metastatic lymph nodes also exhibit peripheral vascular patterns, unlike benign lymph nodes.[9] Cervical lymph node calcification is uncommonly found, but it can signify thyroid cancer infiltration.[13]

Although ultrasound is the imaging modality of choice of thyroid cancer, computed tomography (CT), magnetic resonance imaging (MRI), or positron emission tomography (PET) can be useful in monitoring patients with thyroid cancer and for preoperative planning. These alternated imaging modalities may be useful in the assessment of large, rapidly growing, retrosternal, or invasive tumors to characterize the involvement of extrathyroidal.[6] Fluorodeoxyglucose PET has been known to show metastases in ^{131}I scan-negative thyroid cancer patients with a high accuracy, which is thought to be related to increased glucose metabolism in poorly differentiated carcinoma.[14] The preoperative use of PET remains controversial and has not been thoroughly evaluated. It can be useful in patients with a high tumor stage and less nodal disease than expected or in those with indeterminate nodes on CT or MRI.[15]

Before reviewing the management options for cervical recurrent well-differentiated thyroid cancer, several questions remain unanswered. How often do cervical lymph nodes grow and cause significant local disease? Do local cervical metastases lead to distant metastases? Does removal of these metastatic cervical lymph nodes improve morbidity and mortality? There are no controlled studies evaluating these questions, but the various treatment options will be discussed.[16]

SURGERY

The frequency of locoregional recurrence is anywhere from 5% to 20% in PTC, and more than one-third of reoperations for persistent or recurrent disease are related to insufficient initial thyroid surgery.[17] If a recurrence is easily palpable or visualized on radiography, excision should be strongly considered, because even small lymph node metastases are commonly more extensive than would appear clinically or on imaging.[18] In a study done by Travagli and colleagues in France, 54 patients with persistent or recurrent disease in the neck after surgery for thyroid cancer were enrolled to undergo a combination protocol of radioiodine and probe-guided surgery. Interestingly, in 14 patients, lymph node metastases were not initially visualized by the surgical probe or postoperative ^{131}I whole-body scan, but were found upon histologic dissection. This argues for neck dissection for recurrent thyroid cancer as a means to detect hidden metastases. However, the clinical significance of these smaller metastases in long-term outcomes and prognosis remains controversial.

Al-Saif and colleagues[19] retrospectively analyzed 95 patients with a neck dissection for recurrent or persistent PTC in the cervical lymph nodes. This cohort of patients underwent lymphadenectomies, and complete biochemical remission was initially achieved in only 17% of the patients with an undetectable serum thyroglobulin level after 1 cervical neck dissection. After 2 or 3 reoperations, 27% achieved biochemical remission. In those patients who did not reach biochemical remission, there was a significant reduction in serum thyroglobulin levels after both the first and second reoperation, and none of the patients developed detectable distant metastases or died from PTC during a 60-month average follow-up. The efficacy of first reoperation was subsequently observed by Yim and colleagues,[20] who noted that 51% of patients attained biochemical remission with a stimulated thyroglobulin level of less than 1 ng/mL. Those with stimulated thyroglobulin levels greater than 5 ng/mL after the first reoperation had a higher chance of clinical recurrence (the estimated 5-year clinical recurrence-free survival rate was 94 vs 74). Additionally, Clayman and colleagues[21] reported that 71% of patients had an undetectable unstimulated thyroglobulin levels (<3 ng/mL) after reoperation.

The efficacy of cervical neck dissection depends on the how successful the surgery was; the optimal goal appears to be negative thyroid ultrasounds and undetectable thyroglobulin levels. There is clearly a range of patients that achieve this goal, anywhere from 17% to 71%. The potential complications of a reoperation must also be weighed and discussed with the patient. For small metastases, a reasonable approach is radioiodine, but their persistence after 2 or 3 treatments should usually lead to surgery.[22] Conversely, compartmental surgical dissections may not be feasible in compartments that have been previously explored due to extensive scarring, and only a more limited or targeted lymph node resection may be possible.

RADIOACTIVE IODINE THERAPY

Radioactive iodine (RAI) therapy is often used in the initial treatment for PTC. The initial dose of radioactive iodine 131 after total thyroidectomy is primarily utilized for 1 of 3 reasons: (1) remnant ablation, (2) adjuvant therapy, or (3) to treat known or suspected local or distant disease. RAI therapy after total thyroidectomy is the mainstay of treatment for patients with high-risk disease (evidence of distant metastasis, extrathyroidal extension, tumor size >4 cm). For low-risk patients (unifocal or multifocal tumor burden <1 cm without high-risk features), the use of remnant ablation is usually not necessary.[6] Its utility is more controversial for those patients with intermediate-risk disease. Unfortunately the role of RAI therapy for the treatment of persistent or recurrent cervical lymph nodes is sparse and therefore also remains debatable.

Yim and colleagues[23] retrospectively observed 45 patients who underwent reoperation for locoregionally recurrent PTC with a serum thyroglobulin level of greater than 2 ng/mL. Each of these patients had previously undergone initial thyroidectomy followed by high-dose RAI remnant ablation. Of these 45 participants, 23 received adjuvant RAI therapy, and the remaining 22 did not (control group). The main outcome measures included changes in serum thyroglobulin concentration after reoperation and disease-free survival. Only 15% of patients in the adjuvant group and 33% in the control group showed a greater than 50% decrease in the serum thyroglobulin levels from baseline. The study demonstrated that there were no significant differences in mean serum thyroglobulin concentrations in the adjuvant RAI group versus the control group.

When RAI therapy is being considered, one must take into account the complications associated with it, including secondary malignancies, and more transient risks like sialadenitis, nausea, vomiting, or sore throat. The absolute risk of secondary malignancies is low, although statistically significant. Among patients with differentiated thyroid cancer who have received RAI ablation therapy, the standardized incidence ratio of a secondary primary malignancy is 1.18, compared with those who did not receive RAI. The most common secondary malignancies include cancer of the salivary glands, melanoma, kidney cancer, leukemia, and lymphoma.[24]

OBSERVATION

Monitoring patients with low-risk disease but recurrent or persistent cervical thyroid cancer in the lateral lymph nodes is generally a reasonable approach. Support for this approach was found in a retrospective cohort study analyzing 166 patients with PTC (patients with aggressive histology or clinical features were excluded) and at least 1 abnormal lateral neck lymph node on ultrasound noted during a 3.5-year follow-up period. Only 20% of the patients had lymph nodes that grew at least 3 mm; 9% grew at least 5 mm, and 14% actually resolved. There were no local complications related to the abnormal lymph nodes and no disease-related mortality. The authors concluded that lateral neck lymph nodes could be closely monitored through serum thyroglobulin levels along with clinical and radiologic parameters.[25] Of note, there were some limitations to the study, particularly that only 22% of the patients had biopsy-proven papillary thyroid carcinoma in the lymph nodes.

Thyroid bed nodules have shown similar outcomes to lateral neck lymph nodes. In a retrospective review published in 2011, 191 patients with at least 1 thyroid bed nodule were followed for a median of 5 years. Approximately 9% of the patients had an increase in size of at least 1 nodule, and the average initial size of the nodules was 5 mm. The rate of growth was only 1.3 mm/year, indicating that most thyroid bed nodules do not show clinically significant growth over several years of follow-up.[26] Additionally, the presence of bilateral or mediastinal lymph nodes confers a worse prognosis than unilateral lymph nodes in patients with papillary or follicular thyroid cancer.[27]

In a study by Ito and colleagues,[28] the prognosis of PTC after recurrence to the central neck was investigated. The group concluded that those patients with initial recurrence to the thyroid bed or perithyroid tissue had an overall worse prognosis than those who had an initial recurrence to the lymph nodes. However, if the lymph node was greater than 3 cm, there was an increased mortality over 10 years. Thus, the size of the lymph node metastasis may be a crucial prognostic factor guiding decision making, as is genotype. BRAF-positive tumors should be treated more aggressively rather than being solely monitored. Clearly, further studies are needed to assess the clinical significance of slow-growing lymph nodes and their impact on mortality over time.

ETHANOL INJECTION

Another feasible alternative treatment to surgery, RAI ablation, and observation is percutaneous use of ethanol injections into lymph nodes containing well-differentiated thyroid cancer. This technique has been employed since the 1980s for the palliative treatment of small hepatocellular carcinomas, and is now being more widely used for additional tumors. In 2011, Heilo and colleagues[29] published a retrospective study assessing the efficacy of ultrasound-guided percutaneous ethanol injection as a treatment for metastatic cervical lymph nodes from PTC. They enrolled 63 patients with a total of 109 lymph nodes over a 38.4-month follow-up, and 93% of the ethanol-injected lymph nodes decreased in size, with 84% showing a complete resolution. Of the 38 patients with elevated serum thyroglobulin levels before treatment, 30 patients had undetectable serum thyroglobulin levels after injection. In another study, 29 metastatic lymph nodes were injected with ethanol in 14 patients. The average sonographic follow-up was 18 months, and all the treated lymph nodes decreased in volume, from a mean of 492 mm^3 before percutaneous injection to 76 mm^3 at 1 year and 20 mm^3 at 2 years.[30]

Percutaneous ethanol injection may be useful for patients with a limited number of metastatic lymph nodes who are not amenable to surgery or RAI ablation. The procedure carries low risk and far less invasive than neck re-exploration; additionally, it can be repeated without technical difficulty, has less of a health care burden given its cheaper cost, and has a short recovery time.[31] Conversely, if the ethanol leaks out of the desired cervical lymph node site, it can lead to neck pain and infrequently hoarseness, hypoparathyroidism, and tissue fibrosis. Thus, percutaneous ethanol ablation should be limited to tertiary care centers with experience.

SUMMARY

There are several approaches to patients with recurrent cervical lymph node metastases. Many factors should be taken into consideration when deciding upon the best treatment regimen, including patient comorbidities, patient age, number and location of metastatic lymph nodes, and other high-risk features. For those patients with low-risk disease and a minimal number of metastatic lymph nodes, observation alone is a reasonable strategy. There is insufficient evidence to recommend monitoring alone, but it appears that the growth of cervical lymph nodes or thyroid bed nodules is unusual.

According to the ATA guidelines, surgery is favored for locoregional recurrences when distant metastases are absent.[6] This is particularly true in patients with multiple or bilateral large cervical lymph nodes who have high-risk clinical disease with an unfavorable prognosis. Surgical consideration is also increased when the lymph nodes appear to be enlarging or are near vital structures (eg, trachea or blood vessels). However, surgery has its limitations and risks, and not all patients are ideal surgical candidates. Adjunctive RAI therapy following surgery does not appear to be more effective than monitoring alone for persistent cervical nodal disease, except in patients with cervical node uptake on 131-I scan. Ethanol ablation is associated with a high response rate and few adverse effects, making it a desirable approach in those patients with a limited number of cervical metastatic lymph nodes.

Ultimately, the treatment strategy should consist of a multidisciplinary approach involving the patient and clinicians. The current literature encompasses mostly small, retrospective analyses; thus large randomized controlled studies are needed to further delineate the optimal treatment regimens.

REFERENCES

1. American Cancer Society. Thyroid cancer overview. 2013. Available at: http://www.cancer.org/cancer/thyroidcancer/overviewguide/thyroid-cancer-overview-key-statistics. Accessed November 1, 2013.
2. Hundahl SA, Cady B, Cunningham MP, et al. Initial results from a prospective cohort study of 5583 cases of thyroid carcinoma treated in the united states during 1996. U.S. and German Thyroid Cancer Study Group. An American College of Surgeons Commission on Cancer Patient Care Evaluation study. Cancer 2000;89(1):202–17.
3. Pacini F, Castagna MG. Approach to and treatment of differentiated thyroid carcinoma. Med Clin North Am 2012;96(2):369–83.
4. Nixon IJ, Shaha AR. Management of regional nodes in thyroid cancer. Oral Oncol 2013;49(7):671–5.
5. Grogan RH, Kaplan SP, Cao H, et al. A study of recurrence and death from papillary thyroid cancer with 27 years of median follow-up. Surgery 2013;154(6):1436–46.
6. American Thyroid Association (ATA) Guidelines Taskforce on Thyroid Nodules and Differentiated Thyroid Cancer, Cooper DS, Doherty GM, et al. Revised American Thyroid Association management guidelines for patients with thyroid nodules and differentiated thyroid cancer. Thyroid 2009;19(11):1167–214.
7. Bardet S, Malville E, Rame JP, et al. Macroscopic lymph-node involvement and neck dissection predict lymph-node recurrence in papillary thyroid carcinoma. Eur J Endocrinol 2008;158(4):551–60.
8. Hartl DM, Leboulleux S, Al Ghuzlan A, et al. Optimization of staging of the neck with prophylactic central and lateral neck dissection for papillary thyroid carcinoma. Ann Surg 2012;255(4):777–83.
9. Giacomini CP, Jeffrey RB, Shin LK. Ultrasonographic evaluation of malignant and normal cervical lymph nodes. Semin Ultrasound CT MR 2013;34(3):236–47.
10. Kuna SK, Bracic I, Tesic V, et al. Ultrasonographic differentiation of benign from malignant neck lymphadenopathy in thyroid cancer. J Ultrasound Med 2006;25(12):1531–7.
11. Sakai F, Kiyono K, Sone S, et al. Ultrasonic evaluation of cervical metastatic lymphadenopathy. J Ultrasound Med 1988;7(6):305–10.
12. Shozushima M, Suzuki M, Nakasima T, et al. Ultrasound diagnosis of lymph node metastasis in head and neck cancer. Dentomaxillofac Radiol 1990;19(4):165–70.
13. Chan JM, Shin LK, Jeffrey RB. Ultrasonography of abnormal neck lymph nodes. Ultrasound Q 2007;23(1):47–54.
14. Chung JK, So Y, Lee JS, et al. Value of FDG PET in papillary thyroid carcinoma with negative 131I whole-body scan. J Nucl Med 1999;40(6):986–92.

15. Hoang JK, Vanka J, Ludwig BJ, et al. Evaluation of cervical lymph nodes in head and neck cancer with CT and MRI: tips, traps, and a systematic approach. AJR Am J Roentgenol 2013;200(1):W17–25.

16. Burman KD. Treatment of recurrent or persistent cervical node metastases in differentiated thyroid cancer: deceptively simple options. J Clin Endocrinol Metab 2012;97(8):2623–5.

17. Kouvaraki MA, Lee JE, Shapiro SE, et al. Preventable reoperations for persistent and recurrent papillary thyroid carcinoma. Surgery 2004;136(6):1183–91.

18. Travagli JP, Cailleux AF, Ricard M, et al. Combination of radioiodine (131I) and probe-guided surgery for persistent or recurrent thyroid carcinoma. J Clin Endocrinol Metab 1998;83(8):2675–80.

19. Al-Saif O, Farrar WB, Bloomston M, et al. Long-term efficacy of lymph node reoperation for persistent papillary thyroid cancer. J Clin Endocrinol Metab 2010; 95(5):2187–94.

20. Yim JH, Kim WB, Kim EY, et al. The outcomes of first reoperation for locoregionally recurrent/persistent papillary thyroid carcinoma in patients who initially underwent total thyroidectomy and remnant ablation. J Clin Endocrinol Metab 2011; 96(7):2049–56.

21. Clayman GL, Shellenberger TD, Ginsberg LE, et al. Approach and safety of comprehensive central compartment dissection in patients with recurrent papillary thyroid carcinoma. Head Neck 2009;31(9):1152–63.

22. Pacini F, Cetani F, Miccoli P, et al. Outcome of 309 patients with metastatic differentiated thyroid carcinoma treated with radioiodine. World J Surg 1994;18(4):600–4.

23. Yim JH, Kim WB, Kim EY, et al. Adjuvant radioactive therapy after reoperation for locoregionally recurrent papillary thyroid cancer in patients who initially underwent total thyroidectomy and high-dose remnant ablation. J Clin Endocrinol Metab 2011;96(12):3695–700.

24. Iyer NG, Morris LG, Tuttle RM, et al. Rising incidence of second cancers in patients with low-risk (T1N0) thyroid cancer who receive radioactive iodine therapy. Cancer 2011;117(19):4439–46.

25. Robenshtok E, Fish S, Bach A, et al. Suspicious cervical lymph nodes detected after thyroidectomy for papillary thyroid cancer usually remain stable over years in properly selected patients. J Clin Endocrinol Metab 2012;97(8):2706–13.

26. Rondeau G, Fish S, Hann LE, et al. Ultrasonographically detected small thyroid bed nodules identified after total thyroidectomy for differentiated thyroid cancer seldom show clinically significant structural progression. Thyroid 2011;21(8):845–53.

27. Mazzaferri EL, Jhiang SM. Long-term impact of initial surgical and medical therapy on papillary and follicular thyroid cancer. Am J Med 1994;97(5):418–28.

28. Ito Y, Higashiyama T, Takamura Y, et al. Prognosis of patients with papillary thyroid carcinoma showing postoperative recurrence to the central neck. World J Surg 2011;35(4):767–72.

29. Heilo A, Sigstad E, Fagerlid KH, et al. Efficacy of ultrasound-guided percutaneous ethanol injection treatment in patients with a limited number of metastatic cervical lymph nodes from papillary thyroid carcinoma. J Clin Endocrinol Metab 2011;96(9):2750–5.

30. Lewis BD, Hay ID, Charboneau JW, et al. Percutaneous ethanol injection for treatment of cervical lymph node metastases in patients with papillary thyroid carcinoma. AJR Am J Roentgenol 2002;178(3):699–704.

31. Hay ID, Charboneau JW. The coming of age of ultrasound-guided percutaneous ethanol ablation of selected neck nodal metastases in well-differentiated thyroid carcinoma. J Clin Endocrinol Metab 2011;96(9):2717–20.

Thyroid Disorders During Pregnancy

Nisha Nathan, MD, Shannon D. Sullivan, MD, PhD*

KEYWORDS

- Thyroid gland physiology • Pregnancy • Hypothyroidism
- Isolated hypothyroxinemia • Autoimmune thyroid disease • Hyperthyroidism

KEY POINTS

- Thyroid gland physiology changes during pregnancy because of the effects of increased levels of thyroid-binding globulin and human chorionic gonadotropin, and enhanced iodine metabolism, so it is important to use trimester-specific reference ranges for thyroid function tests during pregnancy.
- Because of the lack of evidence demonstrating that universal screening for thyroid disorders in pregnancy results in improved population outcomes, several clinical organizations recommend obtaining serum thyroid-stimulating hormone (TSH) early in pregnancy only in women at high risk for overt hypothyroidism.
- All women with overt hypothyroidism and thyroid peroxidase antibody–positive subclinical hypothyroidism should be treated with levothyroxine during pregnancy to maintain serum TSH levels within trimester-specific goal ranges.
- Thionamides are the treatment of choice for Graves' disease during pregnancy.
- When necessary, thyroid nodules detected in pregnancy may be evaluated with thyroid ultrasonography and fine-needle aspiration, both of which are safe to perform at any time during pregnancy.

THYROID GLAND PHYSIOLOGY IN PREGNANCY

Normal pregnancy entails complex changes in thyroid physiology.[1–4] In pregnant women with hypothyroidism, exogenous thyroid hormone replacement requirements typically increase by 25% to 47% to maintain normal concentrations of serum thyroid-stimulating hormone (TSH).[5–7] Several factors account for this.

First, high estrogen states such as pregnancy increase hepatic thyroid-binding globulin (TBG) synthesis[8,9]; furthermore, there is prolonged TBG half-life owing to estrogen-induced sialylation.[10] In pregnancy, TBG levels begin to increase after a few weeks, reach a plateau around midgestation, and remain 2- to 3-fold higher

Department of Endocrinology, Medstar Georgetown University Hospital and Medstar Washington Hospital Center, 110 Irving Street Northwest, Suite 2A-72, Washington, DC 20010, USA
* Corresponding author.
E-mail address: Shannon.d.sullivan@medstar.net

Endocrinol Metab Clin N Am 43 (2014) 573–597
http://dx.doi.org/10.1016/j.ecl.2014.02.008
0889-8529/14/$ – see front matter © 2014 Elsevier Inc. All rights reserved.

endo.theclinics.com

than preconception values until term.[11] The increased concentration of TBG leads to an elevation of total thyroxine (tT4) and total triiodothyronine (tT3) levels.[12] Levels of serum tT4 increase sharply between 6 and 12 weeks of gestation, progress more slowly thereafter, and stabilize around midgestation. The increase in tT3 concentration is more progressive. Both tT4 and tT3 reach their plateau by 20 weeks and are maintained until term.[4]

Second, human chorionic gonadotropin (hCG) is a thyroid regulator in normal pregnancy because the hormone-specific β subunits and the extracellular receptor-binding domains of hCG and TSH share multiple similarities.[13] Consequently, high concentrations of hCG during pregnancy stimulate TSH receptors. In pathologic conditions such as molar pregnancy or choriocarcinoma, this may lead to gestational hyperthyroidism. In normal pregnancy, the placenta produces hCG in the first week after conception and the levels peak at week 10, before decreasing and reaching a plateau by week 20.[12] Between 8 and 14 weeks' gestation, the changes in hCG and TSH levels are mirror images of each other, with a significant negative correlation between the two. Conversely, there is a positive linear relationship between hCG and free thyroxine (fT4) concentrations during early gestation.[12]

Third, maternal glomerular filtration rate increases in pregnancy, resulting in increased renal clearance of iodide, an indirect stimulus to the maternal thyroid machinery.[14] Later in gestation, transplacental passage of iodide to the fetus and placental metabolism of iodothyronines further contribute to relative maternal iodine deprivation and stimulation of the maternal thyroid.[15]

In the nonpregnant condition, an adequate iodine intake is estimated to be 100 to 150 μg/d. Because of the increased iodine demands in pregnancy, all women who are planning pregnancy, are pregnant, or are lactating should ingest a minimum of 250 μg of iodine daily. In North America, this could be achieved by adding a daily multivitamin or prenatal vitamin that contains 150 μg of potassium iodide to an iodine-sufficient diet.[16]

Because thyroid hormone economy differs between healthy pregnant women and healthy nonpregnant women, laboratory-dependent, trimester-specific reference intervals for thyroid function tests (TFTs) are required. Compared with preconception levels, TSH concentrations are lower during pregnancy. TSH is lowest in the first trimester and then increases during the second and third trimesters.[12] Among euthyroid pregnant women additional factors, including age, smoking status,[17] and ethnicity,[18] also contribute to TSH differences. It has been proposed that using ethnic-specific reference ranges can change the diagnosis for 18% of women who were initially labeled as having an abnormal TFT; however, ethnic-specific reference ranges for TSH are not currently endorsed by the Endocrine Society or the American Thyroid Association (ATA), nor are ethnic-specific ranges commonly used in clinical practice.[3,16,19] According to ATA and Endocrine Society guidelines, if laboratory-dependent, trimester-specific reference ranges for TSH are not available, recommended ranges for TSH are 0.1 to 2.5 mIU/L in the first trimester, 0.2 to 3.0 mIU/L in the second trimester, and 0.3 to 3.0 mIU/L in the third trimester.[3,16]

The interpretation of free thyroid hormone levels in pregnancy is more challenging; this is due, at least in part, to the use of different assays and differences in dietary iodine intake among women.[20] The optimal method to assess serum fT4 during pregnancy is measurement of thyroxine (T4) in the dialysate or ultrafiltrate of serum samples by liquid chromatography coupled with tandem mass spectrometry (LC/MS/MS).[21] Unfortunately, this method is too technically complex and expensive for routine use. If LC/MS/MS is not available, other assays can be used, as long as the limitations are considered. Method-specific and trimester-specific reference ranges for fT4 are required. In general, fT4 and free triiodothyronine (fT3) levels increase slightly during the first trimester. fT4 levels subsequently decrease as pregnancy progresses, with a nadir in the third trimester.[20]

It has been suggested that tT4 measurements are more reliable than fT4 measurements during pregnancy. tT4 levels are higher in pregnancy compared with the nonpregnant state, so in general normal tT4 reference ranges can be adjusted by multiplying this range by 1.5.[20] The fT4 index may also be used in pregnancy, as the fT4 index corrects tT4 for TBG. Changes in fT4 index correspond to the changes in fT4 measured by equilibrium dialysis and tandem mass spectrometry.[22]

UNIVERSAL SCREENING VERSUS TARGETED HIGH-RISK CASE FINDING OF THYROID DISORDERS IN PREGNANCY

Universal thyroid function testing will detect an elevated serum TSH level in about 2% to 3% of iodine-sufficient women, of whom about two-thirds will have subclinical hypothyroidism and one-third will have overt hypothyroidism.[23] In the last decade, there has been more attention paid to thyroid dysfunction during pregnancy and its effects on maternal and fetal well-being. As a result, there has been a debate regarding universal screening versus targeted high-risk case finding of thyroid dysfunction during pregnancy. Different studies have shown that targeted high-risk screening failed to detect 28% to 36% of women with hypothyroidism.[24–26] A study at an academic medical center in the Boston area revealed that targeted thyroid testing in high-risk patients would have missed 80% of pregnant women with either overt or subclinical hypothyroidism.[27] This number would likely be even higher in areas outside the United States, such as Europe, which have a higher prevalence of iodine deficiency. For example, 7.2% of pregnant women in Belgium, a country with mild iodine deficiency, had hypothyroidism, compared with about 2% to 3% in the United States.[28] These data make a case for universal screening in all women; however, there are few prospective randomized trials to substantiate the benefits of universal screening. In a randomized controlled trial based in Italy, Negro and colleagues[26] showed that universal screening resulted in a significant decrease (28%) in the occurrence of adverse events in women with elevated thyroid peroxidase (TPO) antibodies and TSH greater than 2.5 mIU/L, who would have otherwise been classified as low risk. However, screening is not universally advocated, as only one study has shown that treatment with levothyroxine (LT4) improves outcomes in women with subclinical hypothyroidism.[23]

Data from one large, prospective, randomized controlled trial is currently pending. The National Institutes of Health (NIH) Maternal Fetal Medicine Thyrotropin Study (TSH Study), to be completed in 2015, is screening pregnant women for thyroid dysfunction and comparing maternal and fetal outcomes between women with subclinical hypothyroidism or isolated hypothyroxinemia treated with LT4 versus placebo during pregnancy. Initial results show there is no difference in IQ in offspring of low-risk women screened for hypothyroidism and treated with LT4 therapy when compared with control women who were not screened and, therefore, not treated. However, it seems that compliance to LT4 might not have been optimal in the study group.[29] Nevertheless, there is expert opinion that although statistical evidence to justify universal screening is lacking, more evidence will be produced in the future in favor of routine testing.[30]

Owing to the lack of consistent evidence to date demonstrating that universal screening improves population outcomes, several clinical organizations, including the ATA, recommend obtaining serum TSH early in pregnancy only in women at high risk for overt hypothyroidism (**Box 1** lists the risk factors). The Endocrine Society

---

Box 1
Screening for serum thyroid-stimulating hormone in early pregnancy in high-risk patients

Risk Factors for Overt Hypothyroidism

History of thyroid dysfunction or prior thyroid surgery

Age older than 30 years

Symptoms of thyroid dysfunction or the presence of goiter

Thyroid peroxidase antibody positivity

Type 1 diabetes mellitus or other autoimmune disorders

History of miscarriage or preterm delivery

History of head and neck radiation

Family history of thyroid dysfunction

Morbid obesity (body mass index $\geq$40 kg/m^2)

Use of amiodarone or lithium, or recent administration of iodinated radiologic contrast

Infertility

Residing in an area of known moderate to severe iodine insufficiency

Adapted from Stagnaro-Green A, Abalovich M, Alexander E, et al. Guidelines of the American Thyroid Association for the diagnosis and management of thyroid disease during pregnancy and postpartum. Thyroid 2011;21(10):1111.

---

could not reach a conclusion; some members advocate for screening of all pregnant women at the time of their first prenatal visit, whereas others align with the ATA views.[16,31]

HYPOTHYROIDISM DURING PREGNANCY

Thyroid hormone deficiency is found in approximately 3% to 7% of women of childbearing age,[2] and an estimated 2% to 3% of women are hypothyroid during pregnancy.[2,3] However, the prevalence of hypothyroidism in pregnancy is likely underestimated because in most studies in which prevalence of thyroid dysfunction in pregnancy has been evaluated, 4.2 mIU/L was used as the upper limit of the TSH reference range. Using the pregnancy specific upper limit for TSH of 2.5 mIU/L, the prevalence of hypothyroidism would increase.[23]

In iodine-sufficient areas, the most common cause of hypothyroidism in pregnancy is Hashimoto thyroiditis. Other causes include prior radioactive iodine and/or surgical ablation of Graves' disease (GD),[32] surgical removal of the thyroid because of multinodular goiter or thyroid cancer, overtreatment of hyperthyroidism with thionamides, medications that alter the absorption or metabolism of LT4, and central defects that inhibit the hypothalamic-pituitary-thyroid axis.

The fetal thyroid gland starts producing small amounts of thyroid hormone at approximately 10 weeks' gestation, until production plateaus at approximately 35 weeks.[12] Thus, particularly in the first trimester of pregnancy, the fetus depends entirely on thyroid hormone from the mother. Maternal hypothyroidism can have devastating consequences if left untreated.

Diagnosis

Overt hypothyroidism is defined by a serum TSH higher than the upper limit of the trimester-specific range and serum fT4 below the trimester-specific reference range, or serum TSH level of at least 10 mIU/L, irrespective of fT4 level. Subclinical hypothyroidism is diagnosed when serum TSH is elevated, but less than 10 mIU/L, and fT4 is within the normal range. Differentiating between the two conditions is important because maternal and fetal outcomes are better established for overt maternal hypothyroidism than for subclinical hypothyroidism. Isolated hypothyroxinemia is defined as a normal TSH level, with fT4 in the lower fifth or tenth percentile of the reference range.[16]

Pregnancy Complications

Maternal hypothyroidism is associated with spontaneous abortion,[33] fetal death,[34] preterm delivery,[34,35] pregnancy-induced hypertension,[36] gestational diabetes,[35] anemia, postpartum hemorrhage,[37] placental abruption and preterm labor,[38] preeclampsia,[39] cesarean section,[40] and very early embryo loss.[41] Su and colleagues[42] showed an increased risk of fetal loss (odds ratio [OR] 13.45, 95% confidence interval [CI] 2.54–71.20), low birth weight (OR 9.05, 95% CI 1.01–80.90), and congenital circulation system malformations (OR 10.44, 95% CI 1.15–94.62) in children of women with clinical hypothyroidism. Kuppens and colleagues[43] showed that breech position was significantly and independently related to high maternal TSH concentration ($\geq$2.5 mIU/L) at 36 weeks' gestation (OR 2.23, 95% CI 1.14–4.39). Higher TSH levels late in pregnancy also increased the risk of external cephalic version failure.[44]

Subclinical hypothyroidism has been associated with a 3-fold increased risk of placental abruption and a 1.8-fold increased risk of preterm labor.[38] In a cohort of euthyroid pregnant women without overt thyroid dysfunction, the risk of child loss attributable to miscarriage or fetal/neonatal death increased with higher levels of maternal TSH in early pregnancy, with an OR of 1.8 for every doubling in TSH concentration in multivariate analyses.[45] By contrast, other studies have failed to reveal an association between subclinical hypothyroidism and adverse pregnancy outcomes,[46,47] but interpretation of these data was limited because of exclusion of a significant number of patients from final analyses.

Adverse Outcomes in Neonates and Offspring

Maternal hypothyroidism has been associated with an increased risk of low birth weight, fetal distress, and impaired neuropsychological development.[33,38,48] Haddow and colleagues[48] described a 7-point IQ deficit in 7- to 9-year-old children born to untreated hypothyroid women when compared with age-matched children born to euthyroid women. Nineteen percent of children of hypothyroid mothers had IQ scores of less than 85, compared with 5% of controls. However, these results should be interpreted with caution. Most women in the study group were multiparous and were older than those in the control group. In addition, the social situations of those studied were unclear. TSH was only measured once in midtrimester, and there was limited follow-up of participants. Another study demonstrated that both mild and severe maternal hypothyroxinemia was associated with a higher risk of expressive language delay of offspring aged 18 to 30 months. Severe hypothyroxinemia also predicted a higher risk of nonverbal cognitive delay.[49] Subclinical hypothyroidism has been associated with increased fetal distress (OR 3.65, 95% CI 1.44–9.26), poor vision development (OR 5.34, 95% CI 1.09–26.16), and neurodevelopmental delay (OR 10.49, 95% CI 1.01–119.19).[42] By contrast, a study by Behrooz and colleagues[50] showed that IQ levels and cognitive performance of children born to LT4-treated hypothyroid mothers was similar between those whose mothers had high TSH levels (mean 11.3 $\pm$ 5.3 mIU/L) and those whose mothers achieved normal TSH concentrations during pregnancy. Similarly, a prospective, randomized controlled trial by

Lazarus and colleagues[51] showed that antenatal screening and maternal treatment of hypothyroidism did not result in improved cognitive function in offspring at 3 years of age. It is known that the first trimester is a crucial period for fetal brain development; thus this study was criticized because the patients did not start thyroid hormone replacement therapy until 13 weeks of gestation or later.[23]

Isolated Hypothyroxinemia

Isolated maternal hypothyroxinemia is identified in 1.3% of pregnant women. Some studies have failed to show a significant association between isolated hypothyroxinemia and adverse perinatal outcomes.[47,52] By contrast, other studies have shown an increased risk of fetal distress, musculoskeletal malformations, and small for gestational age (SGA) infants when hypothyroxinemia was diagnosed in the first 20 weeks of gestation,[42] and impaired mental and motor development at age 1 to 2 years when hypothyroxinemia was diagnosed by 12 weeks of gestation.[53,54] Isolated hypothyroxinemia also predicted a higher risk of expressive language delay at 18 and 30 months of age (OR 1.44, 95% CI 1.09–1.91 and OR 1.80, 95% CI 1.24–2.61, respectively), as well as nonverbal cognitive delay in children (OR 2.03, 95% CI 1.22–3.39).[49]

Treatment

Both the Endocrine Society and the ATA support treating all women with (1) overt hypothyroidism and (2) TPO antibody–positive subclinical hypothyroidism with LT4 during pregnancy to maintain serum TSH in the trimester-specific goal range.[16,31]

It has been shown that TPO antibody–negative pregnant women with TSH greater than 2.5 mIU/L have higher miscarriage rates in comparison with women with a TSH level of 2.5 mIU/L or less. The Endocrine Society recommends LT4 treatment in women with subclinical hypothyroidism irrespective of antibody status, including women who are TPO antibody–negative, because the benefits of treatment outweigh the risks.[31] However, this is not widely accepted in clinical practice. Similarly, data demonstrating a benefit of LT4 therapy in pregnant women with isolated hypothyroxinemia are not yet available, so routine LT4 treatment is currently not recommended in these cases.[55] Nonetheless, the ongoing NIH TSH Trial will provide important data regarding maternal and fetal effects of LT4 treatment in isolated maternal hypothyroxinemia and thereby help guide future evidence-based recommendations.

For women who require LT4 treatment during pregnancy, it is crucial to adjust LT4 doses appropriately to account for physiologic pregnancy-induced changes in thyroid hormone economy. Adequate treatment with LT4 to maintain TSH within the target ranges for pregnancy significantly decreases pregnancy-related complications that occur in inadequately treated hypothyroid women.[35] The etiology of hypothyroidism has a marked effect on the timing and magnitude of LT4 dose adjustments. Women with primary hypothyroidism owing to Hashimoto thyroiditis tend to require smaller dose increases, as do women treated for thyroid cancer, compared with women previously treated for GD, who tend to require the largest dose increases, indicating that a single recommendation might not apply to all patients. Among women with thyroid cancer, it is likely that higher prepregnancy doses of LT4 for the purposes of TSH suppression result in smaller dose increases during pregnancy. On average, among a large group of pregnant women with hypothyroidism of varying etiology, the required increase in LT4 dose was 13% in the first trimester and 26% in the second and third trimesters.[56] Another study showed that an increase in LT4 dose was required in 85% of hypothyroid pregnant women, starting as early as the fifth week of gestation and plateauing by week 16. The mean LT4 requirement increased 47% during the first half of pregnancy in this study.[5]

The goal of treatment is to maintain TSH within trimester-specific reference ranges: 0.1 to 2.5 mIU/L in the first trimester, 0.2 to 3.0 mIU/L in the second trimester, and 0.3 to 3.0 mIU/L in the third trimester.[16] Thyroid function should be normalized as rapidly as possible after conception. TFTs should be measured within 30 to 40 days of the first positive pregnancy test, and then every 4 to 6 weeks throughout pregnancy.[31] The recommended therapy is with oral LT4, which should be taken on an empty stomach ($\geq$45 minutes before consumption of food, beverages, or other medications). In addition, calcium, iron, and prenatal vitamin supplements should be avoided within 4 hours of ingestion of LT4, as these may decrease absorption and lead to inadequate circulating T4 levels.

A high proportion of pregnant women with hypothyroidism who are taking LT4 have suboptimal TSH levels at 11 to 13 weeks of gestation.[39] Because most women do not have their first prenatal obstetric visit until the 8th to 12th week of pregnancy, one strategy to avoid maternal hypothyroidism is to empirically increase the LT4 dose as soon as pregnancy is confirmed. In the Thyroid Hormone Early Adjustment in Pregnancy (THERAPY) trial, an empiric increase by 2 additional LT4 doses per week (29% increase), when instituted immediately on confirmation of pregnancy, significantly reduced the risk of maternal hypothyroidism throughout pregnancy, with a safety profile superior to that of an increase of 3 additional doses per week (43% increase).[57] ATA guidelines endorse this recommendation, or the alternative option of empirically increasing LT4 dose by approximately 25% to 30% on confirmation of pregnancy.[16] After delivery, the patient should be instructed to return to her prepregnancy dose of LT4, and serum TSH should be checked again 6 weeks after delivery, keeping in mind that her immediate postpartum weight–based dose may be slightly higher than her prepregnancy dose, owing to weight gain during pregnancy. If this is a concern, more gradual reduction of LT4 dose based on a TSH measurement 2 weeks after delivery may help avoid unnecessary hypothyroidism in the postpartum period.

Iodine is necessary for the synthesis of thyroid hormone. Thirty percent of the population worldwide remains iodine deficient, with women of childbearing age having the lowest iodine levels.[58] The most recent National Health and Nutrition Examination Survey for Pregnant Women revealed that 21% of women in the United States have low urine iodine, less than 100 μg/L,[2] indicating possible iodine deficiency or insufficiency. Indeed, maintaining the increased iodine requirements in pregnancy has been shown to prevent cretinism and improve motor skills in offspring. The recommended daily iodine dose in pregnancy and lactation is 250 μg of iodine daily. This level may be achieved by supplementing an iodine-sufficient diet with a daily oral prenatal multivitamin containing 150 μg of potassium iodide. Caution should be advised because supplemental iodine is not found in more than 50% of prenatal vitamins in the United States, so women should be advised to take a prenatal vitamin that provides iodine, in addition to ensuring adequate dietary iodine intake.[59] Asking women to use iodinized salt is an easy way to help ensure iodine sufficiency.

EUTHYROIDISM WITH AUTOIMMUNE THYROID DISEASE

TPO and/or thyroglobulin antibodies can be detected in 10% to 20% of women of childbearing age.[60] Several studies have shown an increased risk of pregnancy complications in euthyroid women with thyroid autoimmunity, including preterm delivery,[61] spontaneous miscarriage,[62] very preterm delivery (<34 weeks' gestation),[63] placental abruption,[64] postpartum thyroiditis, and postpartum depression.[65] A 2012 study showed that TPO antibody positivity was associated with higher maternal TSH levels, lower fT4 levels, an 8-fold higher risk of developing subclinical hypothyroidism, and a

26-fold higher risk of developing overt hypothyroidism during pregnancy.[66] A recent meta-analysis showed a significant relationship between miscarriage and thyroid antibody positivity in euthyroid women.[67] A large prospective study in Finland showed that perinatal mortality was 2 to 3 times greater in women who were TPO or thyroglobulin antibody positive when compared with women who were antibody negative, which was likely due, at least in part, to increased rates of preterm delivery among thyroid antibody–positive women.[47] Similarly, a study in the Netherlands showed an association between TPO antibody positivity and a higher risk of attention deficit/hyperactivity problems in offspring (OR 1.77, 95% CI 1.15–2.1; $P = .01$). This risk was not exclusively mediated by maternal thyroid status, thus suggesting a multifactorial association between TPO antibody positivity and behavior.[68] Negro and colleagues[63] conducted a prospective, randomized controlled trial showing that euthyroid, TPO antibody–positive women who received LT4 therapy during pregnancy had a statistically significant decrease in miscarriage and preterm delivery in comparison with placebo-treated women.

There are no consistent studies to show a clear benefit, change in outcome, or cost-effectiveness in universal testing of TSH in all pregnant women. Universal screening is a highly controversial topic, and there is lack of good data to unanimously support it. The 2011 ATA guidelines state that there is insufficient evidence to recommend for or against screening all women for thyroid autoantibodies in the first trimester, or treating euthyroid women who are thyroid antibody–positive with LT4.[16] In guidelines published in 2012, The Endocrine Society Task Force could not reach agreement on thyroid testing recommendations for pregnant women. Some recommended universal screening, whereas others supported an aggressive case-based approach similar to that of the ATA. That being said, at a minimum, serum TSH should be monitored throughout pregnancy every 4 to 6 weeks in the first half of pregnancy, then at least once between 26 and 32 weeks of gestation. LT4 therapy should be initiated if serum TSH is greater than 2.5 mIU/L.[31]

HYPERTHYROIDISM IN PREGNANCY

Overt hyperthyroidism occurs in 0.4% to 1.7% of pregnant women, and GD accounts for 85% to 90% of all cases.[69] Other causes of hyperthyroidism in pregnancy include subacute thyroiditis, toxic multinodular goiter, toxic thyroid adenoma, and excessive LT4 intake.[70] Maternal hyperthyroidism is defined as a low or suppressed serum TSH level in the presence of a high fT4 level based on trimester-specific reference ranges. As described previously, serum TSH levels are normally suppressed in the first trimester because of high levels of hCG, so it is necessary to measure the serum fT4 in conjunction with TSH for an accurate diagnosis.

Gestational Transient Thyrotoxicosis

The most common cause of hyperthyroidism in pregnancy is gestational transient thyrotoxicosis (GTT), a transient period of hyperthyroidism that occurs in 1% to 3% of pregnancies[71] and is caused by elevated hCG levels. GTT is often associated with hyperemesis gravidarum, defined as severe nausea and vomiting that results in weight loss, dehydration, and ketonuria in early pregnancy. Risk factors for GTT include multiple gestations, hydatiform mole, and choriocarcinoma.[70] It is important to distinguish GTT from GD or other forms of hyperthyroidism, such as toxic multinodular goiter, because the course, fetal outcomes, management, and follow-up differ. GTT usually resolves spontaneously by 20 weeks' gestation when hCG levels decline. Treatment with antithyroid drugs is not indicated unless the diagnosis is certain.

Supportive therapy should be provided for hyperemesis gravidarum, such as anti-emetics and intravenous fluids, and hospitalization may be required in severe cases.

Graves' Disease in Pregnancy

Diagnosis

It is important to remember that clinical features of hyperthyroidism may be mistaken for normal symptoms of pregnancy, such as palpitations, heat intolerance, dyspnea, and nervousness. GD may present as a new diagnosis during pregnancy in a woman with no history of hyperthyroidism, as a recurrence of GD that was in remission, or as an exacerbation of stable GD treated with antithyroid drugs (ATDs). Exacerbations of GD that was controlled with ATDs before pregnancy typically occur either early in pregnancy or in the immediate postpartum period.[72]

On physical examination, women with GD usually have a palpable goiter, with or without a bruit. In some instances, Graves' ophthalmopathy is present. Graves' dermopathy may rarely be seen. On laboratory evaluation, TSH is usually lower than the trimester-specific reference range, and fT4 is high. Women with GD usually have positive TSH-receptor antibodies (TRAb), which helps differentiate GD from other forms of hyperthyroidism. The performance of TRAb in the differential diagnosis of overt hyperthyroidism is excellent, with a sensitivity and specificity of 90%.[73] Ultrasonography of the thyroid may also be helpful in certain circumstances; for example, to differentiate between toxic multinodular goiter, a single toxic nodule, or the heterogeneous thyroid echotexture that is consistent with GD. Use of radio-labeled iodine for diagnosis (eg, ^{123}I uptake and scan) is contraindicated in pregnancy and lactation.

Outcomes

Lack of control of hyperthyroidism significantly increases the risk of pregnancy complications and poor fetal outcomes. Millar and colleagues[74] showed that, compared with the risk in nonhyperthyroid women, the risk of low birth weight in infants was 9.24 (95% CI 5.5–15.6) among women with uncontrolled hyperthyroidism during pregnancy, 2.36 (95% CI 1.4–4.1) in women whose hyperthyroidism was controlled at some point during pregnancy, and 0.74 (95% CI 0.2–3.1) in women whose hyperthyroidism was controlled at presentation so that euthyroidism was maintained throughout pregnancy. The risk of severe preeclampsia was also significantly higher among women with uncontrolled hyperthyroidism when compared with hyperthyroid women with controlled thyroid levels during pregnancy (OR 4.7, 95% CI 1.1–19.7).[74]

In addition, in a cohort of 60 women with overt hyperthyroidism in pregnancy, stillbirth was more common in untreated women (50%) than in partially treated (16%) and adequately treated hyperthyroid women (0%).[75] Overt untreated maternal hyperthyroidism is also associated with an increased risk of miscarriage,[76] maternal heart failure during pregnancy,[77] pregnancy-induced hypertension, and fetal growth restriction.[78] Uncontrolled maternal hyperthyroidism may cause central congenital hypothyroidism resulting from impaired maturation of the fetal hypothalamic-pituitary thyroid system in a hyperthyroid fetal environment.[79]

A recent study showed that in mothers with normal TSH and fT4 levels, high to normal maternal fT4 in early pregnancy is associated with an increased risk of SGA newborns (OR 1.10–1.17; $P = .03$).[80] The same study demonstrated that in an iodine-sufficient population, maternal urinary iodine levels greater than 500 µg/L are associated with an increased risk of a hyperthyroid newborn.[81] These data demonstrate that even a mild variation in thyroid function within the normal range can have important fetal consequences. A maternal thyroid-stimulating immunoglobulin value of 5 index units or greater can predict neonatal thyrotoxicosis with sensitivity of 100% and specificity of 76%.[82]

TRAbs cross the placental barrier and, in high titers, can stimulate the fetal thyroid gland, which may result in fetal hyperthyroidism.[83] Fetal thyrotoxicosis causes fetal tachycardia, goiter, oligohydramnios, intrauterine growth retardation, and accelerated bone maturation.[84] When present, neonatal hyperthyroidism typically persists for 24 to 72 hours after delivery in cases of high maternal TRAb titers. However, cases of neonatal thyrotoxicosis persisting for up to 45 days after delivery have been reported.[85] Before delivery, the fetus is protected by ATDs taken by the mother, which also cross the placenta. Neonatal hyperthyroidism is usually a transient condition, lasting between 2 and 3 months. Treatment of the neonate with ATDs is indicated until resolution of the hyperthyroidism.[86] Momotani and colleagues[87] suggest that uncontrolled maternal hyperthyroidism may cause congenital malformations, and although methimazole (MMI) might have teratogenic effects, the benefits of treatment with ATDs outweigh the risks of withholding therapy.

Treatment of Maternal Hyperthyroidism in Pregnancy

Preconception counseling

As previously described, uncontrolled hyperthyroidism affects maternal and fetal outcomes poorly. It is imperative to provide preconception counseling to women with hyperthyroidism so that the best therapeutic option to control the disease before pregnancy can be implemented. In the preconception period, treatment options for GD include radioactive iodine (RAI) ablation, total thyroidectomy, or ATDs. Surgery is a reasonable option in cases of high TRAb titers or in women planning to conceive in the subsequent 2 years, because TRAb titers tend to increase following RAI therapy and take longer to trend downwards.[88] RAI ablation is absolutely contraindicated during pregnancy and lactation because of the high risk of transferring RAI to the fetus with resultant fetal thyroid ablation and congenital hypothyroidism. If RAI ablation is desired near pregnancy, it is advised to delay conception for 6 months.[16] Special considerations should be kept in mind, and are listed in **Box 2**.

Antithyroid drugs

Two ATDs, MMI and propylthiouracil (PTU), both of which cross the placenta, are used to treat hyperthyroidism. The goal of ATD therapy in pregnant women with

---

Box 2
Considerations for radioactive iodine therapy (RAI) in women of childbearing age

1. RAI is absolutely contraindicated during pregnancy and lactation
2. A pregnancy test should be performed on all women of childbearing age before RAI
3. Conception should be delayed by a minimum of 6 months after RAI to allow adequate time for diagnosis and treatment of consequent hypothyroidism
4. Lactation should be delayed for at least 6 months following RAI therapy
5. RAI might increase TSH-receptor antibody (TRAb) titers, and it may take up to 1 year for the titers to decline after RAI. Therefore, if TRAb titers are high before treatment, surgery might be a better option
6. Prepregnancy counseling regarding the need to adjust levothyroxine dose at diagnosis of pregnancy is important

Adapted from Patil-Sisodia K, Mestman JH. Graves hyperthyroidism and pregnancy: a clinical update. Endocr Pract 2010;16(1):118–29.

hyperthyroidism is to maintain maternal serum fT4 at or just above the upper limit of normal for pregnancy using the smallest ATD dose possible. This treatment strategy minimizes the potential for overtreatment, which may result in fetal hypothyroidism[89] and goiter.[90] In this regard, Momotani and colleagues[91] showed a strong relationship between maternal and fetal thyroid function: the rates of transient neonatal hypothyroxinemia were 10% when maternal fT4 was maintained in the upper one-third of the normal range, 36% when maternal fT4 was maintained in the lower two-thirds of the normal range, and 100% when maternal fT4 was maintained below the normal range. There was no relationship between the dose or the type of ATD used and neonatal thyroid function.

In rare cases, use of MMI in the first trimester has been associated with congenital abnormalities, including fetal aplasia cutis,[92] choanal atresia, omphalocele, total situs invertus,[93] esophageal atresia,[94] tracheoesophageal fistula, hypoplastic nipples, and psychomotor delay.[95] Yoshihara and colleagues[96] conducted a retrospective review of pregnant women with GD, and showed that women treated with MMI during pregnancy had a higher rate of major infant anomalies compared with women treated with PTU (4.1% vs 2.1%, respectively; $P = .002$). A significant risk associated with PTU is acute liver failure, resulting in a need for liver transplant in approximately 1 in 10,000 treated adults.[97,98] Therefore, to decrease the risk of congenital abnormalities associated with first-trimester MMI use, women taking MMI before pregnancy should be switched to PTU once pregnancy is confirmed or, alternatively, before conception. After the first trimester, consideration should be given to switching from PTU to an equivalent dose of MMI to avoid maternal liver injury.[16] Clinical experience has demonstrated an approximate conversion ratio from PTU to MMI of 10:1 to 15:1 (eg, 100 mg of PTU = 7.5–10 mg of MMI[99]). When this approach is used, care must be taken to ensure that maternal TSH and fT4 are maintained within the pregnancy-specific reference ranges; therefore, frequent monitoring of TFTs, with dose titration when necessary, is essential. At present there are no controlled studies assessing the benefits and problems with this design of switching from PTU to methimazole after the first trimester of pregnancy.

After delivery, GD may worsen or relapse, necessitating that ATDs are restarted or the dose increased. In the past, women taking ATDs were advised against breastfeeding because little was known about their effects on the newborn when delivered via breast milk. More recent studies, however, have demonstrated that ATDs are safe in lactating women. The use of PTU (as high as 750 mg daily) or methimazole (20–30 mg daily) have not been associated with an increased risk of infant hypothyroidism, and no adverse effects on physical or cognitive childhood development have been observed.[100,101]

Surgery

Thyroidectomy during pregnancy is rarely indicated, but should be considered if a woman with severe hyperthyroidism is resistant to or intolerant of ATDs, or if she requires high doses of ATDs (>30 mg/d of MMI or >450 mg/d of PTU[3]) to control her disease. If surgery is indicated during pregnancy, the optimal time is in the second trimester.[16] The use of β-blockers such as metoprolol and a short course of cold (ie, nonradioactive) iodine are recommended in preparation for surgery.[16] Determination of maternal TRAb titers before surgery is recommended to assess the risk of fetal hyperthyroidism.[102]

β-blockers

β-Blockers can be used temporarily in pregnancy to help control adrenergic symptoms, or in preparation for surgery. Long-term use should be avoided, and has been associated with intrauterine growth retardation, fetal bradycardia, neonatal hypoglycemia, and spontaneous abortion.[103,104] Labetolol, a pregnancy category C medication, is the preferred β-blocker for use during pregnancy and lactation.

Cold iodine

The use of cold iodine during pregnancy should be limited to the acute management of thyroid storm or in preparation for thyroidectomy. Studies have reported neonatal hypothyroidism after maternal exposure to cold iodine, including reports in euthyroid women exposed to iodine-rich foods (such as seaweed), iodine-based medications (such as amiodarone), or contrast media, and reports in hypothyroid pregnant women treated simultaneously with ATD and cold iodine. By contrast, Momotani and colleagues[105] showed improved maternal thyroid function and normal neonatal outcomes after treatment of GD with low doses of cold iodine in pregnancy; thus careful, limited use of cold iodine in the management of GD in pregnancy may be appropriate in select cases.

Radioactive iodine therapy

As discussed previously, RAI is absolutely contraindicated in pregnancy and lactation because of its potentially detrimental effects on the developing fetus, which primarily result from fetal thyroid ablation. In fact, caution should be used when administering RAI to women who have recently breastfed, as their breasts could maintain avid uptake of RAI for at least several weeks after breastfeeding has been discontinued.

Fetal monitoring

Ultrasonography is the mainstay of monitoring for fetal hypothyroidism while treating maternal hyperthyroidism. Pregnant women with TRAbs, elevated thyroid-stimulating immunoglobulin, or being treated with ATDs should be screened for fetal hypothyroidism. Presence of a fetal goiter on ultrasonography is highly suggestive of fetal hypothyroidism.[106] If a fetal goiter is present, ATDs should be reduced or discontinued, keeping in mind that the risks of maternal hyperthyroidism in pregnancy are much less than the risks of fetal hypothyroidism, particularly with regard to fetal and neonatal growth and development. During pregnancy in women with GD, TRAb levels often decrease owing to a state of relative maternal immunosuppression. Decreased TRAb titers may permit decreased ATD doses in the second trimester and, possibly, discontinuation of ATDs in the third trimester. Maternal serum fT4 and TSH levels should be monitored every 2 to 4 weeks at the initiation of ATD therapy, and every 4 to 6 weeks after achieving target levels. ATD dose adjustments should be based on fT4 levels rather than on TSH levels, because TSH may remain suppressed throughout pregnancy. A combination of ATDs and LT4 therapy is not recommended because this complicates monitoring of fetal thyroid function, thereby increasing the risk of fetal goiter and hypothyroidism.[104] A 2013 clinical review suggested that lower TRAb titers accurately predicted short-term relapses of hyperthyroidism after a course of ATDs, but were less effective in predicting long-term outcomes. Because pregnancies in TRAb-negative patients were unlikely to result in fetal thyrotoxicosis, these investigators suggested that TRAb levels should be tested before deciding whether ATDs can be stopped.[73]

Indications for maternal TRAb measurement are listed in **Box 3**. TRAb titers should be measured at 20 to 28 weeks' gestation to determine the risk of fetal hyperthyroidism after delivery.[16] If TRAb titers are high (≥3 times the upper limit of normal), close follow-up of the newborn's thyroid function, optimally in collaboration with a maternal-fetal-medicine specialist, is indicated. Serial fetal ultrasonography is also recommended in women with high TRAb titers and/or active GD. The size of the fetal thyroid

---

Box 3
Indications for TRAb measurement during pregnancy

1. Mothers with active hyperthyroidism

2. Previous history of treatment with RAI

3. Previous history of delivering an infant with hyperthyroidism

4. Thyroidectomy for treatment of hyperthyroidism in pregnancy

Adapted from Laurberg P, Nygaard B, Glinoer D, et al. Guidelines for TSH-receptor antibody measurements in pregnancy: results of an evidence-based symposium organized by the European Thyroid Association. Eur J Endocrinol 1998;139(6):584–6.

---

gland should be evaluated monthly starting at 22 weeks' gestation to ensure early diagnosis of fetal thyroid dysfunction.[84] Sonographic features may be able to predict the nature of fetal thyroid dysfunction: color Doppler pattern of fetal goiter typically has a peripheral vascular pattern in hypothyroidism and a central vascular pattern in hyperthyroidism. Additional clinical findings suggesting the nature of fetal thyroid dysfunction include heart rate (tachycardia may indicate hyperthyroidism and bradycardia may indicate hypothyroidism), bone maturation (advanced in hyperthyroidism and delayed in hypothyroidism), and intrauterine movement (increased in hyperthyroidism and decreased in hypothyroidism).[107]

In the later stages of pregnancy, fetal thyroid function can be studied directly by measuring fetal thyroid hormone levels in the umbilical cord blood obtained by cordocentesis.[108] However, cordocentesis itself carries an increased risk of fetal morbidity and mortality, and thus should be reserved for special circumstances, such as an inability to determine whether the fetus is hypothyroid or hyperthyroid clinically or based on fetal ultrasonography.[16]

Postpartum care

Women with GD may experience relapse or worsening of hyperthyroidism after delivery. When relapse of GD occurs, it most frequently becomes manifest within 4 to 8 months after delivery,[109] so it is important to monitor thyroid function regularly postpartum. It is also necessary to distinguish GD from postpartum thyroiditis (PPT) because treatments will differ. In women who choose not to breastfeed, RAI (^{123}I) uptake and scan may be performed to differentiate GD from PPT. In lactating mothers, RAI is contraindicated, and differentiating GD from PPT may be achieved by measuring TRAb titers, assessing the time course of hyperthyroidism (ie, transient vs chronic), and prior history of maternal GD.

POSTPARTUM THYROIDITIS

PPT is an autoimmune destructive inflammation of the thyroid gland[110] that typically occurs within 1 year postpartum. The classic presentation of PPT starts with transient hyperthyroidism in the first 6 months postpartum, followed by transient hypothyroidism, and then a return to the euthyroid state by 1 year postpartum. Not all women with PPT progress through all the phases of this classic presentation. Lazarus and colleagues[111] reported that among a cohort of women diagnosed with PPT, 19.2% developed hyperthyroidism alone, 49.3% developed hypothyroidism alone, and 31.5% developed hyperthyroidism followed by hypothyroidism. PPT may occur in women with hypothyroidism as a result of Hashimoto thyroiditis if the thyroid gland is not completely atrophic.[112] By convention, hypothyroidism with onset 1 year or later postpartum is not PPT.[113]

Prevalence

The reported prevalence of PPT varies widely across studies, from 1.1% to 16.7% (mean 7.5%).[113] Women with a prior history of PPT have a 70% risk of developing recurrent PPT in future pregnancies.[114] Rates of PPT are higher in women with underlying autoimmune disease: 10% to 25% in women with type 1 diabetes mellitus,[113,115] 14% in women with systemic lupus erythematosus,[116] and 25% in women with autoimmune hepatitis.[117] An estimated 30% to 50% of women with positive thyroid autoantibodies will develop PPT.[110,118,119]

Diagnosis

Screening at initial visit for PPT is recommended in women with a history of thyroid disease, PPT, postpartum depression, or autoimmune disease, and in women with signs or symptoms of hyperthyroidism, hypothyroidism, or depression in the postpartum period. Screening should include measurement of TPO antibody titer, TSH, and fT4. Clinical signs and symptoms of PPT are usually mild and transient, with the hypothyroid phase typically being the most symptomatic. In the hyperthyroid state, differentiating between GD and PPT is important in guiding management. Clinical features unique to GD include a goiter with bruit, ophthalmopathy, and elevated TRAb titers. Biochemically, the T4:T3 ratio is typically elevated in PPT. Thyroid ultrasonography with Doppler flow measurements may be helpful in differentiating PPT from GD (decreased vascular flow in PPT vs increased flow in GD) and does not involve radiation that would necessitate an interruption in breast feeding. RAI uptake and scan can be performed to establish the diagnosis; thyroid ^{123}I uptake is elevated in GD and low or absent in PPT. [123]I is preferred over ^{131}I for thyroid imaging during lactation because of its shorter half-life, allowing nursing to resume several days following administration of [123]I.[16]

Maternal Outcomes

PPT is associated with an increased risk of developing permanent hypothyroidism, which has been estimated to occur in 2% to 21% of affected women. Stagnaro-Green and colleagues[119] reported an even higher incidence of permanent hypothyroidism of 54%. The presence, but not the titers, of TPO antibodies in the first trimester of pregnancy and the degree of hypothyroidism at 6 months postpartum were predictive of permanent hypothyroidism. Because of the increased risk of permanent hypothyroidism following PPT, yearly TSH monitoring is recommended, even in women who return to the euthyroid state.

Data remain inconclusive regarding the correlation between PPT and postpartum depression (PPD). TPO antibody positivity is associated with an increased risk of PPD, independent of maternal thyroid function.[120] Because the risk of PPT is also increased by TPO antibody positivity, one could predict that PPT and PPD are related entities. However, studies investigating a possible link between PPD and PPT have been unable to demonstrate a significant correlation, although studies to date are limited by small patient numbers.[121]

Treatment of Postpartum Thyroiditis

Most women with PPT do not require treatment in the hyperthyroid state, which is generally mild and transient. According to ATA guidelines, propranolol 10 to 20 mg every 6 hours as needed can be used for adrenergic symptoms. Most β-blockers are present in breast milk; however, propranolol is highly bound to proteins in the blood and thus is present in only very low levels in breast milk. ATDs are ineffective in the treatment of PPT, because it is a destructive process and does not involve over-production of thyroid hormone. In the hyperthyroid phase, TSH should be tested every 4 to 8 weeks, even if the patient is asymptomatic. LT4 treatment is indicated when TSH elevation persists for longer than 6 months postpartum, or if symptoms of hypothy-roidism are severe, the patient is breastfeeding, or another pregnancy is desired. Ther-apy should be continued for 6 to 12 months after initiation, followed by an attempt to wean the LT4 by halving the dose every 6 to 8 weeks. If the patient is pregnant, breast-feeding, or trying to conceive, weaning LT4 therapy is not indicated, and therapy should be continued to maintain serum TSH at 0.4 to 2.5 mIU/L.[16]

Various attempts have been made to prevent PPT in women at risk. A single-center randomized controlled trial by Negro and colleagues[122] showed that compared with placebo, selenium supplementation of 200 µg/d during pregnancy significantly decreased the prevalence of PPT in women with positive thyroid antibodies (28.6% vs 48.6%). In another study, the postpartum use of LT4 in women with thyroid auto-immunity (defined as positive TPO antibody titers) did not prevent PPT but, as ex-pected, reduced symptoms of hypothyroidism associated with PPT when it did occur.[123]

EVALUATION OF THYROID NODULES AND THYROID CANCER IN PREGNANCY

Not uncommonly, thyroid nodules and thyroid cancer are diagnosed in women during or around the time of pregnancy, posing important diagnostic and therapeutic di-lemmas when considering the best interests of both the mother and her developing child. Differentiated thyroid cancer (DTC) occurs approximately 3 times more frequently in women than in men, with peak onset in the female reproductive years.[124,125] Many women come under closer medical evaluation around the time of pregnancy than at any other time in their lives, contributing to increased detection and diagnosis of thyroid nodules and DTC. In addition, normal physiologic changes in pregnancy include an increase in maternal thyroid volume, including increased size of thyroid nodules, which further increases detection rates.[126] Management of thyroid nodules and thyroid cancer diagnosed during pregnancy affects both the affected mother and her fetus, so these cases require special consideration to ensure the best overall outcomes.

Because thyroid cancer is most commonly detected within thyroid nodules, thyroid nodules should be evaluated with neck ultrasonography and fine-needle aspiration (FNA), when indicated, to rule out malignancy. During pregnancy, both thyroid ultraso-nography and FNA can be performed safely at any time, without risk of harm to the pregnancy. For this reason, thyroid nodules detected in pregnancy may be evaluated in the same way as in nonpregnant individuals. However, if a suspicious nodule is detected late in pregnancy, and intervention such as surgery ± RAI ablation therapy will undoubtedly be delayed until after delivery, it is reasonable to postpone FNA until after delivery. Detection of a thyroid nodule in a pregnant woman should prompt measurement of serum thyroid hormone levels (TSH, fT4) so that maternal hypothy-roidism or hyperthyroidism can be treated promptly and associated complications prevented.[123]

If thyroid malignancy is diagnosed in a pregnant woman, the recommended course of treatment differs from that in a nonpregnant individual. However, despite these dif-ferences in management, most evidence suggests that DTC diagnosed during or around the time of pregnancy does not affect maternal or fetal morbidity or mortality.

In the same regard, pregnancy does not increase a woman's risk for developing thyroid cancer.

When thyroid cancer is diagnosed during pregnancy, a decision must be made regarding performing total thyroidectomy during the pregnancy or postponing surgical resection until the postpartum period. In low-risk cases of DTC, postponing thyroidectomy until after delivery does not affect the course of disease and eliminates the risks associated with surgery during pregnancy.[123] Risks specific to thyroidectomy that may adversely affect a pregnancy include (1) difficulty resecting the thyroid because of increased gland volume in pregnancy, (2) uncontrolled maternal hypothyroidism postoperatively, and (3) transient or permanent maternal hypocalcemia caused by damage to the parathyroid glands. Anesthesia at any time during pregnancy is complicated by multiple factors, including increased maternal blood volume and cardiac output, and can result in maternal hypotension and fetal hypoperfusion.[127,128] In most cases where thyroidectomy is not performed during pregnancy, monitoring should consist of a repeat neck ultrasonogram each trimester to rule out rapid growth of malignant tissue, with consideration of immediate surgical intervention if this should occur, and close monitoring of maternal TFTs (see later discussion).[123]

In cases of advanced DTC or in undifferentiated forms of thyroid cancer (eg, medullary, anaplastic, or insular variants), which are more aggressive and more likely to progress if intervention is delayed, thyroidectomy may be performed in the second trimester. This time point in gestation is the earliest at which organogenesis is complete and the risk to fetal development is lowest.[123]

Pregnant women with an FNA sample that is suspicious for thyroid cancer do not require surgery unless there is rapid growth of the nodule, compressive symptoms, suspicious lymph nodes, or evidence of metastases. Approximately 30% of nodules that are considered suspicious for thyroid cancer are in fact malignant; however, outcomes are not changed by performing surgery after delivery. In cases of DTC diagnosed during pregnancy, where surgery is deferred, suppressive doses of LT4 should be considered, with a goal TSH level between 0.1 and 0.5 mIU/L.[129]

RAI (^{131}I) ablation is often indicated following total thyroidectomy in patients with DTC to prevent disease recurrence. RAI is absolutely contraindicated during pregnancy and lactation because of the risk of transfer of RAI to the fetal thyroid gland. Exposure of the fetal thyroid to RAI may result in fetal thyroid ablation, if administered after the 12th week of gestation, with resultant devastating effects on early development. If RAI is indicated in a woman who has been diagnosed with DTC during pregnancy, ^{131}I treatment should be initiated as soon as possible in the postpartum period. Breastfeeding should not be initiated or continued for at least 6 months following RAI ablation, so many women will postpone RAI treatment until they have had an opportunity to breastfeed their infant for 3 to 6 months, a delay that usually does not worsen maternal outcomes A ^{123}I scan looking for breast uptake should be performed before administering ^{131}I therapy to women who have recently breastfed.[123,130]

In women who have been diagnosed with DTC before pregnancy, most evidence suggests that pregnancy does not alter the course of disease; that is, long-term prognosis remains the same as the prognosis in cases of DTC diagnosed after pregnancies or in nulligravid women.[131–133] When DTC precedes a pregnancy, TSH suppression with LT4 should be maintained at the same level as it was before pregnancy to minimize disease progression.[129] Most women on suppressive doses of LT4 for DTC will require increased doses during pregnancy consequent to increased maternal and fetal demands (discussed previously).[60] In this regard, there are no clinically significant negative consequences to maternal subclinical hyperthyroidism during pregnancy; therefore, maintaining prepregnancy TSH suppression is acceptable.[123]

Treatment of reproductive-aged women with DTC with RAI does not increase their future risk of infertility or adverse pregnancy outcomes, such as miscarriage. Furthermore, no differences have been demonstrated between children born to mothers or fathers who had previously received RAI ablation in comparison with those who had not, including physical or cognitive development and risk of childhood malignancies.[134]

In summary, thyroid cancer diagnosed during or around the time of pregnancy requires careful consideration of the health of both the mother and her developing child to determine the best course of treatment for optimization of maternal and fetal outcomes. These complex cases should be followed closely during pregnancy and lactation by a team of physicians that includes the patient's obstetrician, an endocrinologist, an endocrine surgeon, nuclear medicine specialists, and the baby's pediatrician. Most evidence suggests that long-term maternal outcomes are not usually adversely affected by delaying definitive treatment until the postpartum period. However, because of the theoretical potential that a delay in treatment may worsen maternal survival, close clinical follow-up during and after pregnancy is paramount to making the optimal clinical decisions.

SUMMARY

- Thyroid gland physiology changes during pregnancy because of the effects of increased TBG and hCG levels, and enhanced iodine metabolism. It is important to use trimester-specific reference ranges for thyroid function tests during pregnancy. TSH reference ranges decrease during pregnancy, especially in the first trimester. tT4 and tT3 levels increase as a result of increased TBG levels. The interpretation of free thyroid hormone levels in pregnancy is more challenging.
- Owing to the lack of evidence demonstrating that universal screening for thyroid disorders in pregnancy results in improved population outcomes, several clinical organizations recommend obtaining serum TSH early in pregnancy only in women at high risk for overt hypothyroidism.
- Iodine sufficiency is crucial in pregnancy. The recommended daily iodine intake in pregnancy and lactation is 250 µg of iodine daily, including 150 µg of supplemental iodine from prenatal vitamins in the form of potassium iodide. One must note that not all prenatal vitamins contain iodine supplementation.
- Hypothyroidism is associated with adverse maternal and fetal outcomes in pregnancy. The data on overt hypothyroidism are more conclusive than those for subclinical hypothyroidism. Adverse effects include spontaneous abortion, fetal death, preterm delivery, gestational hypertension, preeclampsia, postpartum hemorrhage, placental abruption and preterm labor, cesarean section, low birth weight, fetal distress, and impaired neuropsychological development.
- All women with overt hypothyroidism and TPO antibody–positive subclinical hypothyroidism should be treated with LT4 during pregnancy to maintain serum TSH levels within trimester-specific goal ranges. Some advocate empirically increasing the LT4 dose by 25% to 30% when pregnancy is confirmed. At a minimum, serum TSH should be checked every 4 weeks during the first half of the pregnancy, then at least once between 26 and 32 weeks of gestation.
- There is not enough evidence to recommend for or against LT4 treatment in thyroid antibody–negative pregnant women with subclinical hypothyroidism, women with isolated hypothyroxinemia, or euthyroid women who are thyroid antibody positive. In these cases, some specialists recommend monitoring TFTs closely during pregnancy. These investigators err on the side of treatment

in these special cases, as the potential benefits of low-dose LT4 therapy likely outweigh any risks.

- The most common cause of hyperthyroidism in pregnancy is GTT, which results from elevated hCG levels. It is important to distinguish GTT from GD because the course, fetal outcomes, management, and follow-up are different.
- Uncontrolled hyperthyroidism during pregnancy is associated with adverse effects such as low birth weight, stillbirth, preeclampsia, miscarriage, maternal heart failure, maternal gestational hypertension, fetal growth restriction, central congenital hypothyroidism, fetal thyrotoxicosis, and neonatal hyperthyroidism.
- Thionamides are the treatment of choice for GD during pregnancy. To decrease the risk of congenital abnormalities associated with first-trimester MMI use, women taking MMI before pregnancy should be switched to PTU once pregnancy is confirmed or, alternatively, before conception. After the first trimester, consideration should be given to switching from PTU to an equivalent dose of MMI to avoid maternal liver injury. Thionamide dose adjustments should be based on fT4 levels rather than TSH levels, because TSH may remain suppressed throughout pregnancy. Surgery might be indicated in certain cases. β-Blockers and cold iodine can be given for a short duration in preparation for surgery. RAI ablation is contraindicated during pregnancy and lactation. Measurement of maternal TRAb titers is indicated before delivery to determine the risk of fetal hyperthyroidism.
- PPT is an autoimmune destructive inflammation of the thyroid gland that typically occurs within 1 year postpartum. The classic presentation of PPT starts with transient hyperthyroidism in the first 6 months postpartum, followed by transient hypothyroidism, and then a return to the euthyroid state by 1 year postpartum. PPT has been associated with an increased risk of permanent hypothyroidism and a possible link to postpartum depression. Most women with PPT do not require treatment in the hyperthyroid state, which is generally mild and transient. LT4 is indicated in certain cases in the hypothyroid phase.
- Thyroid nodules detected in pregnancy may be evaluated with thyroid ultrasonography and FNA when necessary, which are both safe to perform at any time during pregnancy. When thyroid cancer is diagnosed during pregnancy, a decision regarding definitive treatment must be made. In most cases, delaying thyroidectomy and RAI ablation (if indicated) until the postpartum stage does not alter maternal morbidity or mortality. In high-risk cases, thyroidectomy can be performed in the second trimester. RAI ablation is absolutely contraindicated during pregnancy and lactation. Similarly to nonpregnant individuals with thyroid cancer, TSH suppression with LT4 may be indicated during pregnancy in women with thyroid cancer.

REFERENCES

1. Stagnaro-Green A. Overt hyperthyroidism and hypothyroidism during pregnancy. Clin Obstet Gynecol 2011;54(3):478–87.
2. Hollowell JG, Staehling NW, Flanders WD, et al. Serum TSH, T(4), and thyroid antibodies in the United States population (1988 to 1994): National Health and Nutrition Examination Survey (NHANES III). J Clin Endocrinol Metab 2002; 87(2):489–99.
3. Abalovich M, Amino N, Barbour LA, et al. Management of thyroid dysfunction during pregnancy and postpartum: an Endocrine Society Clinical Practice Guideline. J Clin Endocrinol Metab 2007;92(Suppl 8):S1–47.

4. Glinoer D. The regulation of thyroid function in pregnancy: pathways of endocrine adaptation from physiology to pathology. Endocr Rev 1997;18(3):404–33.

5. Alexander EK, Marqusee E, Lawrence J, et al. Timing and magnitude of increases in levothyroxine requirements during pregnancy in women with hypothyroidism. N Engl J Med 2004;351(3):241–9.

6. Kaplan MM. Monitoring thyroxine treatment during pregnancy. Thyroid 1992; 2(2):147–52.

7. Mandel SJ, Larsen PR, Seely EW, et al. Increased need for thyroxine during pregnancy in women with primary hypothyroidism. N Engl J Med 1990;323(2): 91–6.

8. Glinoer D, McGuire RA, Gershengorn MC, et al. Effects of estrogen on thyroxine-binding globulin metabolism in rhesus monkeys. Endocrinology 1977;100(1):9–17.

9. Glinoer D, Gershengorn MC, Dubois A, et al. Stimulation of thyroxine-binding globulin synthesis by isolated rhesus monkey hepatocytes after in vivo beta-estradiol administration. Endocrinology 1977;100(3):807–13.

10. Ain KB, Mori Y, Refetoff S. Reduced clearance rate of thyroxine-binding globulin (TBG) with increased sialylation: a mechanism for estrogen-induced elevation of serum TBG concentration. J Clin Endocrinol Metab 1987;65(4):689–96.

11. Skjoldebrand L, Brundin J, Carlstrom A, et al. Thyroid associated components in serum during normal pregnancy. Acta Endocrinol 1982;100(4):504–11.

12. Glinoer D, de Nayer P, Bourdoux P, et al. Regulation of maternal thyroid during pregnancy. J Clin Endocrinol Metab 1990;71(2):276–87.

13. Smits G, Govaerts C, Nubourgh I, et al. Lysine 183 and glutamic acid 157 of the TSH receptor: two interacting residues with a key role in determining specificity toward TSH and human CG. Mol Endocrinol 2002;16(4):722–35.

14. Dworkin HJ, Jacquez JA, Beierwaltes WH. Relationship of iodine ingestion to iodine excretion in pregnancy. J Clin Endocrinol Metab 1966;26(12):1329–42.

15. Burrow GN, Fisher DA, Larsen PR. Maternal and fetal thyroid function. N Engl J Med 1994;331(16):1072–8.

16. Stagnaro-Green A, Abalovich M, Alexander E, et al. Guidelines of the American Thyroid Association for the diagnosis and management of thyroid disease during pregnancy and postpartum. Thyroid 2011;21(10):1081–125.

17. Shields B, Hill A, Bilous M, et al. Cigarette smoking during pregnancy is associated with alterations in maternal and fetal thyroid function. J Clin Endocrinol Metab 2009;94(2):570–4.

18. La'ulu SL, Roberts WL. Ethnic differences in first-trimester thyroid reference intervals. Clin Chem 2011;57(6):913–5.

19. Koreevaar TI, Medici M, de Rijke YB, et al. Ethnic differences in maternal thyroid parameters during pregnancy. J Clin Endocrinol Metab 2013;98(9):3678–86.

20. Mandel SJ, Spencer CA, Hollowell JG. Are detection and treatment of thyroid insufficiency in pregnancy feasible? Thyroid 2005;15(1):44–53.

21. Kahric-Janicic N, Soldin SJ, Soldin OP, et al. Tandem mass spectrometry improves the accuracy of free thyroxine measurements during pregnancy. Thyroid 2007;17(4):303–11.

22. Lee RH, Spencer CA, Mestman JH, et al. Free T4 immunoassays are flawed during pregnancy. Am J Obstet Gynecol 2009;200(3):260.e261–6.

23. Stagnaro-Green A, Pearce E. Endocrine disorders in pregnancy. Nature 2012;(8):650–7.

24. Vaidya B, Anthony S, Bilous M, et al. Detection of thyroid dysfunction in early pregnancy: universal screening or targeted high-risk case finding? J Clin Endocrinol Metab 2007;92(1):203–7.

25. Li Y, Shan Z, Teng W, et al. Abnormalities of maternal thyroid function during pregnancy affect neuropsychological development of their children at 25-30 months. Clin Endocrinol 2010;72(6):825–9.
26. Negro R, Schwartz A, Gismondi R, et al. Universal screening versus case finding for detection and treatment of thyroid hormonal dysfunction during pregnancy. J Clin Endocrinol Metab 2010;95(4):1699–707.
27. Chang DL, Leung AM, Braverman LE, et al. Thyroid testing during pregnancy at an academic Boston Area Medical Center. J Clin Endocrinol Metab 2011;96(9): E1452–6.
28. Moreno-Reyes R, Glioner D, Van Oyen H, et al. High prevalence of thyroid disorders in pregnant women in a mildly iodine-deficient country: a population based study. J Clin Endocrinol Metab 2013;98(9):3694–701.
29. Casey BM. A randomized trial of thyroxine therapy for subclinical hypothyroidism or hypothyroxinemia diagnosed during pregnancy. Thyroid dysfunction and pregnancy: miscarriage, preterm delivery and decreased IQ. Booklet of the Research Summit and Spring Symposium of the ATA. Washington, April 16–17, 2009.
30. Lazarus J. Screening for thyroid dysfunction in pregnancy: is it worthwhile? J Thyroid Res 2011;2011:397012. http://dx.doi.org/10.4061/2011/397012.
31. De Groot L, Abalovich M, Alexander E, et al. Management of thyroid dysfunction during pregnancy and postpartum: an endocrine society practice guideline. J Clin Endocrinol Metab 2012;97(8):2543–65.
32. Neale D, Burrow G. Thyroid disease in pregnancy. Obstet Gynecol Clin North Am 2004;31(4):893–905, xi.
33. Abalovich M, Gutierrez S, Alcaraz G, et al. Overt and subclinical hypothyroidism complicating pregnancy. Thyroid 2002;12(1):63–8.
34. Allan WC, Haddow JE, Palomaki GE, et al. Maternal thyroid deficiency and pregnancy complications: implications for population screening. J Med Screen 2000; 7(3):127–30.
35. Stagnaro-Green A. Maternal thyroid disease and preterm delivery. J Clin Endocrinol Metab 2009;94(1):21–5.
36. Leung AS, Millar LK, Koonings PP, et al. Perinatal outcome in hypothyroid pregnancies. Obstet Gynecol 1993;81(3):349–53.
37. Davis LE, Leveno KJ, Cunningham FG. Hypothyroidism complicating pregnancy. Obstet Gynecol 1988;72(1):108–12.
38. Casey BM, Dashe JS, Wells CE, et al. Subclinical hypothyroidism and pregnancy outcomes. Obstet Gynecol 2005;105(2):239–45.
39. Ashoor G, Rotas M, Maiz N, et al. Maternal thyroid function at 11-13 weeks of gestation in women with hypothyroidism treated by thyroxine. Fetal Diagn Ther 2010;28(1):22–7.
40. Cohen N, Levy A, Wiznitzer A, et al. Perinatal outcomes in post-thyroidectomy pregnancies. Gynecol Endocrinol 2011;27(5):314–8.
41. De Vivo A, Mancuso A, Giacobbe A, et al. Thyroid function in women found to have early pregnancy loss. Thyroid 2010;20(6):633–7.
42. Su PY, Huang K, Hao JH, et al. Maternal thyroid function in the first twenty weeks of pregnancy and subsequent fetal and infant development: a prospective population-based cohort study in china. J Clin Endocrinol Metab 2011;96(10):3234–41.
43. Kuppens SM, Kooistra L, Wijnen HA, et al. Maternal thyroid function during gestation is related to breech presentation at term. Clin Endocrinol 2010;72(6):820–4.
44. Kuppens SM, Kooistra L, Hasaart TH, et al. Maternal thyroid function and the outcome of external cephalic version: a prospective cohort study. BMC Pregnancy Childbirth 2011;11:10.

45. Benhadi N, Wiersinga WM, Reitsma JB, et al. Higher maternal TSH levels in pregnancy are associated with increased risk for miscarriage, fetal or neonatal death. Eur J Endocrinol 2009;160(6):985–91.

46. Cleary-Goldman J, Malone FD, Lambert-Messerlian G, et al. Maternal thyroid hypofunction and pregnancy outcome. Obstet Gynecol 2008;112(1):85–92.

47. Mannisto T, Vaarasmaki M, Pouta A, et al. Perinatal outcome of children born to mothers with thyroid dysfunction or antibodies: a prospective population-based cohort study. J Clin Endocrinol Metab 2009;94(3):772–9.

48. Haddow JE, Palomaki GE, Allan WC, et al. Maternal thyroid deficiency during pregnancy and subsequent neuropsychological development of the child. N Engl J Med 1999;341(8):549–55.

49. Henrichs J, Bongers-Schokking J, Schenk J, et al. Maternal function during early pregnancy and cognitive functioning in early childhood: the generation r study. J Clin Endocrinol Metab 2010;95(9):4227–34.

50. Behrooz HG, Tohidi M, Mehrabi Y, et al. Subclinical hypothyroidism in pregnancy: intellectual development of offspring. Thyroid 2011;21(10):1143–7.

51. Lazarus JH, Bestwick J, Channon S, et al. Antenatal thyroid screening and childhood cognitive function. N Engl J Med 2012;366:493–501.

52. Casey BM, Dashe JS, Spong CY, et al. Perinatal significance of isolated maternal hypothyroxinemia identified in the first half of pregnancy. Obstet Gynecol 2007;109(5):1129–35.

53. Pop VJ, Brouwers EP, Vader HL, et al. Maternal hypothyroxinaemia during early pregnancy and subsequent child development: a 3-year follow-up study. Clin Endocrinol 2003;59(3):282–8.

54. Pop VJ, Kuijpens JL, van Baar AL, et al. Low maternal free thyroxine concentrations during early pregnancy are associated with impaired psychomotor development in infancy. Clin Endocrinol 1999;50(2):149–55.

55. Negro R, Soldin OP, Obregon MJ, et al. Hypothyroxinemia and pregnancy. Endocr Pract 2011;17(3):422–9.

56. Loh JA, Wartofsky L, Jonklaas J, et al. The magnitude of increased levothyroxine requirements in hypothyroid pregnant women depends upon the etiology of the hypothyroidism. Thyroid 2009;19(3):269–75.

57. Yassa L, Marqusee E, Fawcett R, et al. Thyroid hormone early adjustment in pregnancy (the THERAPY) trial. J Clin Endocrinol Metab 2010;95(7):3234–41.

58. Andersson M, Karumbunathan V, Zimmerman MB. Global iodine status in 2011 and trends over the past decade. J Nutr 2012;142:744–50.

59. Leung AM, Pearce EN, Braverman LE. Iodine content of prenatal vitamins in the United States. N Engl J Med 2009;360:939–40.

60. Negro R, Formoso G, Mangieri T, et al. Levothyroxine treatment in euthyroid pregnant women with autoimmune thyroid disease: effects on obstetrical complications. J Clin Endocrinol Metab 2006;91(7):2587–91.

61. Negro R. Thyroid autoimmunity and pre-term delivery: brief review and meta-analysis. J Endocrinol Invest 2011;34(2):155–8.

62. Chen L, Hu R. Thyroid autoimmunity and miscarriage: a meta-analysis. Clin Endocrinol 2011;74(4):513–9.

63. Negro R, Schwartz A, Gismondi R, et al. Thyroid antibody positivity in the first trimester of pregnancy is associated with negative pregnancy outcomes. J Clin Endocrinol Metab 2011;96(6):E920–4.

64. Abbassi-Ghanavati M, Casey BM, Spong CY, et al. Pregnancy outcomes in women with thyroid peroxidase antibodies. Obstet Gynecol 2010;116(2 Pt 1):381–6.

65. Pop VJ, de Rooy HA, Vader HL, et al. Microsomal antibodies during gestation in relation to postpartum thyroid dysfunction and depression. Acta Endocrinol 1993;129(1):26–30.

66. Marco M, de Rijke Y, Peeters R, et al. Maternal early pregnancy and newborn thyroid hormone parameters: the generation r study. J Clin Endocrinol Metab 2012;97(2):646–52.

67. Thangaratinum S, Tan A, Knox E, et al. Association between thyroid auto-antibodies and miscarriage and pre-term birth: meta-analysis of evidence. BMJ 2009;342:d2616.

68. Ghassabian G, Bongers-Schokking J, de Rijke Y, et al. Maternal thyroid autoimmunity during pregnancy and the risk of attention deficit/hyperactivity problems in children: the generation r study. Thyroid 2012;22(2):178–86.

69. Glinoer D. Thyroid hyperfunction during pregnancy. Thyroid 1998;8(9):859–64.

70. Patil-Sisodia K, Mestman JH. Graves hyperthyroidism and pregnancy: a clinical update. Endocr Pract 2010;16(1):118–29.

71. Tan JY, Loh KC, Yeo GS, et al. Transient hyperthyroidism of hyperemesis gravidarum. BJOG 2002;109(6):683–8.

72. Amino N, Tanizawa O, Mori H, et al. Aggravation of thyrotoxicosis in early pregnancy and after delivery in Graves' disease. J Clin Endocrinol Metab 1982; 55(1):108–12.

73. Barbesino G, Tomer Y. Clinical review: clinical utility of TSH receptor antibodies. J Clin Endocrinol Metab 2013;98(6):2247–55.

74. Millar LK, Wing DA, Leung AS, et al. Low birth weight and preeclampsia in pregnancies complicated by hyperthyroidism. Obstet Gynecol 1994;84(6):946–9.

75. Davis LE, Lucas MJ, Hankins GD, et al. Thyrotoxicosis complicating pregnancy. Am J Obstet Gynecol 1989;160(1):63–70.

76. Anselmo J, Cao D, Karrison T, et al. Fetal loss associated with excess thyroid hormone exposure. JAMA 2004;292(6):691–5.

77. Sheffield JS, Cunningham FG. Thyrotoxicosis and heart failure that complicate pregnancy. Am J Obstet Gynecol 2004;190(1):211–7.

78. Luewan S, Chakkabut P, Tongsong T. Outcomes of pregnancy complicated with hyperthyroidism: a cohort study. Arch Gynecol Obstet 2011;283(2):243–7.

79. Kempers MJ, van Tijn DA, van Trotsenburg AS, et al. Central congenital hypothyroidism due to gestational hyperthyroidism: detection where prevention failed. J Clin Endocrinol Metab 2003;88(12):5851–7.

80. Medici M, Timmermans S, Visser W. Maternal thyroid hormone parameters during early pregnancy and birth weight: the generation r study. J Clin Endocrinol Metab 2013;98(1):59–66.

81. Medici M, Ghassabian A, Visser W, et al. Women with early pregnancy urinary iodine levels have an increased risk of hyperthyroid newborns: population based generation r study. Clin Endocrinol 2013. [Epub ahead of print]. http://dx.doi.org/10.1111/cen.12321.

82. Peleg D, Cada S, Peleg A, et al. The relationship between maternal serum thyroid-stimulating immunoglobulin and fetal and neonatal thyrotoxicosis. Obstet Gynecol 2002;99(6):1040–3.

83. Zakarija M, McKenzie JM. Pregnancy-associated changes in the thyroid-stimulating antibody of Graves' disease and the relationship to neonatal hyperthyroidism. J Clin Endocrinol Metab 1983;57(5):1036–40.

84. Polak M, Le Gac I, Vuillard E, et al. Fetal and neonatal thyroid function in relation to maternal Graves' disease. Best Pract Res Clin Endocrinol Metab 2004;18(2):289–302.

85. Ogilvy-Stuart AL. Neonatal thyroid disorders. Arch Dis Child Fetal Neonatal Ed 2002;87:F165–71.
86. McKenzie JM, Zakarija M. Fetal and neonatal hyperthyroidism and hypothyroidism due to maternal TSH receptor antibodies. Thyroid 1992;2(2):155–9.
87. Momotani N, Ito K, Hamada N, et al. Maternal hyperthyroidism and congenital malformation in the offspring. Clin Endocrinol 1984;20:695–700.
88. Laurberg P, Bournaud C, Karmisholt J, et al. Management of Graves' hyperthyroidism in pregnancy: focus on both maternal and foetal thyroid function, and caution against surgical thyroidectomy in pregnancy. Eur J Endocrinol 2009; 160(1):1–8.
89. Ibbertson HK, Seddon RJ, Croxson MS. Fetal hypothyroidism complicating medical treatment of thyrotoxicosis in pregnancy. Clin Endocrinol 1975;4(5): 521–3.
90. Ochoa-Maya MR, Frates MC, Lee-Parritz A, et al. Resolution of fetal goiter after discontinuation of propylthiouracil in a pregnant woman with Graves' hyperthyroidism. Thyroid 1999;9(11):1111–4.
91. Momotani N, Noh J, Oyanagi H, et al. Antithyroid drug therapy for Graves' disease during pregnancy. Optimal regimen for fetal thyroid status. N Engl J Med 1986;315(1):24–8.
92. Martinez-Frias ML, Cereijo A, Rodriguez-Pinilla E, et al. Methimazole in animal feed and congenital aplasia cutis. Lancet 1992;339(8795):742–3.
93. Clementi M, Di Gianantonio E, Cassina M, et al. Treatment of hyperthyroidism in pregnancy and birth defects. J Clin Endocrinol Metab 2010;95(11): E337–41.
94. Di Gianantonio E, Schaefer C, Mastroiacovo PP, et al. Adverse effects of prenatal methimazole exposure. Teratology 2001;64(5):262–6.
95. Clementi M, Di Gianantonio E, Pelo E, et al. Methimazole embryopathy: delineation of the phenotype. Am J Med Genet 1999;83(1):43–6.
96. Yoshihara A, Noh J, Yamaguchi T, et al. Treatment of graves' disease with antithyroid drugs in the first trimester of pregnancy and the prevalence of congenital malformation. J Clin Endocrinol Metab 2012 Jul;97(7):2396–403.
97. Bahn RS, Burch HS, Cooper DS, et al. The role of propylthiouracil in the management of Graves' disease in adults: report of a meeting jointly sponsored by the American Thyroid Association and the Food and Drug Administration. Thyroid 2009;19(7):673–4.
98. Kim HJ, Kim BH, Han YS, et al. The incidence and clinical characteristics of symptomatic propylthiouracil-induced hepatic injury in patients with hyperthyroidism: a single-center retrospective study. Am J Gastroenterol 2001;96(1): 165–9.
99. Mandel SJ, Cooper DS. The use of antithyroid drugs in pregnancy and lactation. J Clin Endocrinol Metab 2001;86(6):2354–9.
100. Azizi F, Bahrainian M, Khamseh ME, et al. Intellectual development and thyroid function in children who were breast-fed by thyrotoxic mothers taking methimazole. J Pediatr Endocrinol Metab 2003;16(9):1239–43.
101. Momotani N, Yamashita R, Makino F, et al. Thyroid function in wholly breast-feeding infants whose mothers take high doses of propylthiouracil. Clin Endocrinol 2000;53(2):177–81.
102. Laurberg P, Nygaard B, Glinoer D, et al. Guidelines for TSH-receptor antibody measurements in pregnancy: results of an evidence-based symposium organized by the European Thyroid Association. Eur J Endocrinol 1998;139(6): 584–6.

103. Rubin PC. Current concepts: beta-blockers in pregnancy. N Engl J Med 1981; 305(22):1323–6.
104. Sherif IH, Oyan WT, Bosairi S, et al. Treatment of hyperthyroidism in pregnancy. Acta Obstet Gynecol Scand 1991;70(6):461–3.
105. Momotani N, Hisaoka T, Noh J, et al. Effects of iodine on thyroid status of fetus versus mother in treatment of Graves' disease complicated by pregnancy. J Clin Endocrinol Metab 1992;75(3):738–44.
106. Soliman S, McGrath F, Brennan B, et al. Color Doppler imaging of the thyroid gland in a fetus with congenital goiter: a case report. Am J Perinatol 1994; 11(1):21–3.
107. Huel C, Guibourdenche J, Vuillard E, et al. Use of ultrasound to distinguish between fetal hyperthyroidism and hypothyroidism on discovery of a goiter. Ultrasound Obstet Gynecol 2009;33(4):412–20.
108. Nachum Z, Rakover Y, Weiner E, et al. Graves' disease in pregnancy: prospective evaluation of a selective invasive treatment protocol. Am J Obstet Gynecol 2003;189(1):159–65.
109. Rotondi M, Cappelli C, Pirali B, et al. The effect of pregnancy on subsequent relapse from Graves' disease after a successful course of antithyroid drug therapy. J Clin Endocrinol Metab 2008;93(10):3985–8.
110. Stagnaro-Green A, Roman SH, Cobin RH, et al. A prospective study of lymphocyte-initiated immunosuppression in normal pregnancy: evidence of a T-cell etiology for postpartum thyroid dysfunction. J Clin Endocrinol Metab 1992;74(3):645–53.
111. Lazarus JH, Hall R, Othman S, et al. The clinical spectrum of postpartum thyroid disease. QJM 1996;89(6):429–35.
112. Caixas A, Albareda M, Garcia-Patterson A, et al. Postpartum thyroiditis in women with hypothyroidism antedating pregnancy? J Clin Endocrinol Metab 1999;84(11):4000–5.
113. Stagnaro-Green A. Postpartum thyroiditis. Best Pract Res Clin Endocrinol Metab 2004;18(2):303–16.
114. Lazarus JH, Ammari F, Oretti R, et al. Clinical aspects of recurrent postpartum thyroiditis. Br J Gen Pract 1997;47(418):305–8.
115. Alvarez-Marfany M, Roman SH, Drexler AJ, et al. Long-term prospective study of postpartum thyroid dysfunction in women with insulin dependent diabetes mellitus. J Clin Endocrinol Metab 1994;79(1):10–6.
116. Stagnaro-Green A, Akhter E, Yim C, et al. Thyroid disease in pregnant women with systemic lupus erythematosus: increased preterm delivery. Lupus 2011; 20(7):690–9.
117. Elefsiniotis IS, Vezali E, Pantazis KD, et al. Post-partum thyroiditis in women with chronic viral hepatitis. J Clin Virol 2008;41(4):318–9.
118. Harris B, Othman S, Davies JA, et al. Association between postpartum thyroid dysfunction and thyroid antibodies and depression. BMJ 1992;305(6846):152–6.
119. Stagnaro-Green A, Schwartz A, Gismondi R, et al. High rate of persistent hypothyroidism in a large-scale prospective study of postpartum thyroiditis in southern Italy. J Clin Endocrinol Metab 2011;96(3):652–7.
120. Kuijpens JL, Vader HL, Drexhage HA, et al. Thyroid peroxidase antibodies during gestation are a marker for subsequent depression postpartum. Eur J Endocrinol 2001;145(5):579–84.
121. Lucas A, Pizarro E, Granada ML, et al. Postpartum thyroid dysfunction and postpartum depression: are they two linked disorders? Clin Endocrinol 2001;55(6): 809–14.

122. Negro R, Greco G, Mangieri T, et al. The influence of selenium supplementation on postpartum thyroid status in pregnant women with thyroid peroxidase auto-antibodies. J Clin Endocrinol Metab 2007;92(4):1263–8.
123. Kampe O, Jansson R, Karlsson FA. Effects of L-thyroxine and iodide on the development of autoimmune postpartum thyroiditis. J Clin Endocrinol Metab 1990;70(4):1014–8.
124. Rahbari R, Zhang L, Kebebew E. Thyroid cancer gender disparity. Future Oncol 2010;6(11):1771–9.
125. Aschebrook-Kilfoy B, Ward MH, Sabra MM, et al. Thyroid cancer incidence patterns in the United States by histologic type, 1992-2006. Thyroid 2011;21(2): 125–34.
126. Kung AW, Chau MT, Lao TT, et al. The effect of pregnancy on thyroid nodule formation. J Clin Endocrinol Metab 2002;87(3):1010–4.
127. Kuy S, Roman SA, Desai R, et al. Outcomes following thyroid and parathyroid surgery in pregnant women. Arch Surg 2009;144(5):399–406.
128. Mazzaferri EL. Approach to the pregnant patient with thyroid cancer. J Clin Endocrinol Metab 2011;96(2):265–72.
129. Cooper DS, Doherty GM, Haugen BR, et al. Revised American Thyroid Association management guidelines for patients with thyroid nodules and differentiated thyroid cancer: American Thyroid Association (ATA) Guidelines Taskforce on Thyroid Nodules and Differentiated Thyroid Cancer. Thyroid 2009;19: 1167–214.
130. Sisson JC, Freitas J, McDougall IR, et al. Radiation safety in the treatment of patients with thyroid diseases by radioiodine [131]I: practice recommendations of the American Thyroid Association. Thyroid 2011;21(4):335–46.
131. Hirsch D, Levy S, Tsvetov G, et al. Impact of pregnancy on outcome and prognosis of survivors of papillary thyroid cancer. Thyroid 2010;20(10):1179–85.
132. Leboeuf Rosario PW, Barroso AL, Purisch S. The effect of subsequent pregnancy on patients with thyroid carcinoma apparently free of the disease. Thyroid 2007;17(11):1175–6.
133. Leboeuf R, Emerick LE, Martorella AJ, et al. Impact of pregnancy on serum thyroglobulin and detection of recurrent disease shortly after delivery in thyroid cancer survivors. Thyroid 2007;17(6):543–7.
134. Sioka C, Fotopoulos A. Effects of I-131 therapy on gonads and pregnancy outcome in patients with thyroid cancer. Fertil Steril 2011;95(5):1552–9.

Index

Note: Page numbers of article titles are in **boldface** type.

Moving?

Make sure your subscription moves with you!

To notify us of your new address, find your **Clinics Account Number** (located on your mailing label above your name), and contact customer service at:

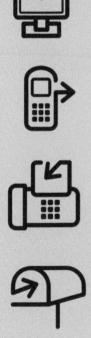

Email: journalscustomerservice-usa@elsevier.com

800-654-2452 (subscribers in the U.S. & Canada)
314-447-8871 (subscribers outside of the U.S. & Canada)

Fax number: 314-447-8029

Elsevier Health Sciences Division
Subscription Customer Service
3251 Riverport Lane
Maryland Heights, MO 63043

ELSEVIER

Printed and bound by CPI Group (UK) Ltd, Croydon, CR0 4YY

03/10/2024

01040491-0013